Liver Cirrhosis: From Pathophysiology to Disease Management

FALK SYMPOSIUM 162

Liver Cirrhosis: From Pathophysiology to Disease Management

Edited by

J. Bosch
University of Barcelona
Barcelona
Spain

A.K. Burroughs
Royal Free Hospital
London
United Kingdom

F. Lammert
University of Bonn
Bonn
Germany

D. Lebrec
Hôpital Beaujon
Clichy
France

T. Sauerbruch
University of Bonn
Bonn
Germany

Proceedings of the Falk Symposium 162 held in Dresden, Germany,
October 13–14 2007

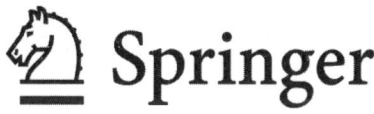

Library of Congress Cataloging-in-Publication Data is available.

ISBN-13 978-1-4020-8655-7

Published by Springer,
PO Box 17, 3300 AA Dordrecht, The Netherlands

Sold and distributed in North, Central and South America
by Springer,
101 Philip Drive, Norwell, MA 02061 USA

In all other countries, sold and distributed
by Springer,
PO Box 322, 3300 AH Dordrecht, The Netherlands

Printed on acid-free paper

All Rights Reserved
© 2008 Springer and Falk Foundation e.V.

No part of the material protected by this copyright notice may be reproduced or utilized in any form or by any means, electronic, mechanical, including photocopying, recording or by any information storage and retrieval system, without written permission from the copyright owners.

Printed and bound in Great Britain by MPG Books Limited, Bodmin, Cornwall.

Contents

	List of principal contributors	ix
	List of chairpersons	xii
	Preface	xiii

SECTION I: PATHOMECHANISMS OF FIBROGENESIS: INITIATION
Chair: SL Friedman, D Häussinger

1	Apoptosis and oncotic necrosis: profibrotic signalling mechanisms of cell death H Jaeschke, J-Y Hong	3
2	The mucosal immune system in the pathogenesis of liver disease B Eksteen, DH Adams	11
3	Immune responses in hepatitis C virus infection U Spengler, J Nattermann, B Langhans, HD Nischalke, D Schulte, C Körner, B Krämer, B Terjung, J Rockstroh, T Sauerbruch	19
4	Inflammatory pathways in liver homeostasis and liver injury T Luedde, F Tacke, C Trautwein	32

SECTION II: PATHOMECHANISMS OF FIBROGENESIS: MEDIATORS
Chair: AM Gressner, F Lammert

5	A complex network of intra- and intercellular mediators regulate cellular activation and transdifferentiation of hepatic stellate cells R Weiskirchen, E Borkham-Kamphorst, SK Meurer, F Drews, S Mohren, J Herrmann, OA Gressner, O Scherner, WN Vreden, E Kovalenko, M Bomble, AM Gressner	45

CONTENTS

6   Genetic determinants of liver fibrogenesis: a systems genetics approach in recombinant inbred mice
R Hall, F Lammert   70

7   Molecular mechanisms of fibrosis progression in non-alcoholic steatohepatitis (NASH)
C Hellerbrand   75

8   New role of bile acid metabolism in intestinal bacteria translocation
M Petruzzelli, A Moschetta   83

SECTION III: CELLULAR RESPONSES TO CHRONIC LIVER INJURY
Chair: D Lebrec, M Pinzani

9   The hepatic stellate cell: a progenitor cell
C Kordes, I Sawitza, D Häussinger   95

10   Role of non-parenchymal cells in portal hypertension
RC Huebert, VH Shah   107

11   Role of angiogenesis in portal hypertension
M Fernandez, M Mejias, E Garcia-Pras, J Bosch   112

12   Current concept of hepatic fibrogenesis in mouse models of liver fibrosis
D Scholten, D Brenner   130

13   Hepatic fibrogenesis and carcinogenesis: Krüppel-like factors and beyond
SL Friedman   144

SECTION IV: CLINICAL MANAGEMENT OF PROGRESSIVE LIVER FIBROSIS
Chair: G Ramadori, C Trautwein

14   Biomarkers of liver fibrosis
D Thabut, M Simon-Rudler   155

15   Clinical evaluation of disease progression in chronic liver disease: towards an integrated system?
M Pinzani, F Vizzutti   163

16   Fibrosis regression and innovative antifibrotic therapies: from bench to bedside
M-L Berres, MM Zaldivar, C Trautwein, HE Wasmuth   173

CONTENTS

SECTION V: CLINICAL MANAGEMENT OF PORTAL HYPERTENSION: PREPRIMARY AND PRIMARY PROPHYLAXIS
Chair: J Heller, F Wong

17 Dynamic increase of intrahepatic vascular resistance in cirrhosis
    A Rodríguez-Vilarrupla, JC García-Pagán 183

18 Remodelling portal hypertension: preprimary prophylaxis
    G Garcia-Tsao 195

19 When and how to scope in portal hypertension
    R de Franchis, A Dell'Era, M Primignani 204

20 Prevention of first variceal bleeding
    P Calès, N Dib, F Oberti 212

SECTION VI: CLINICAL MANAGEMENT OF PORTAL HYPERTENSION: COMPLICATIONS OF CIRRHOSIS
Chair: J Bosch, R Wiest

21 Therapy of acute variceal bleeding
    CK Triantos, AK Burroughs 233

22 Prevention of variceal rebleeding
    D Lebrec 243

23 From sodium retention to refractory ascites: the role of new drugs
    F Wong 248

24 Transjugular intrahepatic portosystemic shunt versus paracentesis: a critical review of randomized studies and meta-analyses
    M Rössle, W Euringer 261

25 Spontaneous bacterial peritonitis – a disease of the gut? Therapeutic implications
    J Fernández, A Cárdenas, P Gines 267

26 Hepatorenal syndrome – a defined entity with a standard treatment?
    AL Gerbes 280

27 From infections to hepatic encephalopathy
    D Häussinger 291

CONTENTS

28 Liver and lung – treatment of hepatopulmonary diseases
   P Schenk   297

29 Allocation in adult liver transplantation: is the Model for
   Endstage Liver Disease the solution?
   DM Heuman   309

30 Emerging future therapies for portal hypertension
   J Bosch, A De Gottardi   318

   Index   325

List of principal contributors

DH Adams
Liver Research Laboratories
MRC Centre for Immune Regulation
5th Floor, Institute for Biomedical
  Research
Wolfson Drive, Medical School
University of Birmingham
Birmingham, B15 2TT
UK

J Bosch
Hepatic Hemodynamic Laboratory
Hospital Clínic-Idibaps and Ciberehd
Villaroel 170
08036 Barcelona
Spain

D Brenner
Department of Medicine
1318A Biomedical Sciences Building
University of California, San Diego
9500 Gilman Drive
La Jolla, CA 92093-0602
USA

AK Burroughs
The Royal Free Sheila Sherlock Liver
  Centre and University Department
  of Surgery
Pond Street
London, NW3 2QG
UK

P Calès
Department of Hepato-
  Gastroenterology
University Hospital and HIFIH
  Laboratory
UPRES EA 3859
49933 Angers Cedex 09
France

A Cárdenas
Institute of Digestive Diseases and
  Metabolism
University of Barcelona
Hospital Clinic - Villaroel 170, Esc 3-2
08036 Barcelona
Spain

M Fernandez
Hepatic Hemodynamic Laboratory
IDIBAPS
Villaroel 170
08036 Barcelona
Spain

R de Franchis
University of Milan
Department of Medical Sciences
Gastroenterology 3 Unit
IRCCS Ospedale Maggiore
  Policlinico
Mangiagalli and Regina Elena
  Foundation
Via Pace 9
20122 Milan
Italy

SL Friedman
Mount Sinai School of Medicine
Division of Liver Diseases
1425 Madison Avenue, Room 11-70C
New York, NY 10029-6574
USA

JC García-Pagán
Hepatic Hemodynamic Laboratory
Liver Unit, Hospital Clinic
Villaroel 170
08036 Barcelona
Spain

LIST OF PRINCIPAL CONTRIBUTORS

G Garcia-Tsao
Digestive Diseases Section
Yale University School of Medicine
333 Cedar Street - 1080 LMP
New Haven, CT 06510
USA

AL Gerbes
Innere Medizin II
Klinikum der Universität München-
 Grosshadern
Marchioninistr. 15
81377 München
Germany

D Häussinger
Heinrich-Heine-Universität
 Düsseldorf
Klinik für Gastroenterologie,
 Hepatologie und Infektiologie
Moorenstrasse 5
40225 Düsseldorf
Germany

C Hellerbrand
Klinik und Poliklinik für Innere
 Medizin I
Klinikum der Universität Regensburg
93042 Regensburg
Germany

DM Heuman
Virginia Commonwealth University
GI Section (111-N) McGuire DVA
 Medical Center
1201 Broad Rock Blvd
Richmond, VA 23249
USA

H Jaeschke
Department of Pharmacology,
 Toxicology and Therapeutics
University of Kansas Medical Center
3901 Rainbow Blvd, MS 1018
Kansas City, KS 66160
USA

C Kordes
Clinic of Gastroenterology,
 Hepatology and Infectiology
Heinrich-Heine-University
Moorenstrasse 5
40225 Düsseldorf
Germany

F Lammert
Department of Medicine II
Saarland University Hospital
Saarland University
Kirrberger Str. 1
66421 Homburg
Germany

D Lebrec
INSERM U773
Centre de Recherche Biomédicale
 Bichât-Beaujon CRB3 and Service
 d'Hépatologie
Hôpital Beaujon
92118 Clichy
France

A Moschetta
University of Bari
Consorzio Mario Negro Sud
Via Nazionale 8/A
66030 Santa Maria Imbaro (CH)
Italy

M Pinzani
Dipartimento di Medicina Interna
Università de Firenze
Viale G.B. Morgagni 85
50134 Firenze
Italy

M Rössle
Praxiszentrum
Bertoldstrasse 48
79098 Freiburg
Germany

T Sauerbruch
Medizinische Klinik und Poliklinik I
Allgemeine Innere Medizin
Sigmund-Freud-Strasse 25
53105 Bonn
Germany

P Schenk
Department of Internal Medicine III
Medical University Vienna
Allgemeines Krankenhaus
Währinger Gürtel 18-20
1090 Vienna
Austria

VH Shah
Gastrointestinal Research Unit
Mayo Clinic and Foundation
200 First Street SW
Rochester, MN 55905
USA

U Spengler
Department of Internal Medicine I
Universitätsklinikum Bonn
Sigmund-Freud-Strasse 25
53127 Bonn
Germany

D Thabut
service d'Hépato-Gastroentérologie
Groupe Hospitalier Pitié-Salpêtrière
47-83 Boulevard de l'Hôpital
75651 Paris Cedex 13
France

C Trautwein
Medical Clinic III
RWTH University Hospital
Pauwelsstrasse 30
52074 Aachen
Germany

HE Wasmuth
Medical Clinic III
University Hospital Aachen
Aachen University
52074 Aachen
Germany

R Weiskirchen
Institute of Clinical Chemistry and
   Pathobiochemistry
RWTH University Hospital
Pauwelsstrasse 30
52074 Aachen
Germany

F Wong
University of Toronto
Toronto General Hospital 9N/983
200 Elizabeth Street
Toronto, M5G 2C4
Ontario
Canada

List of chairpersons

J Bosch
Hepatic Hemodynamic Laboratory
Hospital Clínic-Idibaps and Ciberehd
Villaroel 170
08037 Barcelona
Spain

SL Friedman
Mount Sinai School of Medicine
Division of Liver Diseases
1425 Madison Avenue, Room 11-70C
New York, NY 10029-6574
USA

AM Gressner
Klinische Chemie/Zentrallabor
Universitätsklinikum Aachen
Pauwelsstr. 30
52074 Aachen
Germany

D Häussinger
Heinrich-Heine-Universität
  Düsseldorf
Klinik für Gastroenterologie,
  Hepatologie und Infektiologie
Moorenstrasse 5
40225 Düsseldorf
Germany

J Heller
Medizinische Klinik I
Universitätsklinikum Bonn
Sigmund-Freud-Str. 25
53127 Bonn
Germany

F Lammert
Department of Medicine II
Saarland University Hospital
Saarland University
Kirrberger Str. 1
66421 Homburg
Germany

D Lebrec
INSERM U773
Centre de Recherche Biomédicale
  Bichât-Beaujon CRB3 and Service
  d'Hépatologie
Hôpital Beaujon
Clichy
France

M Pinzani
Dipartimento di Medicina Interna
Università de Firenze
Viale G.B. Morgagni 85
50134 Firenze
Italy

G Ramadori
Gastroenterologie
Universitätskliniken Göttingen
Robert-Koch-Str. 40
37075 Göttingen
Germany

C Trautwein
Medical Clinic III
RWTH University Hospital
52074 Aachen
Germany

R Wiest
Klinik für Innere Medizin I
Klinikum der Universität Regensburg
93042 Regensburg
Germany

F Wong
University of Toronto
Toronto General Hospital 9N/983
200 Elizabeth Street
Toronto, M5G 2C4
Ontario
Canada

Preface

The International Falk Symposium 162 in Dresden is a good example for the promises of history. Sixty years after the misery of the Second World War and the destruction of Dresden and 20 years after a long and threatening Cold War, scientists from more than 50 nations across the world met in a wonderfully reconstructed city to discuss a series of key lectures on the pathophysiology and clinical management of liver cirrhosis.

Liver cirrhosis is a leading cause of morbidity and mortality worldwide. It is the fifth most common cause of death between the age of 25 and 45 years. To date, it is still not possible to inhibit or revert progression of cirrhosis in most patients. Accordingly, clinicians primarily deal with the various complications of cirrhosis, while liver transplantation is only available for selected patients.

There has been tremendous progress in the understanding of liver fibrosis and cirrhosis since the last Falk Symposium devoted to this topic in 2000. Toxins, micro-organisms, autoimmune triggers and metabolic disorders are the main initiators of mechanisms that lead to fibrosis and cirrhosis, with susceptible individuals being more prone to disease due to their genetic background. In the first three sessions of the Falk Symposium 162, we discussed these aspects of liver fibrogenesis as well as the cellular responses to chronic liver injury and novel non-invasive techniques for assessment of fibrosis in patients. On the second day, we focused on preprimary and primary prophylaxis of variceal bleeding and the therapy of other complications, providing a blueprint for future research and clinical management of liver cirrhosis

The chapters of the present book are based on the lectures of the Falk Symposium and provide excellent examples for the advanced but still incomplete knowledge how different fibrogenic stimuli induce recruitment, activation and death of hepatic and bone marrow-derived cells as well as deposition of excess extracellular matrix. These processes alter the architecture of the liver together with a marked change of the vascular bed inside and outside the liver, rendering liver cirrhosis a systemic disorder.

We are grateful to the Falk Foundation, which enabled this symposium of leading experts and key investigators in the field as well as to our co-organizers Jaime Bosch, Andrew Burroughs and Didier Lebrec. With their valuable and stimulating contributions and comments, we managed to set up this high-level symposium, the results of which you have in your hands with this book.

Tilman Sauerbruch
Frank Lammert

Section I
Pathomechanisms of fibrogenesis: initiation

Chair: SL FRIEDMAN and D HÄUSSINGER

1
Apoptosis and oncotic necrosis: profibrotic signalling mechanisms of cell death

H. JAESCHKE and J.-Y. HONG

INTRODUCTION

Liver fibrosis forms part of most chronic liver disease processes including alcoholic and non-alcoholic steatohepatitis, viral and autoimmune hepatitis and obstructive cholestasis[1]. Key features of fibrogenesis include activation of stellate cells and the deposition of excess extracellular matrix, especially the fibril-forming collagens I and III, in the space of Disse[1,2]. These events can lead to a significant impairment of liver function and portal hypertension, and can enhance susceptibility to sepsis. The fibrotic response is initiated and maintained by acute and chronic cell injury. The fibrotic process can be stopped and even reversed by removing the chronic insult, by inducing cell death of activated stellate cells and by promoting degradation of the excess extracellular matrix. Thus, controlling cell death and its profibrotic signalling events are critical therapeutic strategies to prevent or reverse fibrosis.

APOPTOTIC CELL DEATH

During the past decade major advances have been made in the understanding of signalling mechanisms of apoptotic cell death in hepatocytes and other cell types[3–6]. Depending on the initiating signal, two types of apoptosis can be distinguished. In the extrinsic pathway (Figure 1), a ligand, e.g. Fas ligand, binds to its respective death receptor, i.e. Fas receptor. Ligand binding results in trimerization of the receptor, which allows the recruitment of adapter molecules and proenzymes of initiator caspases to form the death-inducing signalling complex (DISC). Assembly of the DISC leads to formation of the active caspase-8 or -10, which cleave the Bcl-2 family member Bid. The truncated form of Bid (tBid) triggers the translocation of Bax to the outer membrane of the mitochondria, where Bax together with other pro-apoptotic Bcl-2 family members (Bak, Bad) form pores in the outer membrane and

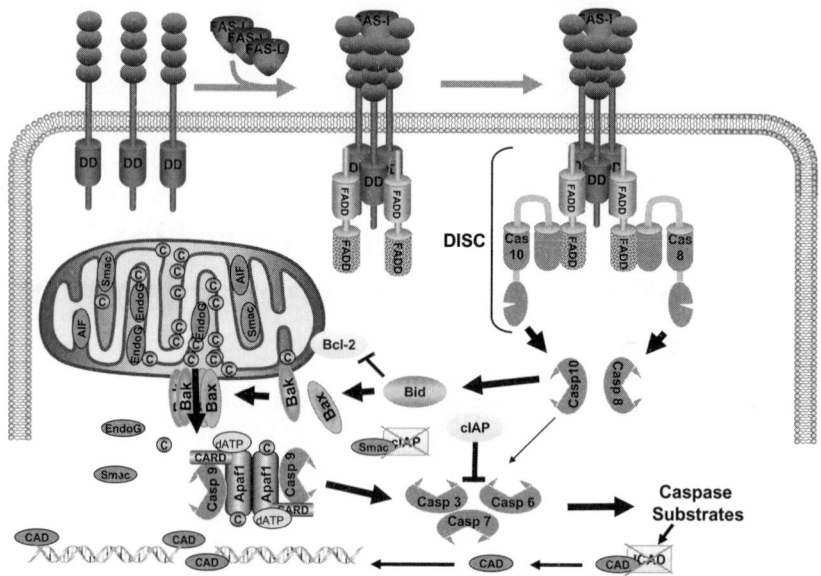

Figure 1 Fas receptor-mediated (extrinsic) pathway of apoptotic signalling in hepatocytes. See text for details. AIF, apoptosis-inducing factor; Apaf1, apoptosis protease-activating factor-1; CAD, caspase-activated DNase; CARD, caspase-activating and -recruiting domain; Casp, caspase; c, cytochrome c; cIAP, cellular inhibitor of apoptosis proteins; DD, death domain; Smac, second mitochondria-derived activator of caspases; DISC, death-inducing signalling complex; EndoG, endonuclease G; FADD, Fas-associated death domain; FAS-L, Fas-ligand; ICAD, inhibitor of CAD. Adapted from ref. 4. Reproduced from ref. 4 with permission of Elsevier

release intermembrane proteins such as cytochrome c, second mitochondria-derived activator of caspases (Smac), apoptosis-inducing factor (AIF) and endonuclease G. An increase of cytochrome c levels in the cytosol leads to the assembly of the apoptosome, which triggers the autocatalytic processing of procaspase-9 to the active enzyme. Caspase-9 processes procaspase-3, the major effector caspase of apoptosis. Hepatocytes also contain inhibitors of apoptosis proteins (IAP), which bind to active caspases and prevent the accidental propagation of the apoptotic signalling cascade. In order to overcome this safety measure within the cell, Smac released from mitochondria binds to IAP and promotes their proteolytic degradation, thereby allowing the uninhibited activation of the caspase cascade. Caspase-3 and other downstream effector caspases such as caspase-6 and -7 cleave numerous substrates within the cell, resulting in the characteristic morphological changes of apoptotic cells[7]. These morphological changes include cell shrinkage, membrane blebbing, chromatin condensation and margination along the nuclear envelope, DNA fragmentation and ultimately formation of apoptotic bodies, which are internalized by neighbouring cells or phagocytosed by hepatic macrophages (Kupffer cells).

In contrast to the extrinsic, receptor-mediated signalling mechanism, the intrinsic pathway is initiated by an internal insult[4,8]. For example, DNA damage can lead to p53 activation and the increased formation of Bax. Alternatively, disturbances of the cellular Ca^{2+} homeostasis can trigger the cleavage of Bid by activation of calpains. These internal initiating events induce the release of cytochrome c from mitochondria and all subsequent signalling mechanisms described previously. In general, if a limited number of cells undergo apoptosis due to a moderate stress, the process can be completed, i.e. the apoptotic bodies can be eliminated without triggering an inflammatory response. However, if the pro-apoptotic stimulus is too severe, and affects many cells, mitochondria undergo the membrane permeability transition pore opening, which causes the collapse of their membrane potential and results in declining cellular adenosine triphosphate (ATP) levels[3,9]. Under these conditions the apoptotic process deteriorates into secondary necrosis with release of cell contents[10]. The important feature of secondary necrosis is that many characteristics of apoptosis, e.g. caspase activation and nuclear changes, are still maintained[11].

ONCOTIC NECROSIS

In the past, oncotic necrosis was considered the consequence of a catastrophic event, which resulted in immediate cell death. Although such a massive insult may occur under special circumstances, the more likely scenario is that a moderate external interference with the cellular homeostasis can induce disturbances within the cell, resulting in ultimate cell death. The external insult triggers a necrotic signalling cascade, which may have certain overlap with apoptotic signalling but is clearly a separate process. An example of this necrotic signalling is liver injury induced by acetaminophen (AAP) overdose (Figure 2)[12]. The injury process is initiated by the formation of a reactive metabolite (N-acetyl-p-benzoquinone imine; NAPQI) through the P450 system. NAPQI can be detoxified by conjugation with glutathione. However, once the cellular glutathione pool is exhausted, excess NAPQI can bind to cellular proteins including mitochondrial proteins. This early cellular stress also causes activation of Bid[12] and c-jun N-terminal kinase[13], which can promote the translocation of Bax to the outer mitochondrial membrane[14]. The mitochondrial translocation of Bax promotes the release of intermembrane proteins. Although cytochrome c and Smac are released from mitochondria after AAP overdose[14], there is no relevant caspase activation, mainly due to the declining cellular ATP levels[15]. On the other hand, mitochondrial release of AIF and endonuclease G results in translocation of these proteins to the nucleus where they induce DNA fragmentation[16,17]. In addition to these signalling events the early mitochondrial dysfunction also results in formation of reactive oxygen species and peroxynitrite[12]. The oxidant stress is mainly responsible for the opening of the mitochondrial membrane permeability transition pore, which leads to the collapse of the mitochondrial membrane potential, mitochondrial swelling and rupture of the outer membrane[18]. At this point mitochondrial release of AIF and endonuclease G and the resulting DNA

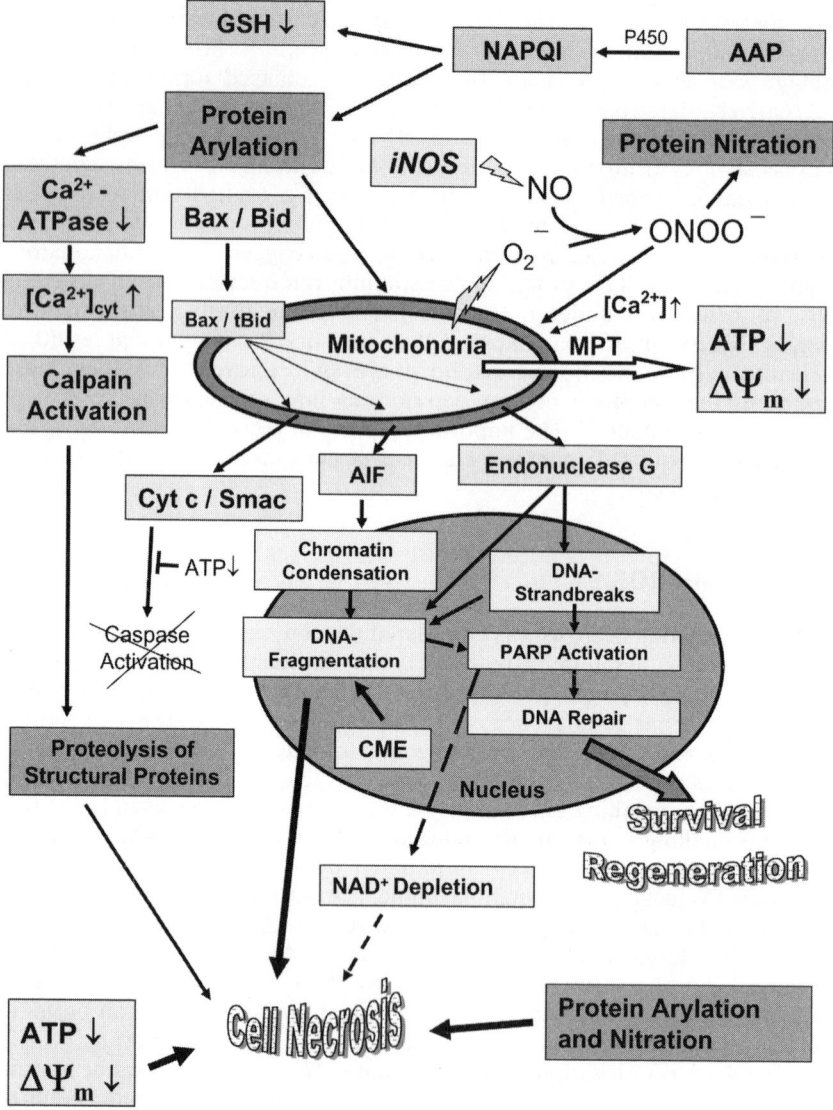

Figure 2 Intracellular signalling mechanisms of oncotic necrosis induced by acetaminophen (AAP) overdose. See text for details. AIF, apoptosis-inducing factor; CMA, nuclear Ca^{2+}/Mg^{2+}-dependent endonuclease; cyt c, cytochrome c; $\Delta\Psi_m$, mitochondrial membrane potential; GSH, reduced glutathione; iNOS, inducible NO synthase; MPT, mitochondrial membrane permeability transition; NAPQI, N-acetyl-p-benzoquinone imine; NO, nitric oxide; O_2^-, superoxide; ONOO$^-$, peroxynitrite; PARP, poly(ADP-ribose) polymerase; Smac, second mitochondria-derived activator of caspases; tBid, truncated form of Bid. Adapted from ref. 12. Reproduced with permission from Oxford University Press

fragmentation is independent of Bax and other Bcl-2 family members[14]. The extensive mitochondrial dysfunction with cessation of ATP production and endonuclease-mediated nuclear DNA fragmentation leads to oncotic necrosis with cell swelling and release of cellular contents (Figure 2). In general, oncotic necrosis in hepatocytes can be induced by a variety of insults including ischaemia–reperfusion, bile acids, and various drugs and chemicals. Although the initiating events may vary, reactive metabolite formation, oxidative stress and mitochondrial dysfunction are common features of many pathophysiological processes[19]. In addition, the intracellular signalling events leading to cell death may be enhanced by triggering an inflammatory response, which can substantially enhance the oxidant stress and aggravate the existing injury[20]. However, the critical message is that not only apoptosis but also oncotic necrosis can be pharmacologically manipulated after the initial insults.

PATHOPHYSIOLOGICAL IMPORTANCE OF APOPTOSIS VERSUS ONCOTIC NECROSIS

Because of overlapping signalling pathways, and the fact that many parameters which investigators use to quantify cell death are not specific for apoptosis or oncotic necrosis, there is a substantial controversy regarding the predominant mode of cell death in various pathophysiologies[3,5,11]. However, it is important to remember that apoptosis is defined by morphology (cell shrinkage, chromatin condensation, formation of apoptotic bodies) and that the activation of executioner caspases is mainly responsible for these characteristic morphological features[7]. Thus, the conclusion that cell death is caused by apoptosis needs to be based on these morphological features together with quantitatively relevant activation of caspases[3,5,11]. Many other parameters including DNA fragmentation (TUNEL assay, DNA ladder, anti-histone ELISA), mitochondrial Bax and Bid translocation, Bid cleavage, mitochondrial cytochrome c release, increased Fas receptor expression, etc., are not specific for apoptosis. These parameters are only useful to define signalling mechanisms once, based on morphological evidence, the mode of cell death has been determined. Although it may seem to be sometimes a futile argument whether to label the cell death as apoptosis or oncotic necrosis, it actually is an important distinction. To resolve an inflammatory or fibrotic process it is necessary to promote apoptosis of activated neutrophils or stellate cells, respectively[21,22]. In this respect it is critical to define whether the chronic cell injury promoting inflammation or fibrosis is due to apoptosis or oncotic necrosis. It would be more challenging to identify therapeutic targets if apoptotic cell death is required for both the promotion of fibrosis and its resolution.

PROFIBROTIC SIGNALLING DURING CELL DEATH

Chronic cell injury and stellate cell activation are critical features of liver fibrogenesis[2]; however, the molecular connection between these events became

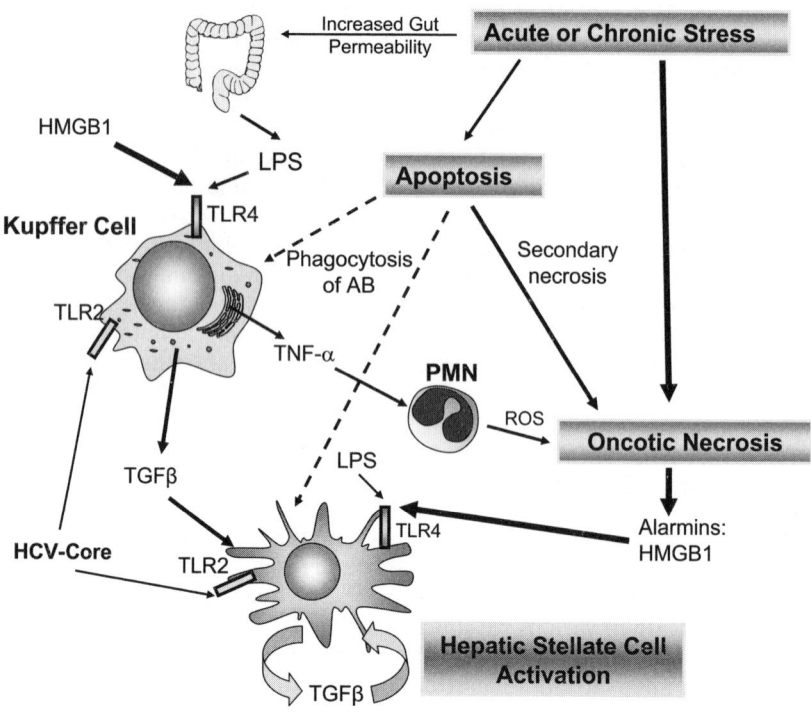

Figure 3 Profibrotic signalling mechanisms of cell death. See text for details. AB, apoptotic bodies; HCV-core, hepatitis C virus core protein; HMGB1, high-mobility group box 1 protein; LPS, lipopolysaccharide, endotoxin; PMN, polymorphonuclear leukocytes; ROS, reactive oxygen species; TGF-β, transforming growth factor β; TLR, toll-like receptor; TNF-α, tumour necrosis factor-α

evident only recently. In the case of apoptotic cell death the main products are apoptotic bodies, which are phagocytosed by macrophages (Kupffer cells) and to a lesser degree also by stellate cells through interaction with the phosphatidyl serine receptor[23,24]. In Kupffer cells the phagocytosis of apoptotic bodies leads to proinflammatory cytokine expression, e.g. tumour necrosis factor alpha (TNF-α), but not to formation of the profibrogenic cytokine transforming growth factor-β$_1$ (TGF-β$_1$)[25]. In contrast, phagocytosis of apoptotic bodies in stellate cells caused the formation of TGF-β$_1$ and collagen α$_1$[24]. Thus, extensive apoptotic cell death triggers stellate activation either directly or indirectly through Kupffer cells, and can promote hepatic fibrosis[24,25].

A hallmark of oncotic necrosis is the release of cell contents including a number of proteins generally termed alarmins[26]. High-mobility group box-1 protein (HMGB1), a nuclear protein, is selectively released by necrotic cells[27]. Interestingly, HMGB1 and other alarmins are recognized by toll-like receptors (TLR) on Kupffer cells and stellate cells[28,29]. Signalling through TLR4, which recognizes HMGB1 and endotoxin, triggers proinflammatory and profibrogenic cytokine formation in Kupffer cells and in stellate cells[30]. Thus, Kupffer cell activation by alarmins and/or phagocytosis of necrotic cell debris contribute to fibrogenesis directly by release of TGF-β, which activates stellate cells, and indirectly by further promoting inflammation (leukocyte infiltration) and cell injury (reactive oxygen and cytokine formation) (Figure 3). Oxidant stress generated extracellularly by inflammatory cells or intracellularly does not induce apoptosis, but causes cell death mainly through oncotic necrosis[31,32] and promotes fibrosis through alarmin signalling. In addition, during viral hepatitis, viral proteins may directly contribute to fibrogenesis through their recognition by the TLR2 receptor on Kupffer and stellate cells[28,29]. In cases where the permeability of the intestinal wall is increased, e.g. ethanol toxicity, or the gut flora is changed, e.g. obstructive cholestasis, endotoxin plays an important role in enhancing inflammatory cell injury and fibrosis[30,33].

SUMMARY

Both apoptosis and oncotic necrosis can indirectly cause stellate cell activation through mediators generated by activated Kupffer cells, which release proinflammatory and profibrotic cytokines in response to TLR signalling induced by alarmins, viral proteins and endotoxin, as well as phagocytosis of apoptotic bodies and necrotic cell debris. Since stellate cells express the same TLR as Kupffer cells, and are able to recognize and phagocytose apoptotic bodies, the same mediators can also directly activate stellate cells and contribute to their continued activation. On the other hand, resolution of inflammation and fibrogenesis depends on the removal of activated leukocytes and stellate cells by apoptosis. Therefore, it is an opportunity, but also a challenge, to selectively inhibit the chronic, profibrotic cell death signalling but induce, or at least not interfere with, apoptosis of stellate cells and leukocytes. A better understanding of the intracellular signalling mechanisms of cell death induced by various insults remains an important goal for the future.

References

1. Bataller R, Brenner DA. Liver fibrosis. J Clin Invest. 2005;115:209–18.
2. Friedman SL. Molecular regulation of hepatic fibrosis, an integrated cellular response to tissue injury. J Biol Chem. 2000;275:2247–50.
3. Jaeschke H, Lemasters JJ. Apoptosis versus oncotic necrosis in hepatic ischemia/reperfusion injury. Gastroenterology. 2003;125:1246-57.
4. Jaeschke H. Mechanisms of liver cell destruction. In: Boyer TD, Wright TL, Manns M, editors. Zakim and Boyer's Hepatology, 5th edn. Philadelphia: Saunders-Elsevier, 2006:37–51.
5. Schulze-Bergkamen H, Schuchmann M, Fleischer B, Galle PR. The role of apoptosis versus oncotic necrosis in liver injury: facts or faith? J Hepatol. 2006;44:984–93.
6. Ding WX, Yin XM. Dissection of the multiple mechanisms of TNF-alpha-induced apoptosis in liver injury. J Cell Mol Med. 2004;8:445–54.
7. Fischer U, Jänicke RU, Schulze-Osthoff K. Many cuts to ruin: a comprehensive update of caspase substrates. Cell Death Differ. 2003;10:76–100.
8. Schattenberg JM, Galle PR, Schuchmann M. Apoptosis in liver disease. Liver Int. 2006;26:904–11.

9. Lemasters JJ, Qian T, He L et al. Role of mitochondrial inner membrane permeabilization in necrotic cell death, apoptosis, and autophagy. Antioxid Redox Signal. 2002;4:769–81.
10. Ogasawara J, Watanabe-Fukunaga R, Adachi M et al. Lethal effect of the anti-Fas antibody in mice. Nature. 1993;364:806–9.
11. Jaeschke H, Gujral JS, Bajt ML. Apoptosis and necrosis in liver disease. Liver Int. 2004;24:85–9.
12. Jaeschke H, Bajt ML. Intracellular signaling mechanisms of acetaminophen-induced liver cell death. Toxicol Sci. 2006;89:31–41.
13. Gunawan BK, Liu ZX, Han D, Hanawa N, Gaarde WA, Kaplowitz N. c-Jun N-terminal kinase plays a major role in murine acetaminophen hepatotoxicity. Gastroenterology. 2006;131:165–78.
14. Bajt ML, Farhood A, Lemasters JJ, Jaeschke H. Mitochondrial bax translocation accelerates DNA fragmentation and cell necrosis in a murine model of acetaminophen hepatotoxicity. J Pharmacol Exp Ther. 2008;324:8–14.
15. Lawson JA, Fisher MA, Simmons CA, Farhood A, Jaeschke H. Inhibition of Fas receptor (CD95)-induced hepatic caspase activation and apoptosis by acetaminophen in mice. Toxicol Appl Pharmacol. 1999;156:179–86.
16. Cover C, Mansouri A, Knight TR et al. Peroxynitrite-induced mitochondrial and endonuclease-mediated nuclear DNA damage in acetaminophen hepatotoxicity. J Pharmacol Exp Ther. 2005;315:879-87.
17. Bajt ML, Cover C, Lemasters JJ, Jaeschke H. Nuclear translocation of endonuclease G and apoptosis-inducing factor during acetaminophen-induced liver cell injury. Toxicol Sci. 2006;94:217–25.
18. Kon K, Kim JS, Jaeschke H, Lemasters JJ. Mitochondrial permeability transition in acetaminophen-induced necrosis and apoptosis of cultured mouse hepatocytes. Hepatology. 2004;40:1170–9.
19. Jaeschke H, Gores GJ, Cederbaum AI, Hinson JA, Pessayre D, Lemasters JJ. Mechanisms of hepatotoxicity. Toxicol Sci. 2002;65:166–76.
20. Jaeschke H, Hasegawa T. Role of neutrophils in acute inflammatory liver injury. Liver Int. 2006;26:912–19.
21. Kobayashi SD, Voyich JM, Burlak C, DeLeo FR. Neutrophils in the innate immune response. Arch Immunol Ther Exp (Warsz). 2005;53:505–17.
22. Elsharkawy AM, Oakley F, Mann DA. The role and regulation of hepatic stellate cell apoptosis in reversal of liver fibrosis. Apoptosis. 2005;10:927–39.
23. Fadok VA, Chimini G. The phagocytosis of apoptotic cells. Semin Immunol. 2001;13:365–72.
24. Canbay A, Taimr P, Torok N, Higuchi H, Friedman S, Gores GJ. Apoptotic body engulfment by a human stellate cell line is profibrogenic. Lab Invest. 2003;83:655–63.
25. Canbay A, Feldstein AE, Higuchi H et al. Kupffer cell engulfment of apoptotic bodies stimulates death ligand and cytokine expression. Hepatology. 2003;38:1188–98.
26. Bianchi ME. DAMPs, PAMPs and alarmins: all we need to know about danger. J Leukoc Biol. 2007;81:1-5.
27. Scaffidi P, Misteli T, Bianchi ME. Release of chromatin protein HMGB1 by necrotic cells triggers inflammation. Nature. 2002;418:191–5.
28. Schwabe RF, Seki E, Brenner DA. Toll-like receptor signaling in the liver. Gastroenterology. 2006;130:1886–900.
29. Szabo G, Mandrekar P, Dolganiuc A. Innate immune response and hepatic inflammation. Semin Liver Dis. 2007;27:339–50.
30. Seki E, De Minicis S, Osterreicher CH et al. TLR4 enhances TGF-beta signaling and hepatic fibrosis. Nat Med. 2007;13:1324–32.
31. Jaeschke H, Ho YS, Fisher MA, Lawson JA, Farhood A. Glutathione peroxidase-deficient mice are more susceptible to neutrophil-mediated hepatic parenchymal cell injury during endotoxemia: importance of an intracellular oxidant stress. Hepatology. 1999;29:443–50.
32. Hong JY, Jaeschke H. Oncotic necrosis and apoptosis mediate liver injury in response to superoxide formation *in vivo* (abstract). Tox Sci. 2008;101(Suppl. 1):171.
33. Hong JY, Sato E, Hiramoto K, Nishikawa M, Inoue M. Mechanism of liver injury during obstructive jaundice: role of nitric oxide, splenic cytokines, and intestinal flora. J Clin Biochem Nutr. 2007;40:184–93.

2
The mucosal immune system in the pathogenesis of liver disease

B. EKSTEEN and D. H. ADAMS

INTRODUCTION

The gastrointestinal tract and accessory organs, which include the salivary glands, liver, pancreas and gall bladder, cooperate to carry out the essential functions of digestion, absorption and metabolism. Ingested foods contain not only complex beneficial molecules such as carbohydrates, proteins and fats, but also potentially harmful pathogens. This poses a very significant challenge to the immune system to limit inappropriate immune responses to harmless food antigens whilst maintaining effective immunity to pathogens[1-3]. The majority of these antigens are processed and controlled by immune responses at the intestinal mucosal barrier and underlying lamina propria; however, translocation of gut antigens to the portal circulation, either through active transport of nutrients or invasive pathogens, means that antigens not dealt with directly in the gut are brought to the liver and this requires a co-ordinated immune response. Immune responses in the gut and liver are individually well described, but the mechanisms that control immunological crosstalk to share knowledge of mutual antigens have only recently become apparent through advances in our understanding of how immune cells are directed to immune compartments in the gut and liver, as well as careful studies into diseases that affect both sites, such as infection, coeliac disease and inflammatory bowel disease (IBD).

ORGANIZATION OF THE GUT IMMUNE SYSTEM

Antigen recognition and acquired intestinal immune responses

The first line of defence against gut pathogens is provided by the mucosal barrier of mucus that is rich in antibacterial substances[4], secreted IgA[5] and commensal bacteria[6]. Invasion is further impeded by the tight junctions of the underlying epithelial cells that prevent bacterial translocation[7]. Gut epithelial cells are also receptors that act as sensors to detect potentially harmful antigens and to trigger innate immune responses[8]. Epithelial cells and some resident haematopoietic cells such as NK cells express nucleotide-binding oligomerization domain (NOD) molecules which act as immune sensors to detect pathogens[9]. Critical mutations that corrupt the function of these immune sensors disrupt our ability to distinguish friend from foe in the gut, and mutations in the NOD2 molecule have been associated with autoimmune gut inflammation in the form of Crohn's disease[10].

Antigens that escape these initial layers of protection and penetrate the mucosal barrier are processed by specialized antigen-presenting cells called dendritic cells (DC) and carried via lymphatics to the draining mesenteric lymph nodes (MLN) where interactions with naive lymphocytes generate antigen-specific immune responses[1,2,11,12]. Together the Peyer's patches and MLN constitute the gut-associated lymphoid tissue (GALT) where naive T and B lymphocytes are not only imprinted by DC to recognize antigen but also to preferentially traffic to the gut to increase their likelihood of finding their cognate antigen[13,14]. A unique feature of gut-derived DC is the ability to convert retinol to retinoic acid which in turn binds with intracellular retinoid receptors in B and T cells to activate transcription of the genes encoding the chemokines receptor, CCR9, and the integrin pairing, $\alpha_4\beta_7$, which induces gut tropism[15].

Gut-specific lymphocyte trafficking

In order for the immune system to target lymphocytes to areas of infection or inflammation it has evolved sets of organ-specific homing molecules that act as molecular postal codes. The gut postal code consists of MAdCAM-1 and the chemokine, CCL25, which are the ligands for the lymphocyte receptors, $\alpha_4\beta_7$ and CCR9, respectively[16]. MAdCAM-1 is widely expressed in mucosal vessels and the intestinal lamina propria[17], whereas CCL25 is found only in the thymus and in the small bowel[16]. Ligation of CCR9 by CCL25 activates $\alpha_4\beta_7$ to adhere to MAdCAM-1 and promotes lymphocyte recruitment to the gut[18,19]. During gut inflammation such as exacerbations of IBD, MAdCAM-1 expression is up-regulated and promotes the sustained recruitment of circulating $\alpha_4\beta_7$+ lymphocytes and the establishment of chronic bowel inflammation. Antibody inhibition of $\alpha_4\beta_7$ and CCR9 reduces inflammation in animal models and this is currently being assessed in patients with IBD[20-22].

DISEASE AFFECTING THE GUT AND LIVER

Coeliac disease

Coeliac disease is an under-recognized cause of liver disease[23]. Increased recognition of coeliac disease through serological detection of antibodies against tissue transglutaminase has established an ever-increasing role for coeliac disease in liver dysfunction[24]. Although the mechanisms that link coeliac disease to liver dysfunction are yet to be described, their importance is underlined by reports in which administration of a gluten-free diet has entirely reversed some forms of liver disease[25]. Abnormal liver enzymes can be detected in up to 60% of patients with a new diagnosis of coeliac disease; conversely up to 10% of patients with unexplained abnormal liver biochemistry will have endomysial antibodies. Liver biopsy in both cases often shows only a non-specific lymphocytic infiltrate, and for the vast majority of patients will resolve on a gluten free-diet[26]. On occasion these infiltrates will persist and have the features of autoimmune liver diseases including autoimmune hepatitis, primary biliary cirrhosis (PBC) and primary sclerosing cholangitis (PSC).

Perhaps the most common liver disease associated with coeliac disease is PBC[27]. Around 3% of patients with coeliac disease will have PBC, and conversely 6–7% of PBC patients will have coeliac disease[26,28]. Unfortunately treatment with a gluten-free diet does not appear to improve liver biochemistry or the progression of PBC. Both PSC and autoimmune hepatitis have been described in a minority of patients with coeliac disease and the condition does not appear to be sensitive to dietary treatment[29,30]. Coeliac disease affecting the liver is, however, not only restricted to autoimmune-mediated liver disease but has also been associated with fatty liver disease[31], iron overload[32], fulminant liver failure and hepatic malignancies. Although these entities vary greatly in their response to treatment with a gluten-free diet, there are case reports of complete resolution of liver failure with dietary treatment for coeliac disease.

IBD and PSC

Liver disease, in the form of autoimmune hepatitis or PSC, is relatively common and develops in 2.4–7.5% of patients with IBD, while 70–85% patients with PSC will suffer from IBD at some point in their lives[33]. The strongest association is with ulcerative colitis (90%), with Crohn's colitis predominating in the remainder. The estimated incidence of PSC is one to six cases per 100 000[34], with men more likely to develop PSC than women[35]. PSC is commonly associated with UC and typically affects the right side of the colon with involvement of the terminal ileum, known as 'backwash ileitis'[36]. PSC can be associated with Crohn's disease when it is invariably associated with extensive large bowel disease[37,38]. PSC is often complicated by the development of cholangiocarcinoma[39,40] and is an independent risk factor for the development of colonic cancer and dysplasia in patients with IBD[41–43]. The only effective treatment for PSC is liver transplantation[44].

This unique relationship between the gut and the liver is further highlighted by the fact that patients can develop PSC for the first time many years after total colectomy for colitis, and colonic inflammation can occur for the first time after patients have undergone liver transplantation for PSC[45]. In contrast to the other extraintestinal manifestations of IBD such as pyoderma and colitis-associated arthropathy, where relapse is closely linked to colonic inflammation and improves on resolution of colitis, PSC follows a course independent of colonic inflammation. Liver dysfunction is often minimal during periods of severe colitis, only to deteriorate once colitis is in remission. These features are also seen post-liver transplantation for PSC when IBD activity is often increased with frequent relapses and increased requirements for immunosuppressive agents. Liver transplantation for PSC also increases the risk of colonic neoplasia in IBD patients even further, and forms the basis for the use of ursodeoxycholic acid (UDCA) and annual colonoscopic surveillance in these patients.

ENTEROHEPATIC LYMPHOCYTE MIGRATION

A plausible explanation for the hepatic dysfunction seen in the context of gut inflammation is that under certain conditions the gut and the liver activate mechanisms that lead to a shared immune response across both sites. Such mechanisms would primarily limit pathogens that have crossed the mucosal barrier and are likely to be encountered in the liver, but at times could become dysregulated and allow autoimmunity to spread from the gut to the liver.

Extraintestinal manifestations of IBD

A common feature of extraintestinal liver disease in IBD and coeliac disease is the presence of heavy lymphocytic infiltrates in the liver. Nearly all of these lymphocytes are long-lived memory cells and are able to rapidly respond to antigenic stimuli. Recent reports would suggest that a proportion of these cells have been generated in the gut during episodes of inflammation and, in the case of IBD and PSC, are aberrantly entering the liver to cause dysfunction. Such a hypothesis could also be extended to the other extraintestinal manifestations; indeed the first evidence linking mucosal T cells with extraintestinal disease came from observations by Salmi and colleagues, who showed that gut-derived lymphocytes could bind to synovial vessels[46]. Binding of gut-activated lymphocytes to vessels in the joint synovium is mediated by generic proinflammatory adhesion receptors such as ICAM-1 and VCAM-1, but not by the gut-specific receptors $\alpha_4\beta_7$-integrin and MAdCAM-1[47]. It still remains unclear why particular tissues are targeted and what factors lead to the induction of inflammation at these sites, but this seems to be closely linked to gut inflammation because extraintestinal disease usually resolves rapidly once bowel inflammation is controlled. Tumour necrosis factor alpha (TNF-α) has been implicated in the pathogenesis of concomitant extraintestinal diseases such as pyoderma gangrenosum and acute seronegative arthritis, and both conditions are exquisitely sensitive to treatment with anti-TNF-α antibodies[48].

This is not the case for the liver complications which arise independent of inflammation in the gut and are unaffected by therapeutic anti-TNF-α antibodies. This paradox makes the hepatic complications of IBD most interesting from the perspective of lymphocyte homing. The fact that liver disease can occur in the absence of a diseased colon implies the link cannot be explained by the release of recently activated effector cells from the gut. However, the existence of a population of long-lived mucosal memory T cells that could be recruited to either the gut or liver might explain this link. Evidence in support of an entero-hepatic lymphocyte pathway in IBD and PSC comes from observations that MAdCAM-1, which is expressed on mucosal vessels[17,49] and is absent from the fetal and normal adult human liver[50], is expressed in inflammatory liver diseases associated with IBD. Hepatic MAdCAM-1 supports *in vitro* $\alpha_4\beta_7$-integrin-mediated lymphocyte adhesion to the liver endothelium[51]. Moreover, VAP-1, which is highly expressed on normal liver endothelium and is detectable only at low levels on normal mucosal vessels, has increased expression in IBD[52,53].

Perhaps the most compelling evidence of enterohepatic homing in PSC comes from the detection of the chemokine CCL25 on endothelium in PSC. CCL25 expression is usually highly restricted to the gut and thymus, and its expression in the liver is almost entirely limited to PSC, where binding to its receptor CCR9 on gut lymphocytes causes $\alpha_4\beta_7$ to bind to MAdCAM-1 on liver endothelium[18]. Up to 20% of the T lymphocytes in PSC express CCR9 and $\alpha_4\beta_7$, which is a unique adhesion molecule combination that can be imprinted only during activation by gut DC and not by DC isolated from liver tissue or liver-draining lymph nodes[13,16]. Thus CCR9 + $\alpha_4\beta_7$ + liver-infiltrating T cells must have been activated in the gut[18]. Liver-infiltrating CCR9 + $\alpha_4\beta_7$ cells are primed to secrete interferon gamma (IFN-γ) on stimulation, suggesting that they can be rapidly expanded into effector cells in the liver[18].

Graft-versus-host disease (GVHD)

Further evidence that, under certain inflammatory conditions, mucosal T cells are preferentially recruited to the liver comes from observations in GVHD. In allogeneic haematopoietic stem-cell transplantation, donor T cells mediate beneficial graft-versus-tumour effects as well as GVHD. Although alloantigens are expressed by all host tissues, GVHD develops in certain organs, including the skin, intestine, liver and thymus. Peyer's patches in the gut appear to be required to activate the host-specific cytotoxic T lymphocyte responses in GVHD, and blocking $\alpha_4\beta_7$-integrin prevents the disease developing[54]. Recent studies in mouse models of GVHD have shown that recipients of $\alpha_4\beta_7$-depleted donor T cells develop significantly less GVHD of the intestines and liver, whereas there was no difference in cutaneous and thymic GVHD between recipients of $\alpha_4\beta_7$-depleted or $\alpha_4\beta_7$-replete T cells[55].

Infections of the gut and liver

Most intrahepatic T cells are primed memory cells, including cells with specificity for persistent viruses, indicating that trafficking of memory T cells through the liver under non-inflammatory conditions might contribute to immune surveillance[56]. It is possible that some memory lymphocytes that are activated in the gut recirculate through the liver to allow memory of mucosal antigens to be shared across both sites. The observation that the intestinal mucosal CD8+ T-cell response to infection with *Listeria monocytogenes* is associated with a marked clonal expansion of memory CD8+ T cells in the liver compared with the spleen is supportive of such a mechanism[57,58]. Pope et al. studied the migration patterns of memory CD8+ T cells that had been activated by gut-restricted antigens; they detected antigen-specific T cells in many extraintestinal sites, including the liver[57]. Such observations are consistent with early transfer studies of Gowans and Knight, in which large lymphocytes mainly migrated to the gut, whereas some cells were also detected in the liver and kidney[59]. However, none of these studies shows that mucosal memory T cells preferentially recirculate through the liver under normal conditions. Indeed studies using adoptive transfer of memory T cells into parabiosis models show that T cells rapidly equilibrate into the liver and that this does not require $\alpha_4\beta_7$ integrins[60].

It is important to recognize that, although there is evidence that memory lymphocytes do recirculate in an enterohepatic pattern, their ability to respond to antigens in the liver might be altered due to the intrinsic tolerogenic immune milieu that exists in the liver. The liver is at best a fairly hostile environment for lymphocytes, with an abundance of potential death signals to clear potentially autoreactive lymphocytes. Thus a large proportion of enteric lymphocytes that enter the liver will die either through neglect or by apoptosis in the liver to limit inappropriate responses to potentially harmless food antigens. Interleukin 10 is a key mediator of liver tolerance, and although this creates an environment that is conducive to tolerating food antigens, it does leave us potentially vulnerable to infections.

Knowledge of the mechanisms that underpin coordinated immune responses between the liver and the gut not only allows us to explain why and how some intestinal diseases are associated with disease at distant extraintestinal sites, but also creates opportunities to intervene and design novel therapies. Potential candidates are undoubtedly the gut addressins, CCL25 and MAdCAM-1 as well as their respective receptors, CCR9 and $\alpha_4\beta_7$. Therapeutic inhibition of both CCR9 and $\alpha_4\beta_7$ is currently in development for the treatment of IBD, but has the potential to be of benefit in treating inflammation at extraintestinal sites such as the liver.

Acknowledgement

This work was supported by grants from the Medical Research Council, Core UK and the European Commission.

References

1. MacDonald TT, Monteleone G. Immunity, inflammation, and allergy in the gut. Science. 2005;307:1920–5.
2. Mowat AM. Anatomical basis of tolerance and immunity to intestinal antigens. Nat Rev Immunol. 2003;3:331–41.
3. Strober W, Fuss IJ, Blumberg RS. The immunology of mucosal models of inflammation. Annu Rev Immunol. 2002;20:495–549.
4. Ayabe T, Satchell DP, Wilson CL et al. Secretion of microbicidal alpha-defensins by intestinal Paneth cells in response to bacteria. Nat Immunol. 2000;1:113–18.
5. Macpherson AJ, Gatto D, Sainsbury E et al. A primitive T cell-independent mechanism of intestinal mucosal IgA responses to commensal bacteria. Science. 2000;288:2222–6.
6. McCracken VJ, Lorenz RG. The gastrointestinal ecosystem: a precarious alliance among epithelium, immunity and microbiota. Cell Microbiol. 2001;3:1–11.
7. Madara JL. Regulation of the movement of solutes across tight junctions. Annu Rev Physiol. 1998;60:143–59.
8. Akira S, Takeda K, Kaisho T. Toll-like receptors: critical proteins linking innate and acquired immunity. Nat Immunol. 2001;2:675–80.
9. Strober W, Murray PJ, Kitani A et al. Signalling pathways and molecular interactions of NOD1 and NOD2. Nat Rev Immunol. 2006;6:9–20.
10. Hugot JP, Chamaillard M, Zouali H et al. Association of NOD2 leucine-rich repeat variants with susceptibility to Crohn's disease. Nature. 2001;411:599–603.
11. Rescigno M, Urbano M, Valzasina B et al. Dendritic cells express tight junction proteins and penetrate gut epithelial monolayers to sample bacteria. Nat Immunol. 2001;2:361–7.

12. Nagler-Anderson C. Man the barrier! Strategic defences in the intestinal mucosa. Nat Rev Immunol. 2001;1:59–67.
13. Mora JR, Iwata M, Eksteen B et al. Generation of gut-homing IgA-secreting B cells by intestinal dendritic cells. Science. 2006;314:1157–60.
14. Mora JR, Bono MR, Manjunath N et al. Selective imprinting of gut-homing T cells by Peyer's patch dendritic cells. Nature. 2003;424:88–93.
15. Iwata M, Hirakiyama A, Eshima Y et al. Retinoic acid imprints gut-homing specificity on T cells. Immunity. 2004;21:527–38.
16. Agace WW. Tissue-tropic effector T cells: generation and targeting opportunities. Nat Rev Immunol. 2006;6:682–92.
17. Briskin M, Winsor-Hines D, Shyjan A et al. Human mucosal addressin cell adhesion molecule-1 is preferentially expressed in intestinal tract and associated lymphoid tissue. Am J Pathol. 1997;151:97–110.
18. Eksteen B, Grant AJ, Miles A et al. Hepatic endothelial CCL25 mediates the recruitment of CCR9+ gut-homing lymphocytes to the liver in primary sclerosing cholangitis. J Exp Med. 2004;200:1511–17.
19. Berg EL, McEvoy LM, Berlin C et al. L-selectin-mediated lymphocyte rolling on madcam-1. Nature. 1993;366:695–8.
20. ChemoCentryx. Traficet EN. http://www.chemocentryx.com 2006.
21. Hamann A, Andrew DP, Jablonski-Westrich D et al. Role of alpha 4-integrins in lymphocyte homing to mucosal tissues *in vivo*. J Immunol. 1994;152:3282–93.
22. Ghosh S. Therapeutic value of alpha-4 integrin blockade in inflammatory bowel disease:the role of natalizumab. Expert Opin Biol Ther. 2003;3:995–1000.
23. Rubio-Tapia A, Murray JA. The liver in celiac disease. Hepatology. 2007;46:1650–8.
24. Freeman HJ. Hepatobiliary and pancreatic disorders in celiac disease. World J Gastroenterol. 2006;12:1503–8.
25. Bardella MT, Vecchi M, Conte D et al. Chronic unexplained hypertransaminasemia may be caused by occult celiac disease. Hepatology. 1999;29:654–7.
26. Volta U, Rodrigo L, Granito A et al. Celiac disease in autoimmune cholestatic liver disorders. Am J Gastroenterol. 2002;97:2609–13.
27. Kingham JG, Parker DR. The association between primary biliary cirrhosis and coeliac disease: a study of relative prevalences. Gut. 1998;42:120–2.
28. Lawson A, West J, Aithal GP et al. Autoimmune cholestatic liver disease in people with coeliac disease: a population-based study of their association. Aliment Pharmacol Ther. 2005;21:401–5.
29. Venturini I, Cosenza R, Miglioli L et al. Adult celiac disease and primary sclerosing cholangitis: two case reports. Hepatogastroenterology. 1998;45:2344–7.
30. Villalta D, Girolami D, Bidoli E et al. High prevalence of celiac disease in autoimmune hepatitis detected by anti-tissue tranglutaminase autoantibodies. J Clin Lab Anal. 2005;19:6–10.
31. Naschitz JE, Yeshurun D, Zuckerman E et al. Massive hepatic steatosis complicating adult celiac disease: report of a case and review of the literature. Am J Gastroenterol. 1987;82:1186–9.
32. Butterworth JR, Cooper BT, Rosenberg WM et al. The role of hemochromatosis susceptibility gene mutations in protecting against iron deficiency in celiac disease. Gastroenterology. 2002;123:444–9.
33. Broome U, Olsson R, Loof L et al. Natural history and prognostic factors in 305 Swedish patients with primary sclerosing cholangitis. Gut. 1996;38:610–15.
34. Chapman RW. Aetiology and natural history of primary sclerosing cholangitis – a decade of progress? Gut. 1991;32:1433–5.
35. Rabinovitz M, Gavaler JS, Schade RR et al. Does primary sclerosing cholangitis occurring in association with inflammatory bowel disease differ from that occurring in the absence of inflammatory bowel disease? A study of sixty-six subjects. Hepatology. 1990;11:7–11.
36. Loftus EV Jr, Harewood GC, Loftus CG et al. PSC–IBD: a unique form of inflammatory bowel disease associated with primary sclerosing cholangitis. Gut. 2005;54:91–6.
37. Helzberg JH, Petersen JM, Boyer JL. Improved survival with primary sclerosing cholangitis. A review of clinicopathologic features and comparison of symptomatic and asymptomatic patients. Gastroenterology. 1987;92:1869–75.

38. Takikawa H, Manabe T. Primary sclerosing cholangitis in Japan – analysis of 192 cases. J Gastroenterol. 1997;32:134–7.
39. Chapman RW. Risk factors for biliary tract carcinogenesis. Ann Oncol. 1999;10(Suppl. 4):308–11.
40. Cullen SN, Chapman RW. The medical management of primary sclerosing cholangitis. Semin Liver Dis. 2006;26:52–61.
41. Kornfeld D, Ekbom A, Ihre T. Is there an excess risk for colorectal cancer in patients with ulcerative colitis and concomitant primary sclerosing cholangitis? A population based study. Gut. 1997;41:522–5.
42. Loftus EVJ, Aguilar HI, Sandborn WJ et al. Risk of colorectal neoplasia in patients with primary sclerosing cholangitis and ulcerative colitis following orthotopic liver transplantation. Hepatology. 1998;27:685–90.
43. Eaden JA, Mayberry JF. Guidelines for screening and surveillance of asymptomatic colorectal cancer in patients with inflammatory bowel disease. Gut. 2002;51(Suppl. 5): V10–12.
44. Neuberger J. Liver transplantation for cholestatic liver disease. Curr Treat Options Gastroenterol. 2003;6:113–21.
45. Grant AJ, Lalor PF, Salmi M et al. Homing of mucosal lymphocytes to the liver in the pathogenesis of hepatic complications of inflammatory bowel disease. Lancet. 2002;359:150–7.
46. Salmi M, Andrew DP, Butcher EC et al. Dual binding capacity of mucosal immunoblasts to mucosal and synovial endothelium in humans: dissection of the molecular mechanisms. J Exp Med. 1995;181:137–49.
47. Salmi M, Rajala P, Jalkanen S. Homing of mucosal leukocytes to joints. Distinct endothelial ligands in synovium mediate leukocyte-subtype specific adhesion. J Clin Invest. 1997;99:2165–72.
48. Juillerat P, Mottet C, Froehlich F et al. Extraintestinal manifestations of Crohn's disease. Digestion. 2005;71:31–6.
49. Connor EM, Eppihimer MJ, Morise Z et al. Expression of mucosal addressin cell adhesion molecule-1 (MAdCAM-1) in acute and chronic inflammation. J Leukoc Biol. 1999;65:349–55.
50. Hillan KJ, Hagler KE, MacSween RN et al. Expression of the mucosal vascular addressin, MAdCAM-1, in inflammatory liver disease. Liver. 1999;19:509–18.
51. Grant AJ, Lalor PF, Hubscher SG et al. MAdCAM-1 expressed in chronic inflammatory liver disease supports mucosal lymphocyte adhesion to hepatic endothelium (MAdCAM-1 in chronic inflammatory liver disease). Hepatology. 2001;33:1065–72.
52. Salmi M, Kalimo K, Jalkanen S. Induction and function of vascular adhesion protein-1 at sites of inflammation. J Exp Med. 1993;178:2255–60.
53. Salter-Cid LM, Wang E, O'Rourke AM et al. Anti-inflammatory effects of inhibiting the amine oxidase activity of semicarbazide-sensitive amine oxidase. J Pharmacol Exp Ther. 2005;315:553–62.
54. Murai M, Yoneyama H, Ezaki T et al. Peyer's patch is the essential site in initiating murine acute and lethal graft-versus-host reaction. Nat Immunol. 2003;4:154–60.
55. Petrovic A, Alpdogan O, Willis LM et al. LPAM (alpha 4 beta 7 integrin) is an important homing integrin on alloreactive T cells in the development of intestinal graft-versus-host disease. Blood. 2004;103:1542–7.
56. Ward SM, Jonsson JR, Sierro S et al. Virus-specific CD8+ T lymphocytes within the normal human liver. Eur J Immunol. 2004;34:1526–31.
57. Pope C, Kim SK, Marzo A et al. Organ-specific regulation of the CD8 T cell response to *Listeria monocytogenes* infection. J Immunol. 2001;166:3402–9.
58. Marzo AL, Vezys V, Williams K et al. Tissue-level regulation of Th1 and Th2 primary and memory CD4 T cells in response to *Listeria* infection. J Immunol. 2002;168:4504–10.
59. Gowans JL, Knight EJ. The route of recirculation of lymphocytes in the rat. Proc R Soc B. 1964;159:257–82.
60. Klonowski KD, Williams KJ, Marzo AL et al. Dynamics of blood-borne CD8 memory T cell migration *in vivo*. Immunity. 2004;20:551–62.

3
Immune responses in hepatitis C virus infection

U. SPENGLER, J. NATTERMANN, B. LANGHANS,
H. D. NISCHALKE, D. SCHULTE, C. KÖRNER, B. KRÄMER,
B. TERJUNG, J. ROCKSTROH and T. SAUERBRUCH

INTRODUCTION

Infection with the hepatitis C virus (HCV) frequently runs a chronic persistent course and thus has been increasingly recognized as a major health problem with an estimated prevalence of 170 million infected people worldwide.

Failure to generate sufficiently effective immune responses is considered a key factor to develop chronic hepatitis C[1,2], whereas effective elimination of HCV infection requires the coordinated function of multiple arms of both innate immunity (interferons, natural killer (NK) cells, NK T cells, $\gamma\delta$-T cells, dendritic cells (DC) and other antigen-presenting cells) and adaptive immunity (antibodies, CD4$^+$ and CD8$^+$ T cells). Circumstantial evidence suggests that activation of the immune system is also a pivotal factor for the pathogenetic processes which lead to progressive tissue injury and ultimately cirrhosis in chronic hepatitis C, because hepatocellular damage coincides with the onset of the immune response during acute infection but not with that of viral replication[3]. Despite failure to achieve viral elimination immune effector mechanisms remain sufficiently effective to mediate liver damage in chronic HCV infection. Nevertheless, the immune system may still contribute importantly to the control of chronic infection preventing excessive levels of HCV replication.

In this chapter we discuss current concepts of how HCV interacts with the host's immune responses to establish and maintain chronic infection, and how in the long term such changes can become pathogenetic factors contributing to secondary complications.

HCV INTERACTIONS WITH THE HOST IMMUNE SYSTEM

Interaction with pathogen-associated molecular pattern (PAMP) receptors

Hepatitis C virus is a positive-sense RNA virus classified as a hepacivirus in the Flaviridae family. Its viral genome encodes a single polyprotein of 3000 amino acids in length, which is cleaved into three structural proteins (HCV core, envelope E1 and E2), six non-structural proteins (HCV NS2, NS3, NS4A, NS4B, NS5A and NS5B) needed for viral replication, and the HCV p7 protein, the function of which has not yet been determined. The various viral components (RNA, viral proteins, and intact virions) can be recognized by the immune system as specific foreign antigens but may also activate innate immunity via distinct cytoplasmic and cell surface receptors. These viral components trigger PAMP receptors, which comprise extracellular (TLR2) and intracellular Toll-like receptors (TLR) 3, 7, 9 as well as the cytoplasmic receptors RIG-I and MDA-5. For instance, TLR 3 and 7 on the cell surface or within membrane-bound cytosolic vesicles may sense for the presence of virus-derived ds-RNA and ss-RNA, respectively[4,5]. PAMP signalling involves recruitment of adaptor proteins and downstream phosphorylation and activation of interferon response factor (IRF) 3 via IKK-ε and TBK1 protein kinases[6–10], as well as activation of the transcription factor NK-κB[5]. Ultimately, activated transcription factors IRF3 and NF-κB up-regulate production of interferons[6] which, after binding to their receptors, activate interferon-inducible genes exerting antiviral and immunoregulatory functions. Importantly, type I and III interferons up-regulate major histocompatibility complex class I molecules and stimulate maturation and differentiation of cytotoxic effector cells[10].

The helicase sensors RIG-I and MDA-5 are cytoplasmic receptors for ds-RNA intermediates formed during replication of RNA viruses[11]. Negative-strand RNA activates RIG-I, which distinguishes endogenous from viral RNA by the presence of a 5′ triphosphate moiety in viral single-stranded RNA[12]. Positive-strand RNA viruses are presumably recognized by the related helicase MDA-5. RNA binding induces a conformational change and exposes paired N-terminal caspase recruitment (CARD) domains in RIG-I and MDA-5, which interact with the adaptor protein Cardif (also termed IPS-1, MAVS or VISA) to initiate downstream phosphorylation of protein kinases IKK-ε and TBK1. Thus, signal transductions in the RIG-I/MDA-5 and TLR pathways converge to induce antiviral and immunoregulatory genes via transcription factors IRF3 and NF-κB[13–16].

HCV protease NS3/NS4A can cleave both the adaptor proteins Cardif[21] and TRIF[17] and also inhibit activation of IKK-ε and TBK1 protein kinases, thus disrupting signal transmission needed for interferon induction. Indeed, first preliminary data indicate that serum levels of type III interferons, the specific receptor of which shows limited expression mainly on hepatocytes, are down-regulated in acute and chronic hepatitis C. Complex interactions between HCV and immunostimulatory pathways are further exemplified by the fact that HCV can interfere with both the interferon signalling JAK-STAT pathway as well as interferon-inducible proteins by a variety of different mechanisms[18].

Interactions of HCV with the tetraspanin CD81

HCV protein E2 and the E2/E1 protein envelope complex can bind to CD81[19,20]. CD81 is a 26 kDa protein member of the tetraspanin superfamily, which is expressed on most human cells up-regulated in response to cellular activation[21]. *In vitro*, ligation of CD81 on NK cells blocked the release of cytolytic granules, interferon-γ production and proliferative responses but induced release of interferon-γ and tumour necrosis factor α in γδ T cell lines[22]. E2/CD81 interactions stimulate RANTES secretion in CD8$^+$ T cells and induce the subsequent internalization of CC chemokine receptor (CCR) 5, thus altering migration of immunocompetent cells[23,24]. In addition, triggering CD81 on DC disrupts their migratory response to CCL21, which normally redirects migration of activated cells towards the lymphoid tissue[25]. Interruption of the physiological re-circulation of DC may account for changes in DC number and function owing to their trapping in the liver[26–30].

Taken together, it is an intriguing hypothesis that HCV–host interactions: (1) blunt antiviral pathways, and (2) trigger unspecific inflammatory mechanisms, possibly creating an intrahepatic milieu facilitating fibrogenesis.

EFFECTS OF HCV ON NATURAL KILLER (NK) CELLS AND CYTOLYTIC EFFECTOR CELLS (CTL)

NK cells play an important part in the first line of defence against viral infections. They rapidly recognize and lyse infected cells and also secrete cytokines which inhibit viral replication and exert immunoregulatory functions. Epidemiological evidence indicates that NK cells constitute a critical element in the initial antiviral response and elimination of HCV[31]. However, functional *ex vivo* studies have yielded conflicting results on the potential roles of NK cells in chronic hepatitis C[32–34].

Activity of NK cells is regulated by the complex interplay of activating and inhibitory NK receptors with their respective ligands such as the killer immunoglobulin (Ig)-like receptor (KIR) family (ligands HLA-A, -B and -C), the CD94-NKG2A/C complex (ligand HLA-E), NKG2D (ligands MIC-A and MIC-B) and the natural cytotoxicity receptors NKp30, NKp44 and NKp46[35]. Binding of distinct HCV peptides to the non-polymorphic MHC class I molecule HLA-E has recently been described resulting in up-regulated expression of HLA-E[36] and altered NK cell functions mediated via interactions of HLA-E with CD94-NKG2A[37]. These *in vitro* results corresponded to up-regulated HLA-E expression on a great variety of different hepatic cell types in biopsies from patients with chronic hepatitis C.

Furthermore, expression of the inhibitory receptor CD94-NKG2A was markedly up-regulated on both intrahepatic NK cells and cytolytic CD8$^+$ T lymphocytes (CTL) in chronic hepatitis C, while expression of activating natural cytotoxicity receptors NKp30 and NKp46 was reduced[38]. This change in balance between activating and inhibitory receptors sensitized cytotoxic effector cells towards overall inhibition upon HLA-E recognition. Of note, up-regulated expression of inhibitory CD94/NKG2A was correlated to CCR5 co-expression in CD8⁺ T lymphocytes, and NKG2A-positive T cells revealed preferential *in vitro* migration towards CCR5 ligands such as RANTES. Since interaction of the HCV envelope protein E2 with CD81 is likely to induce RANTES production in the liver, the observed correlation between CCR5 and NKG2A expression would explain why NKG2A-positive T cells are preferentially recruited into the liver in chronic hepatitis C. These findings have important implications, because failure to generate sufficiently strong cytolytic activity is quite likely to contribute to viral persistence in chronic hepatitis C. Beyond that, blunted cytolytic activity of NK cells in chronic hepatitis C may directly enhance fibrosis, because such cells can no longer down-regulate liver fibrosis by killing activated hepatic stellate cells[39,40].

T CELL ANERGY AND REGULATORY T CELLS

Cell-mediated immunity is considered the key mechanism for resolution of primary HCV infection[41] and involves both CTL, which recognize linear peptides of 8–11 amino acids in length bound to self HLA class I molecules, and CD4⁺ T helper lymphocytes, which recognize longer peptides bound to class II molecules. In acute hepatitis C strong HCV-specific CTL[42,43] and Th1 type CD4⁺ T helper cell responses[44,45] have consistently been reported to result in a self-limited course of HCV infection. Moreover, several groups have reported an inverse relationship between the strength of the CTL response and viral loads in chronic hepatitis C[46–48], supporting the idea that cellular immunity can control HCV infection[49]. Of note, cellular immunity is maintained long-term in those individuals who have successfully eliminated their HCV infection[50].

It has now become clear that a substantial proportion of individuals who eventually develop chronic hepatitis C generate HCV-specific CD4⁺ and CD8⁺ T cell responses during the early acute phase of their infection and transiently gain control over HCV replication[43,51–54]. However, these early T cell responses decline to almost undetectable levels thereafter and initial control over HCV infection is lost. If present, HCV-specific CD4⁺ and CD8⁺ T cells are detected at only low frequency in peripheral blood, although they are somewhat enriched in the liver[55,56]. Importantly T cells in chronic hepatitis C exhibit several characteristic features.

HCV-specific CD8⁺ T cells predominantly carry a CCR7^{high}, perforin^{low} phenotype and fail to exert significant *ex vivo* killing or to secrete interferon-γ[42,57,58]; CD4⁺ T cells show impaired HCV-specific proliferation together with low production of interleukin 2 (IL-2) and interferon-γ[59–62]. Instead, they preferentially produce IL-10 and transforming growth factor beta (TGF-β), indicating a shift in T cell differentiation towards secretion of anti-inflammatory cytokines[60,62–65]. T cell abnormalties in chronic hepatitis C are potentially reversible, since addition of IL-2 or stimulation via TLR2 can restore impaired T cell responses *in vitro*[66–68], and therapeutic restoration of an antiviral Th1 response supports sustained clearance of HCV infection[69]. Appearance of mutations making HCV resistant to T cell recognition, lack of T cell help, T cell exhaustion and induction of regulatory T cells, all have been incriminated to explain T cell dysfunction in chronic hepatitis C.

HCV replicates via an error-prone RNA-dependent RNA polymerase leading to genomic diversity with the potential to generate minor viral variants that can evade immune recognition. Epitopes may be lost, because mutations alter proteasomal processing, binding to MHC molecules or CTL recognition of variant peptides[70]. New epitope variants selected by immune pressure apparently do not elicit strong $CD8^+$ T cell responses, either because they are not immunogenic, the immune system cannot respond to epitopes, which are only slightly modified, or $CD4^+$ T cell help is not sufficient to support expansion of new $CD8^+$ T cells[71].

Escape mutations have been identified only recently in longitudinal studies of acutely infected patients and in single-source outbreaks[72-74]. $CD8^+$ T cell responses are also affected by HCV mutations altering proteasomal processing[75], whereas the role of HCV mutations in evasion from $CD4^+$ T cell responses remains elusive. Of note, however, $CD8^+$ T cell escape mutations occur mainly early after infection in chimpanzees and humans[76], so that delayed acquisition of $CD8^+$ T cell responses cannot explain escape from multispecific CTL responses. Moreover, escape mutations are found in only few epitopes, while all T cell responses decline in chronic hepatitis C[74,77].

However, CTL functions may become impaired because help from $CD4^+$ T cells is lost gradually[53]. The mechanisms which cause loss of $CD4^+$ T cell function in persistent HCV infection remain unclear, because HCV-specific $CD4^+$ T cells are not deleted and their functionality can be restored *in vitro*[66,78,79]. Exhaustion of T cells (clonal deletion/anergy) is a favourite idea to explain altered T cell responses in chronic virus infections. This concept has been derived from experiments in the murine model of lymphocytic choriomeningits virus (LCMV) infection[80], which enables one to study the effects of persistently high levels of viraemia. Initially, mice develop robust T cell responses but fail to eliminate the virus, which is followed by a gradual decline and ultimately complete loss of $CD8^+$ and $CD4^+$ T cell responses. $CD8^+$ T cells in chronic hepatitis C share many features of anergic cells[57,58,81] and, consistent with their loss of function, exhibit immature stages of differentiation[82]. In line with the LCMV model, anergy of $CD8^+$ T cells in chronic hepatitis C is associated with declining virus-specific $CD4^+$ responses[83,84]. Although HCV-specific $CD4^+$ T cells may ultimately become undetectable in chronic hepatitis C[79], it remains unclear if they are actually deleted. Deletion of antigen-specific $CD8^+$ T cells obviously does not occur, since $CD8^+$ T cell responses can be rescued *in vitro* with IL-2 and antigen[85]. Although HCV-specific $CD8^+$ and $CD4^+$ T cells in chronic hepatitis C match several features of the T cell exhaustion model, several issues remain unresolved. For instance, impaired functions of virus-specific $CD8^+$ T cells were also observed after resolution of HCV infection[81], and CMV-specific $CD8^+$ T cells, which exhibit similar changes in phenotype as HCV-specific cells, did not reveal relevant dysfunction[86]. Finally, the cellular and molecular mechanisms underlying T cell exhaustion are not understood in chronic hepatitis C.

Inhibition of T cell responses due to interaction with regulatory T cells is an alternative hypothesis currently under scientific scrutiny. Murine models have provided experimental evidence for naturally occurring $CD4^+CD25^+Foxp3^+$

regulatory T cells (Tregs) and also several types of inducible suppressor T cells to act as inhibitory elements in the regulatory network of the immune system[87]. Regulatory T cells actively control induction and effector functions of other immune cells by suppressing their functional activity via contact-dependent mechanisms as well as by secreting immunosuppressive cytokines such as IL-10 and TGF-β. CD8⁺ T cell lines producing IL-10 in response to HCV antigens provided first evidence for antigen-specific MHC class I-restricted regulatory cells to down-regulate antiviral responses[88]. These initial observations were confirmed by finding CD8⁺ T cells in the livers of patients with chronic hepatitis C which secrete IL-10 and suppress *in vitro* proliferation of liver-derived T cells in an HCV-specific way[89]. Beyond that, numbers of CD4⁺CD25⁺ Tregs had increased in the peripheral blood of patients with chronic hepatitis C, and experimental depletion of CD4⁺CD25⁺ T cells was associated with increased numbers and function of CD8⁺ T cells *in vitro*[90-93]. On the other hand it must be taken into consideration that hyporesponsiveness in chronic hepatitis C is HCV-specific but leaves other responses intact, whereas CD4⁺CD25⁺ Tregs in peripheral blood inhibit responses to cytomegalovirus, Epstein–Barr virus and influenza virus[92,93]. Recently we succeeded in generating T cell clones from patients with chronic hepatitis C, which exert HCV-specific inhibition of reporter cells. All T clones produced IL-10 and expressed Foxp3, GITR and PD1. Of note, expression of other phenotypic markers varied, but the clones clearly differed from natural regulatory T cells. However, the frequency of such cells appeared to be rather low in peripheral blood. Thus, further studies are needed to clarify if preferential compartmentalization concentrates HCV-specific regulatory T cells in the liver and must confirm that such cells actually contribute to the loss of HCV-specific CD8⁺ and CD4⁺ T cell responses observed in chronic hepatitis C.

ACTIVATION OF B CELLS IN CHRONIC HEPATITIS C

Antiviral antibodies usually become detectable within several weeks after acute HCV infection and constitute an important tool for the diagnosis of HCV infection. The role of naturally acquired anti-HCV antibodies for protection is unclear because they cannot prevent reinfection[94,95]. Moreover, in selected cases HCV infection resolved without HCV-specific antibodies[96,97]. On the other hand, adaptive sequence changes in hypervariable region 1 of HCV E2, the putative target of neutralizing antibodies, have been described in acutely HCV-infected individuals and were found to be correlated to the outcome of infection[98], possibly indicating that HCV adapts to the immune selection exerted by HCV antibodies via escape mutations. On the other hand, antibody responses during chronic infection have also been linked to the level of liver injury[99], and anti-E2 antibodies can mediate liver damage via antibody-dependent cellular cytotoxicity after prolonged HCV infection[100].

Antigenic persistence in chronic hepatitis C is a continued stimulus for the immune system, in particular also B lymphocytes. Thus, long-lasting chronic hepatitis C virus infection can lead to immune abnormalities such as autoantibody formation, mixed cryoglobulinaemia and malignant B-cell non-Hodgkin's lymphoma[101-117]. Mixed cryoglobulinaemia is a B-cell proliferative disorder, which shows strong correlation to HCV infection[104,118,119] and is considered to be a potential precursor of HCV-associated B-cell non-Hodgkin's lymphoma.

Recently we and others[120,121] reported that HCV proteins triggered IL-6 and IL-8 production via stimulation of TLR2. Importantly, IL-6 serum levels were elevated in patients chronically infected with HCV, suggesting that TLR2-mediated induction of IL-6 may indeed have *in vivo*-relevance. The concept, that elevated IL-6 serum concentrations may reflect immune stimulation by HCV, is further supported by data from Grungreiff et al., who demonstrated that IL-6 serum concentrations normalized when HCV was eradicated by interferon-alpha treatment[122]. IL-6 serum concentrations were particularly high in patients with HCV-associated cryoglobulinaemia as compared to the other HCV-infected groups. IL-6 is a potent B-cell growth and maturation factor[123,124], and increased B-cell growth could be observed when supernatants of HCV core-stimulated PBMC were transferred to B-cell cultures or when PBMC were directly co-incubated with recombinant HCV core protein[121]. Of note, HCV core-stimulated B-cell proliferation was blocked by neutralizing IL-6 antibody. Thus, there are striking pathogenetic analogies between HCV-associated B-cell proliferative disorders and MALT lymphomas seen in chronic *Helicobacter pylori* infection[59,60], which are triggered by chronic immune stimulation by *H. pylori* antigens, including recognition of *H. pylori*-derived LPS via TLR2[61].

Taken together, immune responses, which in general are overall protective in HCV infection, may eventually lead to severe complications such as lymphoproliferative disorders and malignancy in the long term, and it may be worthwhile discovering whether blocking IL-6 will offer new therapeutic perspectives to prevent or treat HCV-associated lymphoproliferative disorders in patients with long-standing HCV infection.

CONCLUSIONS

In HCV infection a variety of different mechanisms mediated by the host's immune system may play a role in the elimination of infected cells and inflammatory liver damage. HCV-specific cells can now be studied in peripheral blood and the liver owing to novel sensitive techniques such as flow cytometric analysis with HLA-peptide tetramers. Although we can now study how the immune system controls HCV infection, the reasons why immunity frequently fails to successfully eliminate HCV still remain unclear. Certainly, virus-specific $CD4^+$ and $CD8^+$ T cells are involved in clearance of HCV-infected cells, but on the other hand may exert significant liver damage. However, accumulating data indicate that HCV exploits multiple and complex strategies to subvert the host's innate and adaptive immune responses. In its attempt to defend against HCV infection the immune system activates HCV-specific as well as non-specific effector mechanisms, which in principle can eliminate virus-infected cells and are beneficial for the host. However, dysregulation of T cells and continued immune activation will result in persistent liver damage, cirrhosis, lymphoproliferative disorders and ultimately malignancy. The final outcome of immune activation by HCV antigens – viral clearance versus chronic inflammation – is determined during the first few months of infection. Nevertheless, several issues such as the relative contribution from innate and adaptive immunity such as NK cells, NKT cells and $\gamma\delta$ T cells, as well as conventional CD4$^+$ and CD8$^+$ T cells during this decisive phase, remain to be resolved.

References

1. Gale M, Foy EM. Evasion of intracellular host defence by hepatitis C virus. Nature. 2005;436:939–45
2. Bowen DG, Walker CM. Adaptive immune responses in acute and chronic hepatitis C virus infection. Nature. 2005;436:946–52.
3. Farci P, Alter HJ, Shimoda A et al. Hepatitis C virus-associated fulminant hepatic failure. N Engl J Med. 1996;335:631–4.
4. Iwasaki A, Medzhitov R. Toll like receptor control of the adaptive immune responses. Nat Immunol. 2004;5:987–95.
5. Schwabe RF, Seki E, Brenner DA. Toll-like receptor signalling in the liver. Gastroenterology. 2006;130:1886–900.
6. Hertzog PJ, O'Neill LA, Hamilton JA. The interferon in TLR signaling: more than just antiviral. Trends Immunol. 2003;24:534–9.
7. Sharma S, ten Oever BR, Grandvaux N, Zhou GP, Lin R, Hiscott J. Triggering the interferon antiviral response through a novel IKK-related pathway. Science. 2003;300:1148–51.
8. Fitzgerald KA, McWhirter SM, Faia KL et al. IKKε and TBK1 are essential components of the IRF3 signaling pathway. Nat Immunol. 2003;4:491–6.
9. Yamamoto M, Sato S, Hemmi H et al. Role of the adaptor TRIF in the MyD88 independent Toll-like receptor pathway. Science. 2003;301:640–3.
10. Feld JJ, Hoofnagle JH. Mechanism and action of interferon and ribavirin in treatment of hepatitis C. Nature. 2005;436:967–72.
11. Yoneyama M, Kikuchi M, Natsukawa T et al. The RNA helicase RIG-I has an essential function in double-stranded RNA-induced innate antiviral responses. Nat Immunol. 2004;5:730–7.
12. Hornung V, Ellegast J, Kim S et al. 5′-Triphosphate RNA is the ligand for RIG-I. Science. 2006;314:994–7.
13. Kawai T, Takahasi K, Sato S et al. IPS-1 an adaptor triggering RIG-I- and Mda5-mediated type 1 interferon induction. Nat Immunol. 2005;6:981–8.
14. Seth RB, Sun L, Ea CK, Chen ZJ. Identification and characterization of MAVS, a mitochondrial antiviral signaling protein that activates NF-kappaB and IRF3. Cell. 2005;122:669–82.
15. Xu LG, Wang YY, Han KJ, Li LY, Zhai Z, Shu HB. VISA is an adaptor protein required for virus-triggered IFN-beta signaling. Mol Cell. 2005;19:727–40.
16. Meylan E, Curran J, Hofmann K et al. Cardif is an adaptor protein in the RIG-I antiviral pathway and is targeted by hepatitis C virus. Nature. 2005;437:1167–72.
17. Li K, Foy E, Ferreon JC et al. Immune evasion by hepatitis C virus NS3/4A proteasemediated cleavage of the Toll-like receptor 3 adaptor protein TRIF. Proc Natl Acad Sci USA. 2005;102:2992–7.
18. Gale M, Foy EM. Evasion of intracellular host defence by hepatitis C virus. Nature. 2005;436:939–45.
19. Pileri P, Uematsu Y, Campagnoli S et al. Binding of hepatitis C virus to CD81. Science. 1998;282:938–41.
20. Cocquerel L, Kuo CC, Dubuisson J, Levy S. CD81-dependent binding of hepatitis C virus E1E2 heterodimers. J Virol. 2003;77:10677–83.

21. Levy S, Todd SC, Maecker HT. CD81 (TAPA-1): a molecule involved in signal transduction and cell adhesion in the immune system. Annu Rev Immunol. 1998;16:89–109.
22. Tseng CT, Miskovsky E, Houghton M, Klimpel GR. Characterization of liver T-cell receptor gammadelta T cells obtained from individuals chronically infected with hepatitis C virus (HCV): evidence for these T cells playing a role in the liver pathology associated with HCV infections. Hepatology. 2001;33:1312–20.
23. Lichterfeld M, Leifeld L, Nischalke HD et al. Reduced CC chemokine receptor (CCR) 1 and CCR5 surface expression on peripheral blood T lymphocytes from patients with chronic hepatitis C infection. J Infect Dis. 2002;185:1803–7.
24. Nattermann J, Nischalke HD, Feldmann G, Ahlenstiel G, Sauerbruch T, Spengler U. Binding of HCV E2 to CD81 induces RANTES secretion and internalization of CC chemokine receptor 5. J Viral Hepat. 2004;11:519–26.
25. Nattermann J, Zimmermann H, Iwan A et al. Hepatitis C virus E2 and CD81 interaction may be associated with altered trafficking of dendritic cells in chronic hepatitis C. Hepatology. 2006;44:945–54.
26. Kanto T, Hayashi N, Takehara T et al. Impaired allostimulatory capacity of peripheral blood dendritic cells recovered from hepatitis C virus-infected individuals. J Immunol. 1999;162:5584–91.
27. Auffermann-Gretzinger S, Keeffe EB, Levy S. Impaired dendritic cell maturation in patients with chronic, but not resolved, hepatitis C virus infection. Blood. 2001;97:3171–6.
28. Bain C, Fatmi A, Zoulim F, Zarski JP, Trepo C, Inchauspe G. Impaired allostimulatory function of dendritic cells in chronic hepatitis C infection. Gastroenterology. 2001;120:512–24.
29. Kanto T, Inoue M, Miyatake H et al. Reduced numbers and impaired ability of myeloid and plasmacytoid dendritic cells to polarize T helper cells in chronic hepatitis C virus infection. J Infect Dis. 2004;190:1919–26.
30. Ulsenheimer A, Gerlach JT, Jung MC et al. Plasmacytoid dendritic cells in acute and chronic hepatitis C virus infection. Hepatology. 2005;41:643–51.
31. Khakoo SI, Thio CL, Martin MP et al. HLA and NK cell inhibitory receptor genes in resolving hepatitis C virus infection. Science. 2004;305:872–4.
32. Corano J, Toro F, Rivera H, Bianco NE, Deibis L, De Sanctis JB. Impairment of natural killer (NK) cytotoxic activity in hepatitis C virus (HCV) infection. Clin Exp Immunol. 1997;109:451–7.
33. Düesberg U, Schneiders AM, Flieger D, Inchauspé G, Sauerbruch T, Spengler U. Natural cytotoxicity and antibody-dependent cellular cytotoxicity (ADCC) is not impaired in patients suffering from chronic hepatitis C. J Hepatol. 2001;35:650–7.
34. Morishima C, Paschal DM, Wang CC et al. Decreased NK cell frequency in chronic hepatitis C does not affect *ex vivo* cytolyti killing. Hepatology. 2006;43:573–80.
35. Moretta L, Moretta A. Unravelling natural killer cell function: triggering and inhibitory human NK receptors. EMBO J. 2004;23:255–9.
36. Nattermann J, Nischalke HD, Hofmeister V et al. The HLA-A2 restricted T cell epitope HCV core 35-44 stabilizes HLA-E expression and inhibits cytolysis mediated by natural killer cells. Am J Pathol. 2005;166:443–53.
37. Jinushi M, Takehara T, Tatsumi T et al. Negative regulation of NK cell activities by inhibitory receptor CD94/NKG2A leads to altered NK cell-induced modulation of dendritic cell functions in chronic hepatitis C virus infection. J Immunol. 2004;173:6072–81.
38. Nattermann J, Feldmann G, Ahlenstiel G, Langhans B, Sauerbruch T, Spengler U. Surface expression and cytolytic function of natural killer cell receptors is altered in chronic hepatitis C. Gut. 2006;55:869–77.
39. Radaeva S, Sun R, Jarugga B, Nguyen VT, Tian Z, Gao B. Natural killer cells ameliorate liver fibrosis by killing activated stellate cells in NKG2D-dependent and tumor necrosis factor-related apoptosis-inducing ligand-dependent manners. Gastroenterology. 2006;130:435–52.
40. Melhem A, Muhanna N, Bishara A et al. Anti-fibrotic activity of NK cells in experimental liver injury through killing of activated HSC. J Hepatol. 2006;45:60–71.
41. Bowen DG, Walker CM. Adaptive immune responses in acute and chronic hepatitis C virus infection. Nature. 2005;436:946–52.

42. Lechner F, Wong DK, Dunbar PR et al. Analysis of successful immune responses in persons infected with hepatitis C virus. J Exp Med. 2000;191:1499–512.
43. Thimme R, Oldach D, Chang KM, Steiger C, Ray SC, Chisari FV. Determinants of viral clearance and persistence during acute hepatitis C virus infection. J Exp Med. 2001;194:1395–406.
44. Missale G, Bretoni R, La Monaca V et al. Different clinical behaviours of acute hepatitis C virus infection are associated with different vigor of the antiviral cell-mediated immune response. J Clin Invest. 1996;98:706–14.
45. Diepolder HM, Zachoval R, Hoffmann RM et al. Possible mechanism involving T-lymphocyte response to non-structural protein 3 in viral clearance in acute hepatitis C virus infection. Lancet. 1995;346:1006–7.
46. Rehermann B, Chang KM, McHutchinson J et al. Differential cytotoxic T-lymphocyte responsiveness to the hepatitis B and C viruses in chronically infected patients. J Virol. 1996;70:7092–102.
47. Hiroishi K, Kita H, Kojima M et al. Cytotoxic T lymphocyte response and viral load in hepatitis C virus infection. Hepatology. 1997;25:705–12.
48. Nelson DR, Marousis CG, Davis GL et al. The role of hepatitis C virus specific cytotoxic T lymphocytes in chronic hepatitis C. J Immunol. 1997;158:1473–81.
49. Koziel MJ, Wong DKH, Dudley D, Houghton M, Walker BD. Hepatitis C virus-specific cytolytic T lymphocyte and T helper cell responses in seronegative persons. J Infect Dis. 1997;176:859–66.
50. Takaki A, Wiese M, Maertens G et al. Cellular immune responses persist and humoral responses decrease two decades after recovery from a single-source outbreak of hepatitis C. Nat Med. 2000;6:578–82.
51. Lechner F, Gruener NH, Urbani S et al. $CD8^+$ T lymphocyte responses are induced during acute hepatitis C virus infection but are not sustained. Eur J Immunol. 2000;30:2479–87.
52. Cox AL, Mosbruger T, Lauer GM, Pardoll D, Thomas DL, Ray SC. Comprehensive analyses of $CD8^+$ T cell responses during longitudinal study of acute human hepatitis C. Hepatology. 2005;42:104–12.
53. Gerlach JT, Diepolder HM, Jung MC et al. Recurrence of hepatitis C virus after loss of virus-specific CD4(+) T-cell response in acute hepatitis C. Gastroenterology. 1999;117:933–41.
54. Folgori A, Spada E, Pezzanera M et al. Early impairment of hepatitis C virus specific T cell proliferation during acute infection leads to failure of viral clearance. Gut. 2006;55:1012–19.
55. He XS, Rehermann B, Lopez-Labrador FX et al. Quantitative analysis of hepatitis C virus-specific CD8(+) T cells in peripheral blood and liver using peptide-MHC tetramers. Proc Natl Acad Sci USA. 1999;96:5692–7.
56. Grabowska AM, Lechner F, Klenerman P et al. Direct *ex vivo* comparison of the breadth and specificity of the T cells in the liver and peripheral blood of patients with chronic HCV infection. Eur J Immunol. 2001;31:2388–94.
57. Gruener NH, Lechner F, Jung MC et al. Sustained dysfunction of antiviral $CD8^+$ T lymphocytes after infection with hepatitis C virus. J Virol. 2001;75:5550–8.
58. Wedemeyer H, He XS, Nascimbeni M et al. Impaired effector function of hepatitis C virus-specific $CD8^+$ T cells in chronic hepatitis C virus infection. J. Immunol. 2002;169:3447–58.
59. Lechmann M, Ihlenfeldt HG, Braunschweiger I et al. T and B cell responses to different hepatitis C virus antigens in patients with chronic hepatitis C and healthy anti-HCV positive blood donors without viremia. Hepatology. 1996;24:790–5.
60. Woitas R, Lechmann M, Jung G, Kaiser R, Sauerbruch T, Spengler U. CD30 induction and cytokine profiles in HCV core-specific peripheral blood T lymphocytes. J Immunol. 1997;159:1012–18.
61. Lechmann M, Woitas RP, Langhans B et al. Decreased frequency of HCV core-specific peripheral blood mononuclear cells with type 1 cytokine secretion in chronic hepatitis C. J Hepatol. 1999;31:971–8.
62. Ulsenheimer A, Gerlach JT, Gruener NH et al. Detection of functionally altered hepatitis C virus-specific CD4 T cells in acute and chronic hepatitis C. Hepatology. 2003;37:1189–98.
63. Tsai S-L, Liaw Y-F, Chen M-H, Huang C-Y, Kuo GC. Detection of type 2-like T-helper cells in hepatitis C virus infection: implication for hepatitis C chronicity. Hepatology. 1997;25:449–58.

64. Reiser M, Marousis CG, Nelson DR et al. Serum interleukin 4 and interleukin 10 levels in patients with chronic hepatitis C virus infection. J Hepatol. 1997;26:471–8.
65. Cacciarelli T, Martinez OM, Gish RG, Villanueva JC, Krams SM. Immunoregulatory cytokines in chronic hepatitis C virus infection: pre- and posttreatment with interferon alfa. Hepatology. 1996;24:6–9.
66. Semmo N, Day CL, Ward SM et al. Preferential loss of IL-2-secreting CD4$^+$ T helper cells in chronic HCV infection. Hepatology. 2005;41:1019–28.
67. Langhans B, Braunschweiger I, Schweitzer S et al. Lipidation of T helper sequences from hepatitis C virus core significantly enhances T-cell activity *in vitro*. Immunology. 2001;102:460–5.
68. Langhans B, Braunschweiger I, Nischalke HD, Nattermann J, Sauerbruch T, Spengler U. Presentation of the HCV-derived lipopeptide LP20-44 by dendritic cells enhances function of *in vitro*-generated CD4$^+$ T cells via up-regulation of TLR2. Vaccine. 2006;24:3066–75.
69. Cramp ME, Rossol S, Chokshi S, Carucci P, Williams R, Naoumov NV. Hepatitis C virus-specific T-cell reactivity during interferon and ribavirin treatment in chronic hepatitis C. Gastroenterology. 2000;118:346–55.
70. Bowen DG, Walker CM. Mutational escape from CD8$^+$ T cell immunity: HCV evolution, from chimpanzees to man. J Exp Med. 2005;201:1709–14.
71. Meyer-Olson D, Shoukry NH, Brady KW et al. Limited T cell receptor diversity of HCV-specific T cell responses is associated with CTL escape. J Exp Med. 2004;200:307–19.
72. Cox AL, Mosbruger T, Mao Q et al. Cellular immune selection with hepatitis C virus persistence in humans. J Exp Med. 2005;201:1741–52.
73. Timm J, Lauer GM, Kavanagh DG et al. CD8 epitope escape and reversion in acute HCV infection. J Exp Med. 2004;200:1593–604.
74. Ray SC, Fanning L, Wang XH, Netski DM, Kenny-Walsh E, Thomas DL. Divergent and convergent evolution after a common-source outbreak of hepatitis C virus. J Exp Med. 2005;201:1753–9.
75. Seifert U, Liermann H, Racanelli V et al. Hepatitis C virus mutation affects proteasomal epitope processing. J Clin Invest. 2004;114:250–9.
76. Erickson AL, Kimura Y, Igarashi S et al. The outcome of hepatitis C virus infection is predicted by escape mutations in epitopes targeted by cytotoxic T lymphocytes. Immunity. 2001;15:883–95.
77. Urbani S, Amadei B, Cariani E et al. The impairment of CD8 responses limits the selection of escape mutations in acute hepatitis C virus infection. J Immunol. 2005;175:7519–29.
78. Diepolder HM, Gerlach JT, Zachoval R et al. Immunodominant CD4$^+$ T-cell epitope within nonstructural protein 3 in acute hepatitis C virus infection. J Virol. 1997;71:6011–19.
79. Day CL, Lauer GM, Robbins GK et al. Broad specificity of virus-specific CD4$^+$ T-helper-cell responses in resolved hepatitis C virus infection. J Virol. 2002;6:12584–95.
80. Moskophidis D, Laine E, Zinkernagel M. Peripheral clonal deletion of antiviral memory CD8$^+$ T cells. Eur J Immunol. 1993;23:3306–11.
81. Gruener NH, Lechner F, Jung MC et al. Sustained dysfunction of antiviral CD8$^+$ T lymphocytes after infection with hepatitis C virus. J Virol. 2001;75:5550–8.
82. Appay V, Dunbar PR, Callan M et al. Memory CD8$^+$ T cells vary in differentiation phenotype in different persistent virus infections. Nat Med. 2002;8:379–85.
83. Zajac AJ, Blattman JN, Murali-Krishna K et al. Viral immune evasion due to persistence of activated T cells without effector function. J Exp Med. 1998;188:2205–13.
84. Khanolkar A, Fuller MJ, Zajac AJ. CD4 T cell-dependent CD8 T cell maturation. J Immunol. 2004;172:2834–44.
85. Lauer GM, Ouchi K, Chung RT et al. Comprehensive analysis of CD8(+)-T-cell responses against hepatitis C virus reveals multiple unpredicted specificities. J Virol. 2002;76:6104–13.
86. Lucas M, Vargas-Cuero AL, Lauer GM et al. Pervasive influence of hepatitis C virus on the phenotype of antiviral CD8$^+$ T cells. J Immunol. 2004;172:1744–53.
87. Chang K-M. Regulatory T cells and the liver: a new piece of the puzzle. Hepatology. 2005;41:700–2.
88. Koziel MJ, Dudley D, Afdhal N et al. HLA class I-restricted cytotoxic T lymphocytes specific for hepatitis C virus. Identification of multiple epitopes and characterization of patterns of cytokine release. J Clin Invest. 1995;96:2311–21.

89. Accapezzato D, Francavilla V, Paroli M et al. Hepatic expansion of a virus-specific regulatory CD8(+) T cell population in chronic hepatitis C virus infection. J Clin Invest. 2004;113:963–72.
90. Sugimoto K, Ikeda F, Stadanlick J, Nunes FA, Alter HJ, Chang KM. Suppression of HCV-specific T cells without differential hierarchy demonstrated *ex vivo* in persistent HCV infection. Hepatology. 2003;38:1437–48.
91. Cabrera R, Tu Z, Xu Y et al. An immunomodulatory role for CD4(+)CD25(+) regulatory T lymphocytes in hepatitis C virus infection. Hepatology. 2004;40:1062–71.
92. Boettler T, Spangenberg HC, Neumann-Haefelin C et al. T cells with a CD4+CD25+ regulatory phenotype suppress *in vitro* proliferation of virus-specific CD8$^+$ T cells during chronic hepatitis C virus infection. J Virol. 2005;79:7860–7.
93. Rushbrook SM, Ward SM, Unitt E et al. Regulatory T cells suppress *in vitro* proliferation of virus-specific CD8$^+$ T cells during persistent hepatitis C virus infection. J Virol. 2005;79:7852–9.
94. Farci P, Alter HJ, Govindarajan S et al. Lack of protective immunity against reinfection with hepatitis C virus. Science. 1992;258:135–40.
95. Lai ME, Mazzoleni AP, Argiolu F et al. Hepatitis C virus in multiple episodes of acute hepatitis in polytransfused thalassaemic children. Lancet. 1994;343:388–90.
96. Cooper S, Erickson AL, Adams EJ et al. Analysis of a successful immune response against hepatitis C virus. Immunity. 1999;10:439–49.
97. Post JJ, Pan Y, Freeman AJ et al. Clearance of hepatitis C viremia associated with cellular immunity in the absence of seroconversion in the hepatitis C incidence and transmission in prison study (HITS) cohort. J Infect Dis. 2004;189:1846–55.
98. Farci P, Shimoda A, Coiana A et al. The outcome of acute hepatitis C predicted by the evolution of the viral quasispecies. Science. 2000;288:339–44.
99. Farci P, Quinti I, Farci S et al. Evolution of hepatitis C viral quasispecies and hepatic injury in perinatally infected children followed prospectively. Proc Natl Acad Sci USA. 2006;103:8475–80.
100. Nattermann J, Schneiders AM, Leifeld L et al. Serum antibodies against the hepatitis C virus E2 protein mediate antibody-dependent cellular cytotoxicity (ADCC). J Hepatol. 2005;42:499–504.
101. De Vita S, Sacco C, Sansonno D et al. Characterization of overt B-cell lymphomas in patients with hepatitis C virus infection. Blood. 1997;90:776–82.
102. Gisbert JP, Garcia-Buey L, Arranz R et al. The prevalence of hepatitis C virus infection in patients with non-Hodgkin's lymphoma. Eur J Gastroenterol Hepatol. 2004;16:135–8.
103. Karavattathayyil SJ, Kalkeri G, Liu HJ et al. Detection of hepatitis C virus RNA sequences in B-cell non-Hodgkin lymphoma. Am J Clin Pathol. 2000;113:391–8.
104. Gharagozloo S, Khoshnoodi J, Shokri F. Hepatitis C virus infection in patients with essential mixed cryoglobulinemia, multiple myeloma and chronic lymphocytic leukemia. Pathol Oncol Res. 2001;7:135–9.
105. Mayo MJ. Extrahepatic manifestations of hepatitis C infection. Am J Med Sci. 2003;325:135–48.
106. Gisbert JP, Garcia-Buey L, Pajares JM, Moreno-Otero R. Prevalence of hepatitis C virus infection in B-cell non-Hodgkin's lymphoma: systematic review and meta-analysis. Gastroenterology. 2003;125:1723–32.
107. De Vita S, Zagonel V, Russo A et al. Hepatitis C virus, non-Hodgkin's lymphomas and hepatocellular carcinoma. Br J Cancer. 1998;77:2032–5.
108. Montella M, Crispo A, Frigeri F et al. HCV and tumors correlated with immune system: a case–control study in an area of hyperendemicity. Leuk Res. 2001;25:775–81.
109. Mele A, Pulsoni A, Bianco E et al. Hepatitis C virus and B-cell non-Hodgkin lymphomas: an Italian multicenter case–control study. Blood. 2003;102:996–9.
110. Imai Y, Ohsawa M, Tanaka H et al. High prevalence of HCV infection in patients with B-cell non-Hodgkin's lymphoma: comparison with birth cohort- and sex-matched blood donors in a Japanese population. Hepatology. 2002;35:974–6.
111. Pioltelli P, Gargantini L, Cassi E et al. Hepatitis C virus in non-Hodgkin's lymphoma. A reappraisal after a prospective case–control study of 300 patients. Lombart Study Group of HCV-Lymphoma. Am J Hematol. 2000;64:95–100.

112. Paydas S, Ergin M, Tanriverdi K et al. Detection of hepatitis C virus RNA in paraffin-embedded tissues from patients with non-Hodgkin's lymphoma. Am J Hematol. 2004;76:252–7.
113. Engels EA, Chatterjee N, Cerhan JR et al. Hepatitis C virus infection and non-Hodgkin lymphoma: results of the NCI-SEER multi-center case–control study. Int J Cancer. 2004;111:76–80.
114. Morton LM, Engels EA, Holford TR et al. Hepatitis C virus and risk of non-Hodgkin lymphoma: a population-based case–control study among Connecticut women. Cancer Epidemiol Biomarkers Prev. 2004;13:425–30.
115. de Sanjose S, Nieters A, Goedert JJ et al. Role of hepatitis C virus infection in malignant lymphoma in Spain. Int J Cancer. 2004;111:81–5.
116. Bronowicki JP, Bineau C, Feugier P et al. Primary lymphoma of the liver: clinical-pathological features and relationship with HCV infection in French patients. Hepatology. 2003;37:781–7.
117. Takai S, Tsurumi H, Ando K et al. Prevalence of hepatitis B and C virus infection in haematological malignancies and liver injury following chemotherapy. Eur J Haematol. 2005;74:158–65.
118. Sene D, Limal N, Cacoub P. Hepatitis C virus-associated extrahepatic manifestations: a review. Metab Brain Dis. 2004;19:357–81.
119. Dammacco F, Sansonno D, Piccoli C, Tucci FA, Racanelli V. The cryoglobulins: an overview. Eur J Clin Invest. 2001;31:628–38.
120. Dolganiuc A, Oak S, Kodys K et al. Hepatitis C core and nonstructural 3 proteins trigger toll-like receptor 2-mediated pathways and inflammatory activation. Gastroenterology. 2004;127:1513–24.
121. Feldmann G, Nischalke HD, Nattermann J et al. Induction of interleukin-6 by hepatitis C virus core protein in hepatitis C-associated mixed cryoglobulinemia and B-cell non-Hodgkin's lymphoma. Clin Cancer Res. 20061;12:4491–8.
122. Grungreiff K, Reinhold D, Ansorge S. Serum concentrations of sIL-2R, IL-6, TGF-beta1, neopterin, and zinc in chronic hepatitis C patients treated with interferon-alpha. Cytokine. 1999;11:1076–80.
123. Hirano T, Akira S, Taga T, Kishimoto T. Biological and clinical aspects of interleukin 6. Immunol Today. 1990;11:443–9.
124. Friederichs K, Schmitz J, Weissenbach M, Heinrich PC, Schaper F. Interleukin-6-induced proliferation of pre-B cells mediated by receptor complexes lacking the SHP2/SOCS3 recruitment sites revisited. Eur J Biochem. 2001;268:6401–7.
125. Seve P, Renaudier P, Sasco AJ et al. Hepatitis C virus infection and B-cell non-Hodgkin's lymphoma: a cross-sectional study in Lyon, France. Eur J Gastroenterol Hepatol. 2004;16:1361–5.
126. Correa P. Gastric neoplasia. Curr Gastroenterol Rep. 2002;4:463–70.
127. Mandell L, Moran AP, Cocchiarella A et al. Intact gram-negative *Helicobacter pylori*, *Helicobacter felis*, and *Helicobacter hepaticus* bacteria activate innate immunity via toll-like receptor 2 but not toll-like receptor 4. Infect Immun. 2004;72:6446–54.

4
Inflammatory pathways in liver homeostasis and liver injury

T. LUEDDE, F. TACKE and C. TRAUTWEIN

INTRODUCTION

The liver is an exceptional organ in terms of its metabolic, synthetic and detoxifying function. It has the unique potential to regenerate after tissue loss and, for instance, plays an important role in the regulation of blood glucose or blood lipids. All these and many other functions represent the organ's ability to execute the proper reaction towards the body's demands and keeping it in homeostasis. The central function of the liver for homeostasis and inflammatory responses is also underscored by its sole anatomical location, allowing continuous blood supply not only from the arterial system (hepatic arteries) but also from the gastrointestinal tract via the portal vein (Figure 1). Circulating blood cells, e.g. from the innate or adaptive immune system, are pressed through a network of sinusoids allowing contact to a variety of intrahepatic cell populations such as parenchymal liver cells (hepatocytes), endothelial cells, liver-resident macrophage (Kupffer cell) or lymphocyte (mainly NKT cells) populations, hepatic stellate cells and others (Figure 1)[1]. Communication between these cell types and the regulation of hepatic functions is primarily achieved by cytokines. Cytokines are small molecular weight messengers secreted by one cell to alter the behaviour of the cell itself (autocrine messenger), a closely related cell (paracrine messenger) or cells in different organs (endocrine messenger)[2]. This chapter will highlight some of the relevant cytokines and mediators for liver homeostasis and will discuss the manifold consequences of cytokine-driven activation of hepatocellular signalling pathways in liver homeostasis and injury.

CYTOKINES AND CYTOKINE RECEPTORS IN THE LIVER

Besides direct effects of immune cells on hepatocytes, inflammatory pathways in the liver are primarily regulated by cytokines. Cytokine action is generally mediated by the interaction of cellular receptors which signal internally to the nucleus, and external factors which are able to bind these receptors. These

INFLAMMATORY PATHWAYS IN LIVER HOMEOSTASIS AND INJURY

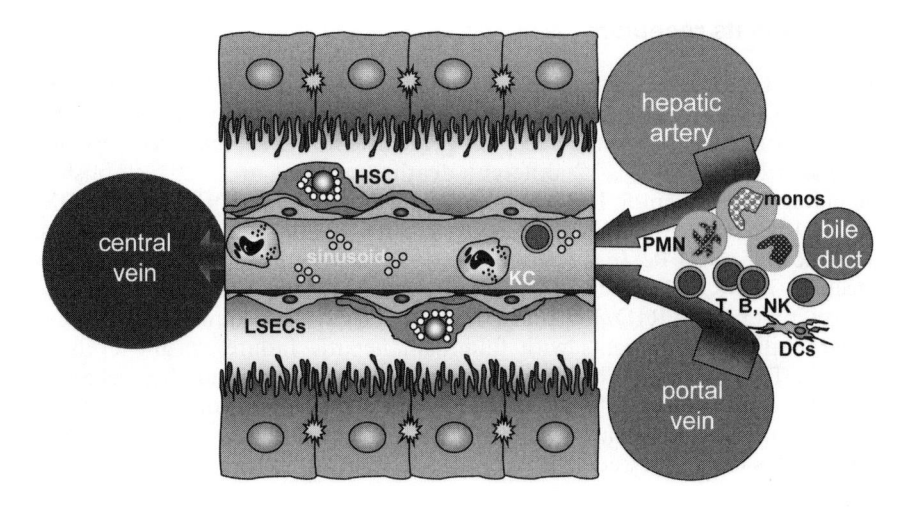

Figure 1 Intrahepatic cell populations. The healthy liver comprises about 60–80% hepatocytes; the other intrahepatic cell populations include biliary cells, liver sinusoidal endothelial cells (LSEC) lining the liver sinusoids, Kupffer cells (KC), and hepatic stellate cells (HSC) in the Disse space between hepatocytes and LSEC. In addition, many immune cells are found in the liver, mainly entering from the circulation via hepatic arteries and portal vein branches, including neutrophils (PMN), monocytes (monos), dendritic cells (DC) and lymphocytes (T, B, NK, NKT cells)

networks have evolved early in evolution; pathways with strong homology to human cytokine networks are already found in *Drosophila* and molluscs[3], for example in *Drosophila*, nuclear factor (NF)-κB-like transcription factors are activated in order to combat infections; this represents one major role of cytokine networks in higher organisms such as humans. Maintaining the ordered balance between proliferation and controlled cell death (apoptosis) during embryonic development and organogenesis is another important function of cytokines in physiological conditions. Since these functions are preserved in the adult organism, a disturbance of the critical balance might have deleterious effects[2]. Dysregulated cytokine actions after liver injury can result in excessive apoptosis, a key finding in various acute and chronic liver diseases, e.g. viral and autoimmune hepatitis, cholestatic disease, alcoholic or drug/toxin-induced liver injury. Among the manifold cytokines relevant for liver homeostasis and injury, we will highlight important findings on tumour necrosis factor alpha (TNF-α) and interleukin 6 (IL-6), as these represent two extensively studied pathways with exceptional significance in the liver. Studies in patients and animal models have strongly indicated that death receptor ligands such as TNF-α or Fas ligand (FasL) are involved in the induction of apoptosis and in triggering destruction of the liver[4]. The IL-6 cytokine family, on the other hand, may have essential functions in protecting the liver during acute or chronic injury[5,6].

TNF-α and its receptors

TNF and FasL belong to a family of nine ligands (TNF, lymphotoxin-α, TNF-β, FasL, OX40L, CD40L, CD27L, CD30L, 4-1BBL and lymphotoxin-β) that activate structurally related receptor proteins known as the TNF receptor superfamily. Currently, 12 different death receptors are well established including TNF receptor 1 (TNF-R1, Figure 2), TNF-R2, TNF-RP, Fas, OX-40, 4-1BB, CD40, CD30, CD27, pox virus PV-T2, PV-A53R gene products, and the p75 NGFR. In addition, the apoptosis-signalling receptors death receptor 3 (DR3), DR4 and DR5, their ligand TRAIL, and a non-signalling decoy receptor TRID/DcR are recently identified members of these superfamilies[7]. In patients with fulminant hepatic failure, serum levels of TNF-α, TNF-R1 and TNF-R2 are markedly increased, and these changes directly correlated with disease activity. In explanted livers of these patients, infiltrating mononuclear cells expressed large amounts of TNF-α and hepatocytes overexpressed TNF-R1[4].

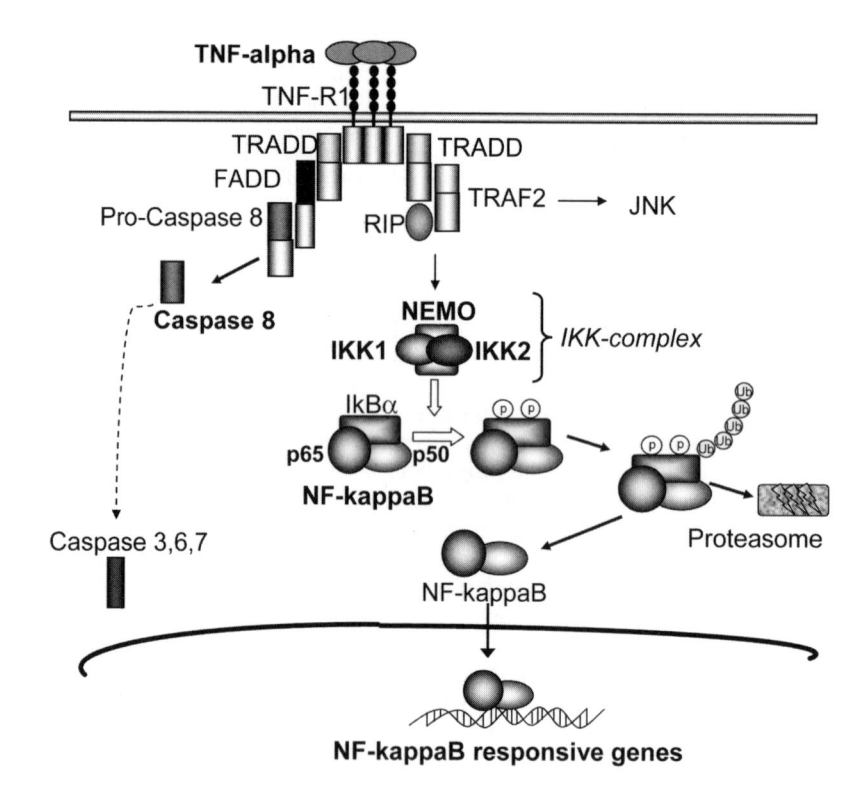

Figure 2 TNF-α signalling in the liver. TNF-α binds to its receptors, e.g. TNF-R1, and can thereby activate the pro-apoptotic caspase cascades (via TRADD, FADD and cleavage of pro-caspase 8) or the anti-apoptotic NF-κB pathway (via activation of the IKK complex resulting in phosphorylation of IκBα, subsequent translocation of NF-κB to the nucleus and expression of NF-κB responsive genes). For details, please see main text

IL-6 and its receptor

IL-6 belongs to a family of cytokines comprising IL-6, IL-11, leukaemia inhibitory factor (LIF), oncostatin M, ciliary neurotropic factor, novel neurotrophin-1/B cell stimulating factor-3 and cardiotropin 1[8]. IL-6 binds directly to hepatocytes by interacting with an 80-kDa membrane glycoprotein (gp80) that complexes with a signal-transducing molecule named gp130 (Figure 3)[3]. Serum and intrahepatic levels of IL-6 are elevated in patients with acute and chronic liver diseases[5].

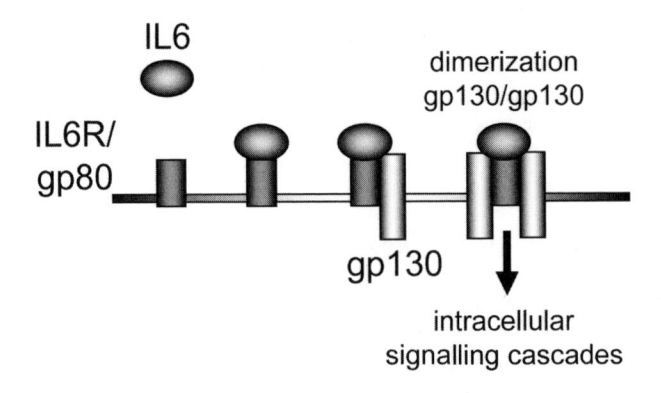

Figure 3 Interleukin 6 and its receptors. Interleukin 6 (IL-6) binds to the IL-6R/gp80, e.g. on hepatocytes. IL-6-gp80 then complexes with the signal transducing molecule gp130. Dimerization of two gp130 molecules activates intracellular signalling cascades

INTRACELLULAR PATHWAYS CONTROLLING LIVER HOMEOSTASIS AND INFLAMMATION

TNF-α signalling in the liver

In many instances hepatic failure might result from an imbalance between damaging and protective signals that are very tightly regulated under physiological conditions. As mentioned above, TNF-α and related cytokines are key players in liver homeostasis as they can activate both proapoptotic (mainly caspases) and anti-antiapoptotic (mainly NF-κB) pathways in hepatocytes (Figure 2).

Activation of proapoptotic signalling cascades

FasL and TNF-α facilitate programmed cell death in a similar manner by activation of caspases. The most important target of both pathways orchestrating cellular death is the aspartate-specific cysteine protease or caspase cascade, consisting of *initiator* caspases such as caspases 8 and 9 and *executioner* caspases, e.g. caspase 3, 6 and 7. Since proteolytic cleavage generates the mature caspases, one way in which these enzymes are activated is via the action of proteases, including other caspases. TNF-α signals through two distinct cell surface receptors, TNF-R1 and TNF-R2, of which TNF-R1 initiates the majority of TNF-α's biological activities. Binding of TNF-α to its receptor leads to the release of the inhibitory protein silencer of death domains (SODD) from TNF-R1's intracellular domain. This results in the recognition of the intracellular TNF-R1 domain by the adaptor protein TNF receptor-associated death domain (TRADD), which in turn recruits Fas-associated death domain (FADD). FADD recruits caspase-8 to the TNF-R1 complex, where it becomes activated and initiates the protease cascade leading to activation of executioner caspases and apoptosis (Figure 2). In contrast to TNF-dependent signalling, FasL can interact directly with the death domain of FADD without recruiting TRADD. In several studies involvement of mitochondria and the release of cytochrome c in the apoptotic process has been demonstrated, and this was also shown for FasL and TNF-α-mediated apoptosis in the liver[3].

Activation of the NF-κB pathway

Next to the activation of caspases, binding of TNF-α to its receptor also leads to the activation of the NF-κB pathway (Figure 2). NF-κB is a dimer of members of the Rel family of DNA-binding proteins. The mammalian NF-κB family includes five cellular DNA-binding subunits proteins: p50 (NF-κB1), p52 (NF-κB2), c-Rel (Rel), p65 (RelA) and RelB[9]. The NF-κB DNA-binding subunits share an N-terminal Rel homology domain (RHD). This region is responsible for DNA-binding, dimerization, nuclear translocation and interaction with the inhibitory IκB proteins[10].

TNF-induced activation of NF-κB relies on the phosphorylation of two conserved serines (S32 and S36 in human IκBα) in the N-terminal regulatory domain of IκBs. After phosphorylation the IκB undergo a second post-translational modification: polyubiquitination by a cascade of enzymatic reactions, followed by the degradation of IκB proteins by the proteasome, thus releasing NF-κB from its inhibitory IκB-binding partner, so it can translocate to the nucleus and activate transcription of NF-κB-dependent target genes[11,12]. Since the enzymes that catalyse the ubiquitination of IκB are constitutively active, the only regulated step in NF-κB activation appears to be in most cases the phosphorylation of IκB molecules.

A high-molecular-weight complex, called 'IKK-complex', that mediates the phosphorylation of IκB has been purified and characterized (Figure 2). This complex consists of three tightly associated IκB kinase (IKK) polypeptides: IKK1 (also called IKKα) and IKK2 (IKKβ) are the catalytic subunits of the kinase complex and have very similar primary structures with 52% overall similarity[13–15]. Moreover, it contains a regulatory subunit called NEMO (NF-κB Essential Modulator), IKKγ or IKKAP-1[13,16]. *In vitro*, IKK1 and IKK2 can form homodimers and heterodimers. Both IKK1 and IKK2 are able to phosphorylate IκB *in vitro*, but IKK2 has a higher kinase activity *in vitro* compared with IKK1[13,17–20].

Activation of the IKK complex upon TNF-α stimulation involves IKK recruitment to the TNF-R1[21–23]. Besides TNF-R1, this process involves TNF-receptor-associated-factor 2 (TRAF2) and the death-domain kinase receptor-interacting protein (RIP). In response to TNF-α treatment, TRAF2 recruits the IKK complex to TNF-R1 via the interaction of the RING-finger motifs of TRAF2 with the leucin-zipper motif of both IKK1 and IKK2[21,23]. RIP can directly interact with NEMO and mediate IKK activation, although the enzymatic activity of RIP is not required for this process[22]. The mechanism by which recruitment of the IKK complex to the TNF receptor leads to IKK activation is not clear, but might involve NEMO-induced autophosphorylation of the IKK complex. Moreover, ubiquitination of multiple factors that regulate the IKK complex, such as TRAF6/TAK1 or c-IAP1, an inhibitor of apoptosis that is also part of the TNF receptor complex, modulate the activity of the NF-κB pathway[12].

Consequences of NF-κB activation in the liver

Numerous studies have shown that NF-κB provides survival signals in the context of death receptor-induced apoptosis in the liver. This process is assumed to involve the transcriptional induction of various apoptotic suppressors[24]. Evidence that NF-κB governs critical anti-apoptotic proteins comes from well-described animal models. Injection of TNF-α into mice and addition of TNF-α to hepatic cells resulted in activation of nuclear translocation and of DNA binding of NF-κB[25], and hepatocytes are resistant to apoptosis induced by TNF-α or LPS, a potent inductor for endogenous TNF-α in the liver, unless they are treated with inhibitors of transcription of (anti-apoptotic) proteins such as cycloheximide or actinomycin D[26–28]. Knockout mice lacking the p65 subunit of NF-κB die between days E15 and E16 post-coitum as a result of fetal hepatocyte apoptosis[29]. This is caused by increased sensitivity towards TNF-α, since *TNF/p65* double-deficient mice are rescued from embryonic lethality[30].

Genetic experiments have also highlighted the differential functions of the IKK subunits in TNF-α-mediated liver apoptosis. Mice lacking IKK1 die shortly after birth and display a phenotype marked by thickening of skin and limb as well as skeletal defects. IKK2-deficient mice die *in utero* approximately at embryonic day 12.5 as a result of massive apoptosis in the liver, and fibroblasts from these mice show no activation of NF-κB in response to TNF-α. A similar phenotype was noted in mice lacking the regulatory subunit NEMO, which also die from massive apoptosis in the liver and show a defect in NF-κB activation upon TNF-α stimulation in their primary murine embryonic fibroblasts. Therefore, at least during embryogenesis, IKK2 and NEMO appear to be the critical subunits for NF-κB activation and protection of liver cells from proinflammatory cytokines such as TNF-α[31].

The role of the IKK subunits in the adult animal is less well understood. Conditional knockout mice based on the cre/loxP system have emerged as new powerful tools to study gene functions in the adult animal *in vivo*[31,32]. In a recent study we could show that hepatocyte-specific ablation of IKK2 did not lead to a strongly impaired activation of NF-κB or increased apoptosis after

TNF-α stimulation, probably because IKK1 homodimers can take over this function in the absence of IKK2 in the adult mouse[33]. In contrast, conditional hepatocyte-specific knockout of NEMO resulted in complete block of NF-κB activation and massive hepatocyte apoptosis, underlining that NEMO is the only irreplaceable IKK subunit for prevention of TNF-α-mediated liver apoptosis[34].

Besides its anti-apoptotic function in TNF-α-mediated liver apoptosis, NF-κB appears to be also critically involved in other models of experimental liver injury. NF-κB DNA-binding occurs quickly upon hepatic ischaemia–reperfusion (I/R) injury[35], but the mechanism of NF-κB activation has long been obscure in this model. It has also long been unclear whether NF-κB-dependent signalling withholds a protective or damaging role in I/R injury. We could show that hepatocyte-specific conditional knockout mice for IKK2 show a defect in NF-κB activation after I/R[33]. Inhibition of NF-κB activation in conditional IKK2-deficient mice protects from liver injury due to I/R[33], thus underlining that, depending on the experimental model, the NF-κB pathway does not serve as a survival pathway, but instead can aggravate hepatocyte death and liver damage. However, complete abolishment of NF-κB activation in conditional NEMO-knockout mice resulted in massive hepatic inflammation and apoptosis after I/R injury[34].

IL-6 SIGNALLING IN THE LIVER

IL-6 binds to the gp80/IL-6 receptor on hepatocytes that then complex with the signal transducer gp130 (Figure 3). Binding of gp130 leads to dimerization of the intracellular domains of two gp130 molecules, which promotes association with receptor-associated Janus kinases (JAK; JAK1, JAK2, and TYK). The JAK become activated and phosphorylate different tyrosine residues on the gp130 molecule. Depending on the location of the phosphorylated tyrosines, signal transducers and activators of transcription (STAT) proteins (mainly STAT-3) and also the Ras/mitogen-activated protein (MAP) kinase pathway become activated and trigger numerous downstream effects mediated by the signalling of IL-6 and related cytokines (Figure 4)[8].

An important role of IL-6-dependent signalling in the liver is the induction of the acute-phase response[36], and STAT-3 participates in its transcriptional activation. In patients with fulminant hepatic failure or with chronic liver diseases, IL-6 expression in serum and liver tissue correlates with disease progression[5,6]. In experimental models of liver injury, mice deficient for the gp130 receptor in hepatocytes show an abolished acute-phase response and an increased susceptibility to LPS-induced liver failure or to bacterial infections[6,37]. In the model of ConA-induced hepatitis, pretreatment with IL-6 can protect mice from liver injury. This protection from ConA-induced liver damage requires gp130 signalling in hepatocytes and is mediated via the gp130/STAT-3 signalling cascade, resulting in the up-regulation of other cytokines such as the IL-8 orthologue KC (gro-alpha) and serum amyloid A-2 (SAA-2)[38]. Gp130-signalling in non-parenchymal cells is, on the other hand, essential for mediating protective IL-6/gp130 effects during experimental

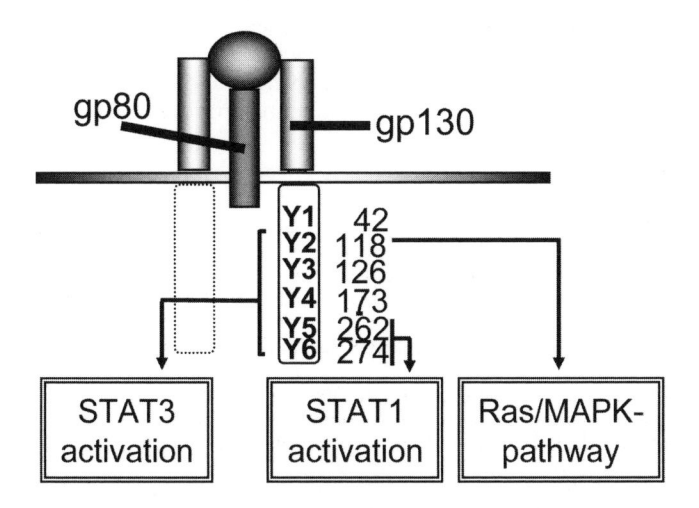

Figure 4 IL-6 signalling in the liver. The complex of IL-6, gp80 (IL-6R) and two gp130 molecules mediates IL-6 signalling via phosphorylation of tyrosine (Y) residues of the intracellular gp130 molecule. Depending on the location of the phosphorylated tyrosines, signal transducers and activators of transcription (STAT) proteins (mainly STAT-3) and also the Ras/mitogen-activated protein (MAP) kinase pathway become activated and trigger the downstream effects

chronic liver diseases and liver fibrogenesis[5]. Studies are ongoing to translate findings of hepatoprotective effects of IL-6/gp130 into novel therapeutic approaches in acute and chronic liver diseases[3].

CONCLUSION

A growing number of studies have implicated immune cells, cytokines and cytokine-dependent pathways in the development of liver failure, chronic liver disease, hepatic inflammation and liver carcinogenesis. Resident and infiltrating immune cells have been linked to progression, but also to restriction and regression of liver injury. Parenchymal and non-parenchymal survival pathways such as NF-κB or IL-6 withhold a protective function in many experimental liver disease models, and thus are an attractive target for a pharmacological intervention. However, many experimental models highlighted dual functions of these key players, namely beneficial or adverse effects. For instance, blockage of monocyte infiltration into the liver may limit disease progression, but would negatively affect the resolution of liver fibrosis. Thus, an inflammatory immune cell is not necessarily detrimental in any context. Also, an inhibition of NF-κB in the liver can have different outcomes depending on the experimental model applied: protecting from apoptosis in a model of TNF-dependent cell death versus aggravating cellular necrosis in a model of ischaemia–reperfusion injury. Thus, a survival pathway is not necessarily protective in any context. Dissecting the cellular and molecular inflammatory pathways during liver homeostasis and during liver injury will hopefully provide the basis for novel therapeutic approaches in the near future.

References

1. Racanelli V, Rehermann B. The liver as an immunological organ. Hepatology. 2006;43: S54–62.
2. Luedde T, Liedtke C, Manns MP, Trautwein C. Losing balance: cytokine signaling and cell death in the context of hepatocyte injury and hepatic failure. Eur Cytokine Netw. 2002;13:377–83.
3. Luedde T, Trautwein C. Intracellular survival pathways in the liver. Liver Int. 2006;26:1163–74.
4. Streetz K, Leifeld L, Grundmann D et al. Tumor necrosis factor alpha in the pathogenesis of human and murine fulminant hepatic failure. Gastroenterology. 2000;119:446–60.
5. Streetz KL, Tacke F, Leifeld L et al. Interleukin 6/gp130-dependent pathways are protective during chronic liver diseases. Hepatology. 2003;38:218–29.
6. Streetz KL, Wustefeld T, Klein C et al. Lack of gp130 expression in hepatocytes promotes liver injury. Gastroenterology. 2003;125:532–43.
7. Schulze-Osthoff K, Ferrari D, Los M, Wesselborg S, Peter ME. Apoptosis signaling by death receptors. Eur J Biochem. 1998;254:439–59.
8. Streetz KL, Luedde T, Manns MP, Trautwein C. Interleukin 6 and liver regeneration. Gut. 2000;47:309–12.
9. Ghosh S, May MJ, Kopp EB. NF-kappa B and Rel proteins: evolutionarily conserved mediators of immune responses. Annu Rev Immunol. 1998;16:225–60.
10. Ghosh S, Karin M. Missing pieces in the NF-kappaB puzzle. Cell. 2002;109(Suppl.):S81-96.
11. Karin M. How NF-kappaB is activated: the role of the IkappaB kinase (IKK) complex. Oncogene. 1999;18:6867–74.
12. Yamamoto Y, Gaynor RB. IkappaB kinases: key regulators of the NF-kappaB pathway. Trends Biochem Sci. 2004;29:72–9.
13. Mercurio F, Murray BW, Shevchenko A et al. IkappaB kinase (IKK)-associated protein 1, a common component of the heterogeneous IKK complex. Mol Cell Biol. 1999;19:1526–38.
14. Regnier CH, Song HY, Gao X, Goeddel DV, Cao Z, Rothe M. Identification and characterization of an IkappaB kinase. Cell. 1997;90:373–83.
15. DiDonato JA, Hayakawa M, Rothwarf DM, Zandi E, Karin M. A cytokine-responsive IkappaB kinase that activates the transcription factor NF-kappaB. Nature. 1997;388:548–54.
16. Rothwarf DM, Zandi E, Natoli G, Karin M. IKK-gamma is an essential regulatory subunit of the IkappaB kinase complex. Nature. 1998;395:297–300.
17. Delhase M, Hayakawa M, Chen Y, Karin M. Positive and negative regulation of IkappaB kinase activity through IKKbeta subunit phosphorylation. Science. 1999;284:309–13.
18. Mercurio F, Zhu H, Murray BW et al. IKK-1 and IKK-2: cytokine-activated IkappaB kinases essential for NF-kappaB activation. Science. 1997;278:860–6.
19. Woronicz JD, Gao X, Cao Z, Rothe M, Goeddel DV. IkappaB kinase-beta: NF-kappaB activation and complex formation with IkappaB kinase-alpha and NIK. Science. 1997;278:866–9.
20. Zandi E, Rothwarf DM, Delhase M, Hayakawa M, Karin M. The IkappaB kinase complex (IKK) contains two kinase subunits, IKKalpha and IKKbeta, necessary for IkappaB phosphorylation and NF-kappaB activation. Cell. 1997;91:243–52.
21. Devin A, Cook A, Lin Y, Rodriguez Y, Kelliher M, Liu Z. The distinct roles of TRAF2 and RIP in IKK activation by TNF-R1: TRAF2 recruits IKK to TNF-R1 while RIP mediates IKK activation. Immunity. 2000;12:419–29.

22. Zhang SQ, Kovalenko A, Cantarella G, Wallach D. Recruitment of the IKK signalosome to the p55 TNF receptor: RIP and A20 bind to NEMO (IKKgamma) upon receptor stimulation. Immunity. 2000;12:301–11.
23. Devin A, Lin Y, Yamaoka S, Li Z, Karin M, Liu Z. The alpha and beta subunits of IkappaB kinase (IKK) mediate TRAF2-dependent IKK recruitment to tumor necrosis factor (TNF) receptor 1 in response to TNF. Mol Cell Biol. 2001;21:3986–94.
24. Liu ZG, Hsu H, Goeddel DV, Karin M. Dissection of TNF receptor 1 effector functions: JNK activation is not linked to apoptosis while NF-kappaB activation prevents cell death. Cell. 1996;87:565–76.
25. FitzGerald MJ, Webber EM, Donovan JR, Fausto N. Rapid DNA binding by nuclear factor kappa B in hepatocytes at the start of liver regeneration. Cell Growth Differ. 1995;6:417–27.
26. Lehmann V, Freudenberg MA, Galanos C. Lethal toxicity of lipopolysaccharide and tumor necrosis factor in normal and D-galactosamine-treated mice. J Exp Med. 1987;165:657–63.
27. Leist M, Gantner F, Bohlinger I, Germann PG, Tiegs G, Wendel A. Murine hepatocyte apoptosis induced *in vitro* and *in vivo* by TNF-alpha requires transcriptional arrest. J Immunol. 1994;153:1778–88.
28. Leist M, Gantner F, Naumann H et al. Tumor necrosis factor-induced apoptosis during the poisoning of mice with hepatotoxins. Gastroenterology. 1997;112:923–34.
29. Beg AA, Baltimore D. An essential role for NF-kappaB in preventing TNF-alpha-induced cell death. Science. 1996;274:782–4.
30. Doi TS, Marino MW, Takahashi T et al. Absence of tumor necrosis factor rescues RelA-deficient mice from embryonic lethality. Proc Natl Acad Sci USA. 1999;96:2994–9.
31. Pasparakis M, Luedde T, Schmidt-Supprian M. Dissection of the NF-kappaB signalling cascade in transgenic and knockout mice. Cell Death Differ. 2006;13:861–72.
32. Luedde T, Beraza N, Trautwein C. Evaluation of the role of nuclear factor-kappaB signaling in liver injury using genetic animal models. J Gastroenterol Hepatol. 2006;(Suppl. 3):S43–6.
33. Luedde T, Assmus U, Wustefeld T et al. Deletion of IKK2 in hepatocytes does not sensitize these cells to TNF-induced apoptosis but protects from ischemia/reperfusion injury. J Clin Invest. 2005;115:849–59.
34. Beraza N, Ludde T, Assmus U, Roskams T, Vander BS, Trautwein C. Hepatocyte-specific IKK gamma/NEMO expression determines the degree of liver injury. Gastroenterology. 2007;132:2504–17.
35. Zwacka RM, Zhang Y, Zhou W, Halldorson J, Engelhardt JF. Ischemia/reperfusion injury in the liver of BALB/c mice activates AP-1 and nuclear factor kappaB independently of IkappaB degradation. Hepatology. 1998;28:1022–30.
36. Trautwein C, Boker K, Manns MP. Hepatocyte and immune system: acute phase reaction as a contribution to early defence mechanisms. Gut. 1994;35:1163–6.
37. Wuestefeld T, Klein C, Streetz KL et al. Lack of gp130 expression results in more bacterial infection and higher mortality during chronic cholestasis in mice. Hepatology. 2005;42:1082–90.
38. Klein C, Wustefeld T, Assmus U et al. The IL-6-gp130-STAT3 pathway in hepatocytes triggers liver protection in T cell-mediated liver injury. J Clin Invest. 2005;115:860–9.

Section II
Pathomechanisms of fibrogenesis: mediators

Chair: AM GRESSNER and F LAMMERT

5
A complex network of intra- and intercellular mediators regulate cellular activation and transdifferentiation of hepatic stellate cells

R. WEISKIRCHEN, E. BORKHAM-KAMPHORST, S. K. MEURER,
F. DREWS, S. MOHREN, J. HERRMANN, O. A. GRESSNER,
O. SCHERNER, W. N. VREDEN, E. KOVALENKO, M. BOMBLE and
A. M. GRESSNER

HEPATIC STELLATE CELLS IN NORMAL AND FIBROTIC LIVER

Hepatic stellate cells (HSC) present a highly dynamic phenotype with diverse functions in normal liver. They are crucial in controlling vitamin A metabolism and homeostasis, influence the sinusoidal blood flow, synthesize a plurality of extracellular matrix constituents, are part of complex intercellular networks, and synthesize important mediators such as erythropoietin, constituents of the plasminogen activation system, and a broad set of different cytokines and chemokines. Most recently it was demonstrated that they encompass antigen-presenting functions presenting specific antigenic peptides to $CD8^+$ and $CD4^+$ T cells and further mediate cross-priming of $CD8^+$ T cells[1]. However, the most amazing features of HSC biology emerged in studies investigating hepatic fibrogenesis, a process in which quiescent HSC adopt proliferative attributes and transdifferentiate into myofibroblasts (MFB). Accompanying this process of phenotypical diversification, typical marker proteins such as α-smooth muscle actin (α-SMA) and a fibrotic matrix rich in type I collagen are synthesized[2]. Furthermore, the activities of a multitude of different regulatory signalling cascades are modified that activate autocrine or paracrine pathways. The underlying mechanisms are manifold, including an overall augmented production of respective cytokines and a distinct up-regulation of cytokine receptors. Moreover, it recently became evident that the activity of various cytokines is influenced by specialized modifier proteins (e.g. CTGF) and receptors (e.g. endoglin) and that the biological activities of some cytokines are absorbed by opposing cytokines. In this chapter we will summarize recent findings on transforming growth factor beta (TGF-β), its biological antagonist bone morphogenetic protein-7 (BMP-7), and the known isoforms of the platelet-derived growth factor (PDGF) in promoting the fibrogenic response in injured liver. These cytokines are part of a regulatory network influencing the health status of the liver (Figure 1). In addition, we will give some defined examples how the activity of TGF-β is modulated by proteins affecting its secretion, biological processing, and/or receptor binding.

THE SIMPLE IS BECOMING COMPLEX: THE TGF-β/SMAD SIGNALLING NETWORK IN HSC AND MFB

The major soluble profibrogenic trigger of fibrogenesis in liver is TGF-$β_1$ that is a key regulator of extracellular matrix (ECM) assembly and remodelling. The signal transduction of TGF-β in HSC is initiated by proteolytic activation (see next section) and binding of the ligand to a hetero-oligomeric complex composed of the signalling receptors type II (TβRII) and type I serine/threonine kinases which are commonly known as activin receptor-like kinase (ALK). Binding of TGF-β to TβRII leads to recruitment and phosphorylation of ALK5, which transfers the signal via phosphorylation to the receptor-regulated Smads (R-Smad), R-Smad2 and R-Smad3 (Figure 2). R-Smads in complex with the common Smad4 (co-Smad) translocate into the nucleus to regulate the expression of TGF-β target genes. The contemporary induction of the inhibitory Smad7 in turn switches off this signalling cascade by blocking further R-Smad activation[3].

The functional relevance of TGF-β for the processes of activation and transdifferentiation has been addressed for more than two decades. It was previously shown that the Smad-dependent responses of HSC are modulated when they become MFB. Most apparently, the potential of TGF-β to inhibit HSC/MFB proliferation, to trigger ECM production and to activate Smad7 expression, is reduced when cells have acquired the fully transdifferentiated phenotype[4,5]. Although strongly dependent on culture conditions, it was found that the surface expression of TβRII and ALK5, and the capacity to bind TGF-β, are decreased during the transdifferentiation process[4,5]. It was suggested that the intracellular signalling in response to TGF-β is mediated by R-Smad2 and R-Smad3 in HSC and, coinciding with reduced receptor availability, that this pathway is abrogated in MFB[5,6]. Because Smad3 is necessary for maximal expression of collagen type I and inhibition of HSC proliferation, it was further assumed that Smad3 is the key regulator in hepatic fibrogenesis[7]. This perhaps doubtful view must be somewhat revised because it was found that the activation of Smad3 by ALK5 and its subsequent DNA binding capacity is drastically reduced in MFB[5,8]. However, based on data from investigations in scleroderma fibroblasts, it has beeen shown that Smad3 has a central role in the initiation of the fibrotic response, but may not be required for the maintenance of the fibrotic phenotype[9]. Moreover, the finding that phospho-Smad3 is absent at early time points in cultured HSC supports the notion that Smad3 is not

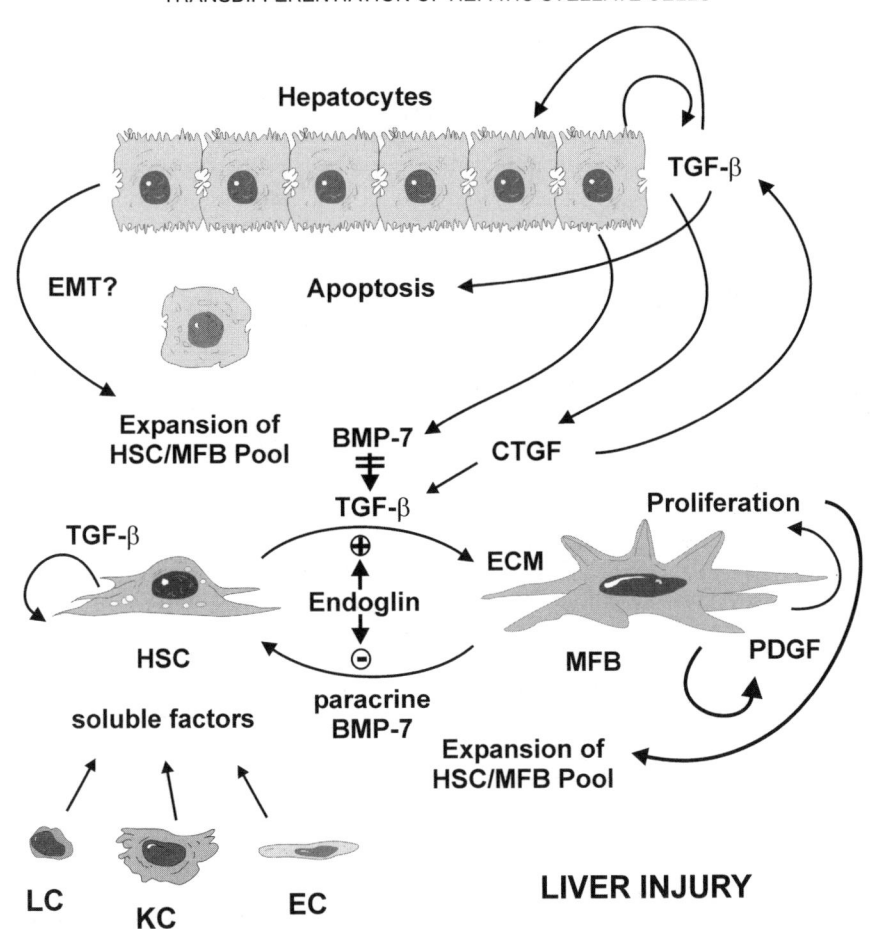

Figure 1 Transdifferentiation of HSC in injured liver tissue, a process influenced by diverse factors and cell types. Generally, liver injury is initiated by hepatocyte damage that is associated with release of TGF-β. Subsequently this cytokine induces hepatocyte apoptosis and expression of target genes (e.g. CTGF). TGF-β and its biological modifier (CTGF) subsequently induce the activation and transdifferentiation of HSC into MFB, resulting in a net accumulation of ECM. The HSC/MFB pool is expanded by proliferation that is mainly triggered by the activity of PDGF and transition of hepatocytes into profibrogenic cells, a process that is termed epithelial-to-mesenchymal transition (EMT). Furthermore, the process of fibrogenesis is locally modulated by soluble factors that are released by infiltrating lymphocytes (LC), Kupffer cells (KC) and endothelial cells (EC). The activity of TGF-β is further influenced by opposing factors (e.g. BMP-7, endoglin)

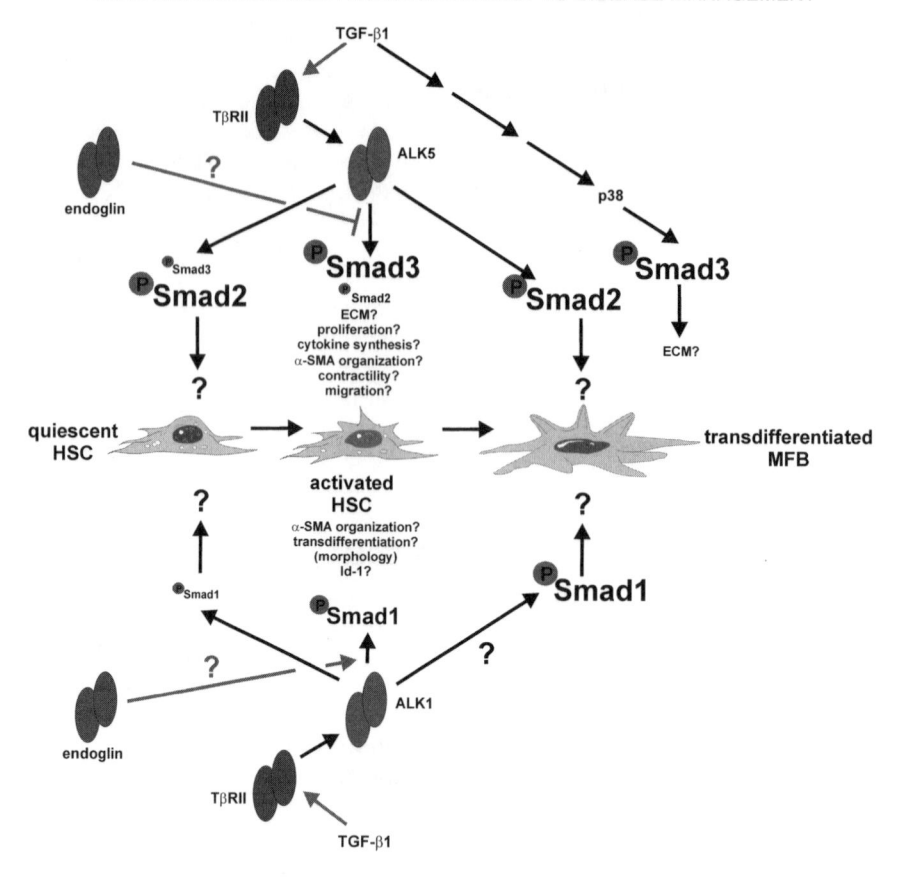

Figure 2 Smad signalling pathways active during transdifferentiation of HSC to MFB. Depicted are the two signalling branches, i.e. ALK5/Smad2/Smad3 and ALK1/Smad1, which are activated by TGF-β in HSC and MFB, respectively. The so-far-assigned functions of the Smads with respect to the activation state are indicated. For detailed information see text

involved in HSC activation, a finding that is substantiated by the observation that HSC taken from Smad3-deficient mice showed normal α-SMA expression[7]. It was further shown that Smad3 is primarily phosphorylated in activated HSC when ECM synthesis is going to be established, confirming the above-mentioned role of Smad3 in the control of ECM expression[10]. In addition, Smad3 mediates inhibition of proliferation, enhances migration and regulates the organization of the cytoskeleton in early and late activated HSC[11]. In contrast, the role of Smad2 in HSC is less well defined. Smad2 is primarily activated in quiescent HSC and the constitutive C-terminal phosphorylation that is found in MFB or in chronic liver disease[12] was found to be independent of TGF-β[10]. This constitutive activation may be linked to proliferation, since the transient overexpression of a dominant negative Smad2 variant caused a higher proliferation rate in transdifferentiated cells[11].

However, the function of Smads is not solely regulated by the corresponding type I receptor. In MFB, which show negligible amounts of ALK5 phosphorylated Smad3 (see above), Smad3 was found to be phosphorylated in the linker region by p38 MAP kinase in a TGF-β-dependent manner. Smad3 that is phosphorylated at this site translocates in complex with Smad4 into the nucleus and binds to Smad binding elements (SBE). Furthermore, linker- but not C-terminally phosphorylated Smad3 was found in isolated MFB that were isolated from livers of chronically injured rats. These findings substantiate the postulated autocrine stimulation of MFB by TGF-β and further prove that MFB do not entirely escape from the control of TGF-β[8].

In addition to its capability to influence the activity of the classical TGF-β Smads (i.e. Smad2 and Smad3), TGF-β is likewise competent to activate a member (i.e. Smad1) of the 'BMP Smads' that is increasingly phosphorylated during the process of transdifferentiation. The contribution of TGF-β to control Smad1 activation in HSC is controversially discussed. While there are reports demonstrating that TGF-β significantly inhibits Smad1 gene expression in HSC in a time- and dose-dependent manner[13], recent reports have shown that TGF-β strongly induces Smad1 phosphorylation[14]. Smad1 is a substrate of the ALK1 receptor which is expressed in HSC and MFB. Signalling by ALK1/Smad1 in response to TGF-β facilitates the induction of the transcription factor inhibitor of differentiation1 (Id1) that enhances the activation of HSC and influences α-SMA organization[14].

In HSC the precise analysis of the interdependence and exact functionalities of the two well-defined TGF-β-activated signalling pathways, i.e. ALK5/Smad3 and ALK1/Smad1, is currently in progress. Experimental data from endothelial cells point towards an antagonistic relationship of these signalling pathways, in which they exclusively regulate different cellular and functional features[15]. Even more interesting is the finding that HSC express high levels of the accessory receptor endoglin[16]. This receptor was shown to inhibit ALK5/Smad3 and enhance ALK1/Smad1 signalling in endothelial cells[17] and therefore may represent a general switch which governs the fine-tuning of TGF-β signals in HSC/MFB.

NOVEL ASPECTS OF TGF-β SECRETION AND ACTIVATION IN HSC

The complex regulation of the TGF-β bioavailability includes its intracellular synthesis as a pre-pro-protein, the proteolytic processing by a furin-like protease and the final assembly into a latent complex in which the mature TGF-β dimer is associated with the latency-associated peptide and bound to the latent transforming growth factor-β binding protein (LTBP)[18]. By this means stored in the ECM, multiple effector mechanisms lead to the release of mature TGF-β that initiate the above-mentioned signalling processes by assembling receptor complexes and the following phosphorylation of downstream transcription factors.

Therefore, the concentration of biological active TGF-β is arising from the amount of secreted latent TGF-β that becomes activated out of the latent complex. Several mechanisms such as conformational rearrangements triggered by thrombospondin-1, or the cleavage by the serine protease plasmin, were proposed for the activation process of latent TGF-β[19,20], whereas the export of the latent complex from the producing cell is only incompletely known. Three out of four LTBP isoforms, termed LTBP-1, -3 and -4, are able to interact more or less effectively with TGF-β_1 (see ref. 21). This covalent interaction takes place via the third of the characteristic 8-cysteine-motifs[21,22]. The N-terminal hinge region and parts of the C-terminal region of the high molecular weight and glycosylated LTBP are responsible for the interaction with the ECM[23–25]. The complexity of the LTBP gene family is further increased by the existence of different promoters within the LTBP-1 gene resulting in the generation of short (LTBP-S) and long (LTBP-L) forms. Moreover, alternative splicing and differential proteolytic processing further increase the variability of LTBP proteins (Figure 3A). However, the influence of the different LTBP-1 splice variants described in humans and mice on TGF-β secretion is still unclear[26–32]. At present three different isoforms have been isolated in humans, while only one modification was described in mouse. In a recent study, we analysed in more detail the occurrence of splice variants in mice. Based on the assumption that potential splice donor and acceptor sites within the LTBP-1 mRNA may be functionally relevant, we have carried out a comprehensive analysis in which we tested if assumed splice variants were detectable by RT-PCR. Using this strategy we could determine several transcript variants that could predict curtailed proteins in which the reading frame remained preserved (Figure 3B). Some of the expected variants were found in many different organs, while others have a more restricted expression pattern (not shown). While the Δ56, Δ53, and Δ42 variants have potential homologues in humans that were previously described, the Δ90 variant lacking 90 amino acids is presently unknown in other species, suggesting that in future a more extended panel of LTBP-1 splice variants will be identified in other species.

Moreover, first *in vitro* and *in vivo* analysis using models in which LTBP-1 is absent showed that LTBP-1 has an essential influence on overall TGF-β activity[33]. When we comparatively subjected wild-type mice and mice lacking functional LTBP-1 protein to bile duct ligature (BDL), we found that livers of mice lacking LTBP-1 were less prone to liver fibrogenesis indicated by an overall decreased deposition of fibrillar collagen (Figure 4). These experiments demonstrated that the LTBP-1 protein is an essential mediator in TGF-β functionality.

CONNECTIVE TISSUE GROWTH FACTOR, A MODIFIER OF THE FIBROGENIC RESPONSE

Connective tissue growth factor (CTGF/CCN2) is a 36–38 kDa cysteine-rich, heparin-binding and secreted protein, which was originally identified in the conditioned medium of human umbilical vein endothelial cells[34]. It belongs to a family of six highly conserved secreted proteins that specifically associate with the ECM[35]. The human *CTGF* gene is located on chromosome 6q23.1 and encompasses approximately 3 kbp. It encodes a protein of multimodular

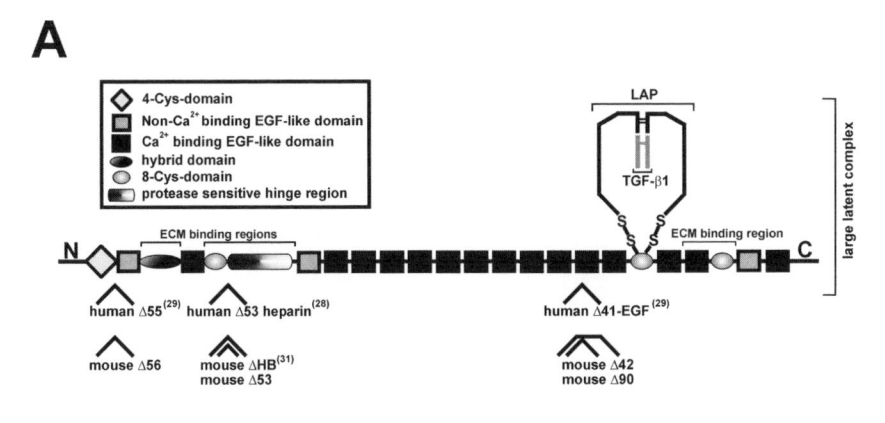

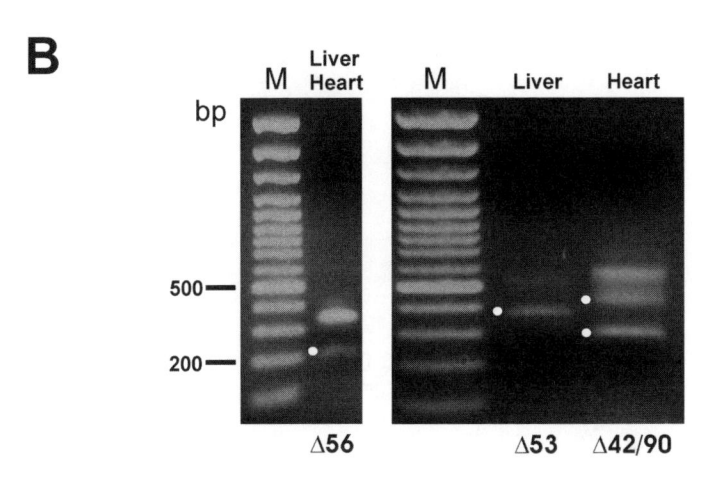

Figure 3 Splice variants of the human and murine LTBP-1 gene. **A**: LTBP-1 protein structure and positions of already characterized splice variants (*upper row*) previously published[28,29,31] and novel splice variants identified in our investigation (*lower row*). **B**: RT-PCR of mRNAs extracted from murine heart and liver. Expected PCR products (*upper fragments*) and products generated by the existence of new splice variants lacking the indicated numbers of amino acids (*lower bands with white dots*) were separated by agarose gel electrophoresis

organization including a secretory signal, an IGF binding protein domain, a von Willebrand factor domain, a thrombospondin type I domain, and a cysteine knot motif (Figure 5). The *CTGF* promoter contains several regulatory elements (i.e. AP-1, TATA-box, SP1-box) as well as a specific TGF-β response element which is included in the CTGF promoter but not in those of other CCN family members[36].

In fibroblasts the profibrogenic master cytokine TGF-β is the most important transcriptional activator of CTGF and, from a functional aspect, CTGF is regarded as a downstream mediator of TGF-β effects[37]. It was

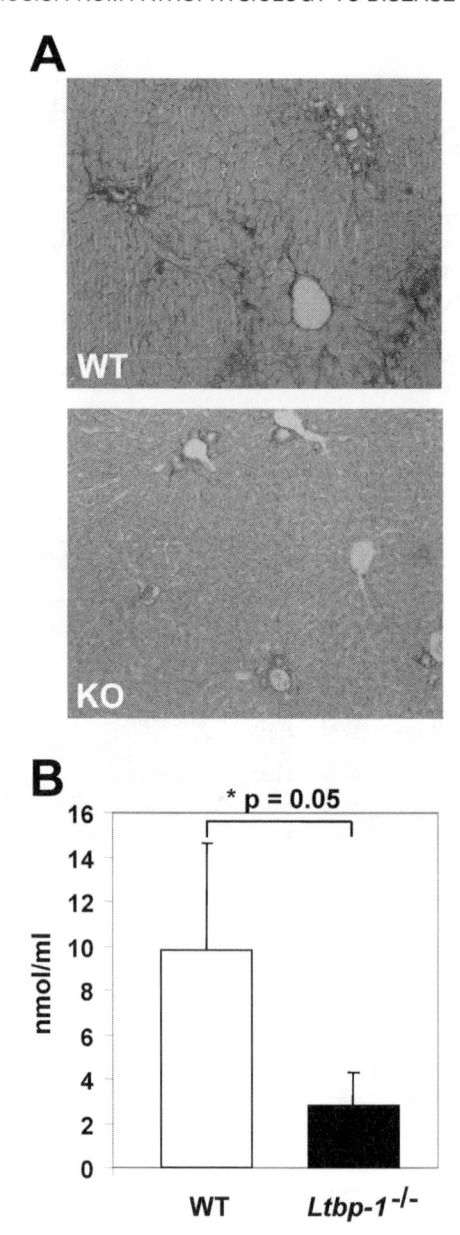

Figure 4 Mice lacking LTBP-1 are less prone to liver fibrogenesis. **A**: Sirius red stain of liver slices taken from wild-type and LTBP-1 nulls that were subjected to BDL for 4 weeks. **B**: The hydroxyproline content of respective liver samples from BDL animals was determined by a HPLC method

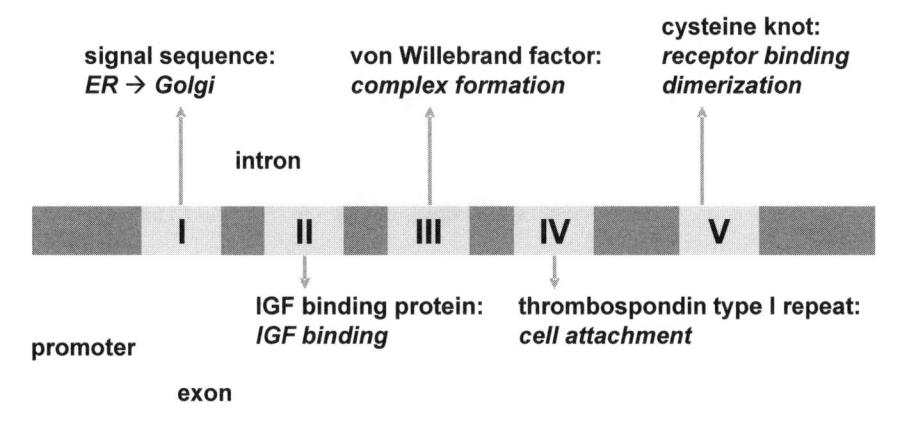

Figure 5 Genomic organization of the *CTGF* gene. The gene encoding CTGF comprises five exons encoding functionally different domains of the CTGF protein (modified after ref. 39)

claimed that many of the profibrogenic characteristics of TGF-β are mediated via an induction of CTGF expression with subsequent stimulation of fibroblast activity and matrix production.

Involved in the mediation of TGF-β-dependent CTGF expression are the profibrogenic pSmad3 and ERK1/2[38]. The common mediator Smad4 is also involved, whereas pSmad2 and the CREB-binding protein/p300 do not participate[9]. More recent work[39] has proven that, besides TGF-β/Smad3/Smad4, Ras/MEK/ERK signalling as well as protein kinase C and A also contribute to the basal, TGF-β-dependent CTGF expression in fibroblasts[40,41]. The functional Smad binding site in the *CTGF* gene is located between nucleotides −173 and −166 and consists of a CAGACGAA sequence[9]. The *CTGF* promoter furthermore contains a binding site for the Ets-1 transcription factor whose activity is regulated by Sp1, suggesting that this zinc finger protein transcription factor is involved in the constitutive expression of CTGF via Ets-1[42,43].

The pathophysiological significance of CTGF for liver fibrosis is clear. Particularly, recent *in vivo* experiments using si-RNA approaches in experimental liver fibrosis have shown that CTGF silencing has a strikingly antifibrotic and thus potentially therapeutic effect[44]. Furthermore, other models of fibrosis indicate a strong pathogenetic synergism between TGF-β and CTGF[45,46]. CTGF was further supposed[47] to be an extracellular trapping protein for BMP and TGF-β$_1$. According to this functionality, CTGF physically interacts with BMP-4 and TGF-β$_1$ via the CR domain, and thus antagonizes BMP-4 activity by inhibition of receptor binding, whereas the receptor binding of TGF-β$_1$ is sensitized. As BMP and TGF-β are the major opponents in the regulation of the epithelial–mesenchymal transition (EMT)[47], CTGF would thus act profibrogenically by shifting the balance towards mesenchymal activity. However, the role of EMT in the pathophysiology of liver fibrosis is still under critical discussion[48,49] and is a promising field of

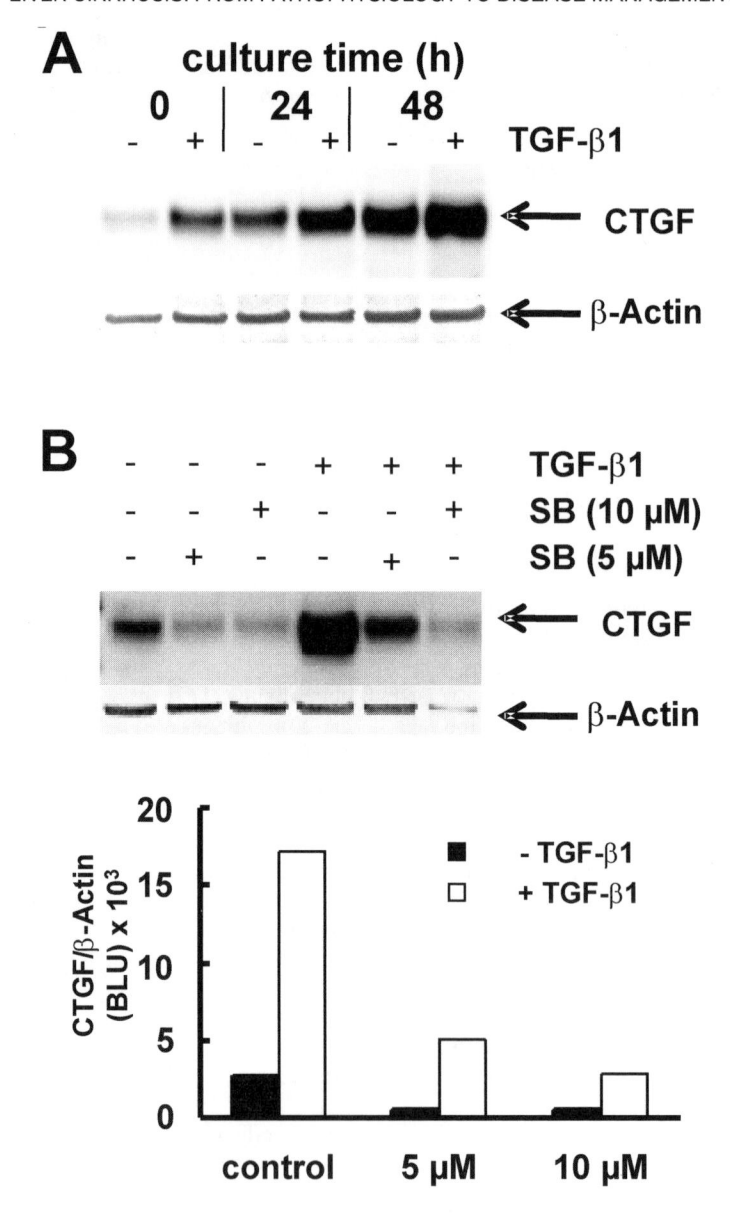

Figure 6 CTGF expression is dependent on the ALK5 receptor system in hepatocytes. **A**: A time-dependent increase of CTGF, spontaneous and in response to TGF-β stimulation. **B**: A dose-dependent modulation of CTGF expression in response to specific, intracellular ALK5-receptor inhibition (SB-431542) in the presence or absence of TGF-β

research in the future. In particular the question of which consequences result from an overexpression of CTGF, is currently unanswered.

Recently, we found that the expression of CTGF in HSC is only slightly affected by TGF-β but stimulated by endothelin-1, independently from Smad2/3 phosphorylation[50]. In addition, CTGF expression is not regulated during transdifferentiation to MFB in culture. These results are in contrast to cultured hepatocytes, where CTGF expression is strongly stimulated by TGF-β$_1$ (Figure 6A). But also under entirely TGF-β-free culture conditions, a time-dependent hepatocellular CTGF expression can be observed which correlates with increased intracellular activation of latent TGF-β, manifested in a cycloheximide-insensitive accumulation of active TGF-β within the hepatocyte under these culture conditions (unpublished observation).

Sequential inhibition of extracellular TGF-β signalling, as well as of TGF-β-activated kinase-1 (TAK1), provides evidence that spontaneous CTGF expression as a result of intracellular TGF-β activation does not necessarily take place via extracellular, autocrine signalling but may also happen intracellularly (within the hepatocyte). Intracellular activation of ALK4/ALK5 seems to play a central role in this process, as an abrogation of CTGF expression and Smad2 but not Smad3 phosphorylation is observed following specific blockade of the intracellular kinase domain of the ALK4/ALK5 subtypes of TGF-β receptor type I by the SB-431542 inhibitor (Figure 6B).

Smad2-specific signalling is found during ALK4-mediated activin A signalling[51]. Inhibitors of external activin A signalling such as follistatin or neutralizing activin A antibodies do not interfere with CTGF expression under serum free conditions. The final role of activin A in the physiology of spontaneous CTGF expression, however, still needs to be elucidated.

In conclusion these data suggest, that during cellular stress, both intracellular TGF-β and activin A are able to trigger specific, ALK4/5- and Smad2-dependent signalling pathways within the hepatocyte leading to CTGF expression. This might play an important role in the pathogenesis of hepatocellular damage by amplification of TGF-β receptor interactions and apoptosis during early liver impairment that subsequently contributes to the pathogenesis of fibrosis. Further characterization of this pathway will provide hints for potential therapeutic intervention and for optimizing culture conditions to maintain long-term viability of hepatocytes and for cell replacement therapy.

BMP SIGNALLING IN HSC/MFB

BMP form their own multifunctional group within the TGF-β superfamily[52,53]. To date there are more than 20 different members of this BMP family known, which are initially identified through their involvement in the formation of bone and cartilage[54]. Regarding their homology they are further divided into individual subgroups. HSC express BMP-4, BMP-6 and BMP-9[55–57]. While the expression of BMP-6 is induced by TGF-β$_1$ (see ref. 56), BMP-9 is able to influence its own expression in autocrine- and paracrine-stimulatory loops[55]. Signalling of BMP proceeds, similar to TGF-β, via type I and type II receptors and is based on a serine/threonine kinase. There are at least three type I receptors which are able to bind BMP, namely BMP-R-IA (ALK3), BMPR-IB (ALK6) and ActR-IA (ALK2)[58–60]. Besides these type I receptors there are three type II receptors, which are able to bind BMP (Figure 7), namely BMPR-II, ActR-II and ActR-IIB[61,62]. Comparable to TGF-β signalling, BMP ligands bind to a heterodimeric complex of type I and type II receptors. Within this complex the type II receptor is able to phosphorylate the type I receptor, and subsequently this receptor is able to phosphorylate intracellular mediators of the BMP pathway, which are either the R-Smad, such as Smad1, Smad5 and Smad8 or the mitogen-activated protein kinase (MAPK). For instance BMP-4 phosphorylates Smad1 in HSC, but can also initiate the phosphorylation of the extracellular-signal regulated kinases 1/2 (ERK1/2)[57]. BMP-7 is also capable of mediating signals via Smad1 as well as via p38 as a member of the MAPK pathway[63]. In this process special anchor proteins (e.g. CD44) are necessary to present Smad1 to the BMP receptors. After phosphorylation of the R-Smads they bind to Smad4 and are finally directed into the nucleus in order to activate the expression of BMP target genes[64,65]. BMP signalling can be further modulated by endoglin (CD105), which is commonly known as a TGF-β type III receptor. Endoglin binds both, TGF-β1 and BMP-7, but regarding these two cytokines endoglin has controversial functions.

Endoglin has an inhibitory effect on the TGF-β pathway[17,66] and conversely, a stimulatory effect on BMP-7 signalling[67]. Once the translocation of the phosphorylated R-Smads and Co-Smads is completed, endogenous target genes are activated. The classical endogenous target genes for members of the BMP family in mesenchymal cells are the inhibitors of differentiation (Id). Id-1, Id-2 as well as Id-3 are directly induced by the members of the BMP family[68–72]. Another target gene in HSC, which is up-regulated in response to BMP-2, BMP-4 and BMP-7, is Smad6. Smad6 belongs to the group of inhibitory Smads (I-Smad) and is part of a negative feedback loop. Similar to TGF-β stimulation, which results in increased expression of Smad7, BMP induce negative feedback loops[73]. While the inhibitory Smad6 exclusively inhibits BMP-2, BMP-4 and BMP-7, Smad7 is able to affect both the TGF-β and the BMP pathways[74]. The inhibitory function of the I-Smads is based on two different mechanisms. Either they are binding to the type I receptor, thus competing with the R-Smads, or they guide the E3 ubiquitin ligases Smurf1 and Smurf2 to the activated type I receptor, resulting in their degradation[75,76].

Even though phosphorylation of Smad3 is accepted as the key player in regulating ECM synthesis in HSC[7], phosphorylation of Smad1 is also

---

Figure 7 (opposite) BMP signalling pathway in HSC/MFB. BMP signalling is initiated by binding of BMP to type II receptors (BMPR-II, ActR-II, ActR-IIB) that subsequently transfer the signal to the type I receptors (ALK2, 3, and 6). Once activated the signal is propagated via phosphorylation of Smad1/5/8 proteins that bind to the common Smad4, translocate to the nucleus and initiate target gene expression (e. g. Id-1, -2, -3, Smad6, Snail). Smad1 was found to interact with the cytoplasmic domain of CD44, suggesting that this surface marker has essential functions in recruiting Smad for receptor phosphorylation

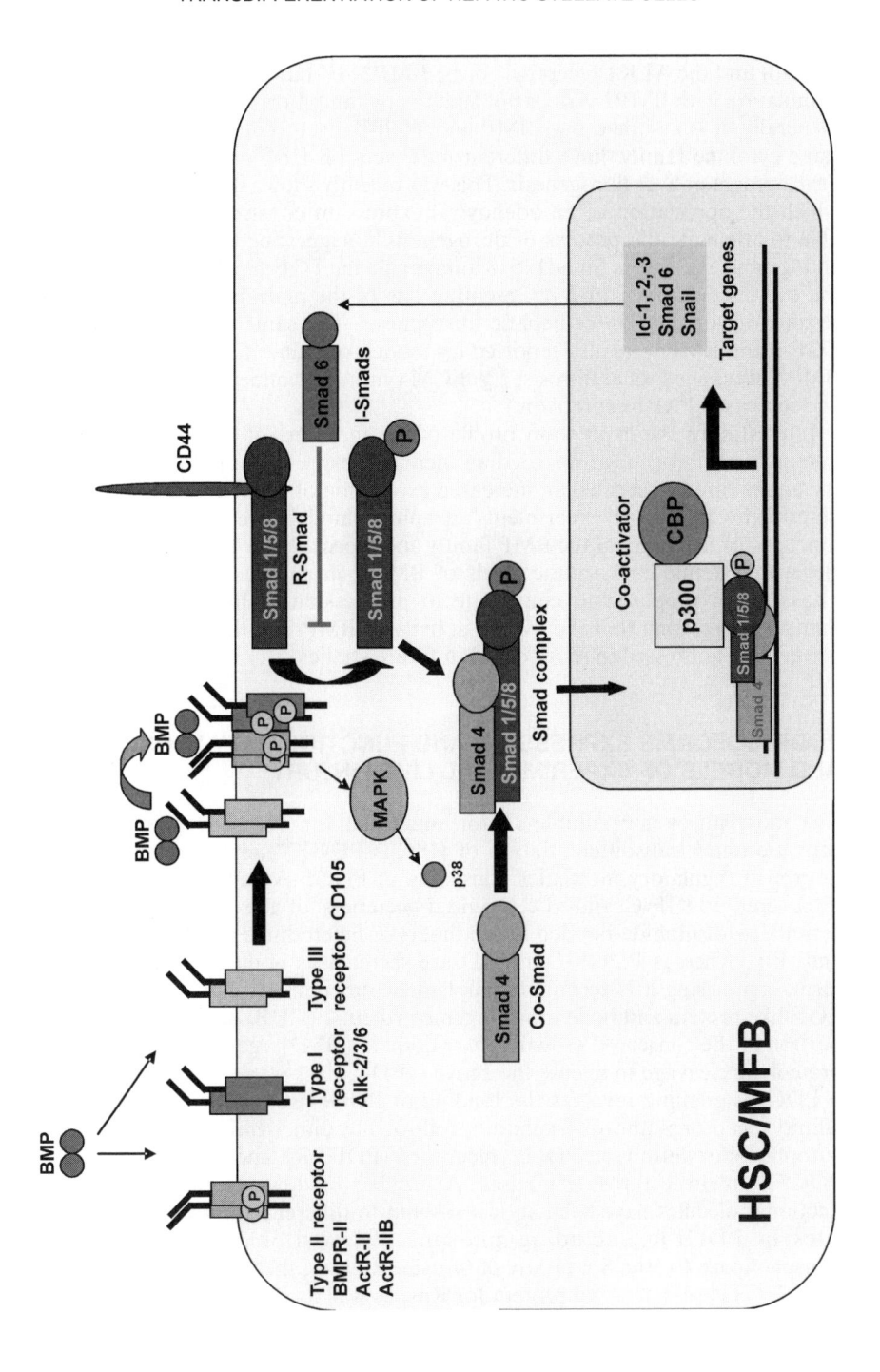

TRANSDIFFERENTIATION OF HEPATIC STELLATE CELLS

important within this process. Phosphorylation of Smad1 is induced either by TGF-β_1 and the ALK1 receptor[14] or by BMP2/4[57] but, in contrast to TGF-β_1, stimulation with BMP2/4 does not lead to any inhibition of cell proliferation[13]. Generally, it is assumed that BMP and TGF-β, even though belonging to the same cytokine family, have different influences on HSC and therefore on the development of liver fibrogenesis. This was recently shown in the BDL model in which the application of an adenoviral expression construct for BMP-7 was able to attenuate the process of fibrogenesis[65], suggesting that BMP-7 and its endogenous mediators Smad1/5/8 antagonize the TGF-β pathway. In this way the overexpression of Id-2 representing one of the main BMP-7 target genes resulted in attenuation of hepatic fibrogenesis. The same opposing effects of TGF-β and BMP were also reported for models of kidney fibrogenesis in which BMP-7 weakened renal fibrosis, e.g. ECM synthesis, connective tissue deposits and increased PAI-1 expression[77].

Interestingly, the expression profile of the members of the BMP family in human liver fibrogenesis revealed an increased expression of BMP-7, whereas the animal model revealed an increased expression of BMP-2[57,78]. Finally, it is noteworthy that most experiments in animal models predict an antifibrotic function for members of the BMP family and especially for BMP-7. Contrarily, elevated systemic and hepatic levels of BMP-7 in patients with chronic liver disease were proposed to contribute to progression of liver fibrosis in humans, suggesting that the overall activity of BMP-7 in the fibrotic response needs to be addressed in more detail in future studies[79].

PDGF ISOFORMS EXPRESSION AND FUNCTIONALITY IN HSC/MFB AND MODELS OF EXPERIMENTAL LIVER INJURY

The most mitogenic soluble factor identified for the process of cellular activation and transdifferentiation of HSC is PDGF[80], representing a family of growth regulatory molecules consisting of PDGF-A and -B and the newly discovered PDGF-C and -D. Original members of the PDGF family are secreted as disulphide-bonded homodimers or heterodimers (PDGF-AA, -AB, and -BB), whereas PDGF-C and -D are secreted as homodimers in a latent form, comprising a N-terminal complement subcomponents C1r/C1s, urchin EGF-like protein and bone morphogenic protein-1 (CUB) domain in the front portion of the conserved growth factor domain (GFD), requiring extracellular proteolytic cleavage to release the active GFD[81-83].

PDGF signalling involves the binding of PDGF isoforms to specific high-affinity receptor α- and/or β-subunits, followed by dimerization and subsequent autophosphorylation of PDGF receptors (PDGFR) and activation of the PDGFR intrinsic tyrosine kinases. A number of downstream signal transduction molecules have been shown to bind to different autophosphorylation sites in PDGFR, including phosphatidylinositol 3-kinase (PI3-K), phospholipase C-, the Src family of tyrosine kinases, the tyrosine phosphatase SHP-2, GTPase-activating protein for Ras, as well as other adaptor molecules (reviewed in ref. 84).

PDGF mitogenic signalling in HSC requires activation of phospholipase C- and PI 3-K, in addition to a major role for Ras activation followed by a kinase cascade including Raf-1, MEK and ERK. ERK activation is followed by nuclear translocation and phosphorylation of several transcription factors, including activator protein-1, Elk-1, SAP and increased expression of c-fos[85,86].

The β-isoform of the PDGF receptor (PDGFRβ), which binds PDGF-B, is up-regulated mainly during HSC activation in CCl_4- and BDL-induced liver injury models[87]. In rats the relative mRNA expressions of all PDGF isoforms and receptors were up-regulated after BDL (Figure 8A). PDGF-A, -B and -D expression showed significantly higher values compared to the increases of PDGF-C, while PDGF-D and PDGFRβ protein also increased markedly. Immunostaining revealed PDGF-D localization along the fibrotic septa of the periportal and perisinusoidal areas[88].

Besides PDGF-B, PDGF-D is the second most potent PDGF isoform in PDGFRβ signalling in HSC/MFB, as evidenced by PDGFRβ autophosphorylation and activation of the downstream signalling molecules ERK1/2-, JNK-, p38 MAPK, and PKB/Akt, while PDGF-C effects were minimal (Figure 8B).

PDGF-D exerted mitogenic and fibrogenic effects in both cultured HSC and MFB comparable to PDGF-B, but PDGF-A and -C showed only marginal effects (Figure 8C). The mitogenic effects of PDGF-B and -D are both inhibited by the soluble PDGFRβ (sPDGFRβ), a specific PDGF-B scavenger[89], indicating that PDGF-D is a specific ligand for PDGFRβ and in fact supporting our previous experiment showing sPDGFRβ to attenuate liver fibrosis in BDL rat models[90].

Compared to other PDGF isoforms the expression of PDGF-C was only slightly increased during ongoing BDL, contradicting previous reports showing the occurrence of spontaneous liver fibrosis in PDGF-C transgenic mice[91]. Possibly the less profiled up-regulation of PDGF-C may result from weaker inflammatory responses in the BDL liver compared to other toxic or infective liver fibrosis models consisting of predominant inflammatory cells, including platelets containing PDGF-C in α-granule.

Higher levels of PDGF-B chain mRNA were detected in the bile duct segments of cholestatic rats compared to controls, while PDGF-B was found to localize in the bile duct epithelial cells. The latter PDGF-B is considered the major chemotactic mediator of HSC towards bile duct segments, thus contributing to the development of periductular fibrosis in cholestatic disorders. This process was inhibited by neutralizing anti-PDGF antibodies and STI-571, a PDGF receptor tyrosine kinase inhibitor[92].

PDGF-B overexpression causes liver fibrosis without significantly up-regulating of TGF-$β_1$, suggesting that the fibrogenic effect of PDGF might be a TGF-β-independent mechanism[93] and predicting that anti-PDGF therapeutic strategies are an attractive alternative to interfere with the fibrogenic response. Several reports show PDGF antagonists, such as a dominant negative sPDGFRβ[90] and PDGF-kinase inhibitors[94,95] to be promising technologies in the attenuation of liver fibrogenesis when applied during the initiation phase[96]. In ongoing liver injury, however, other mediators seem to compensate for the inhibited PDGF effect. Dual suppression of PDGF

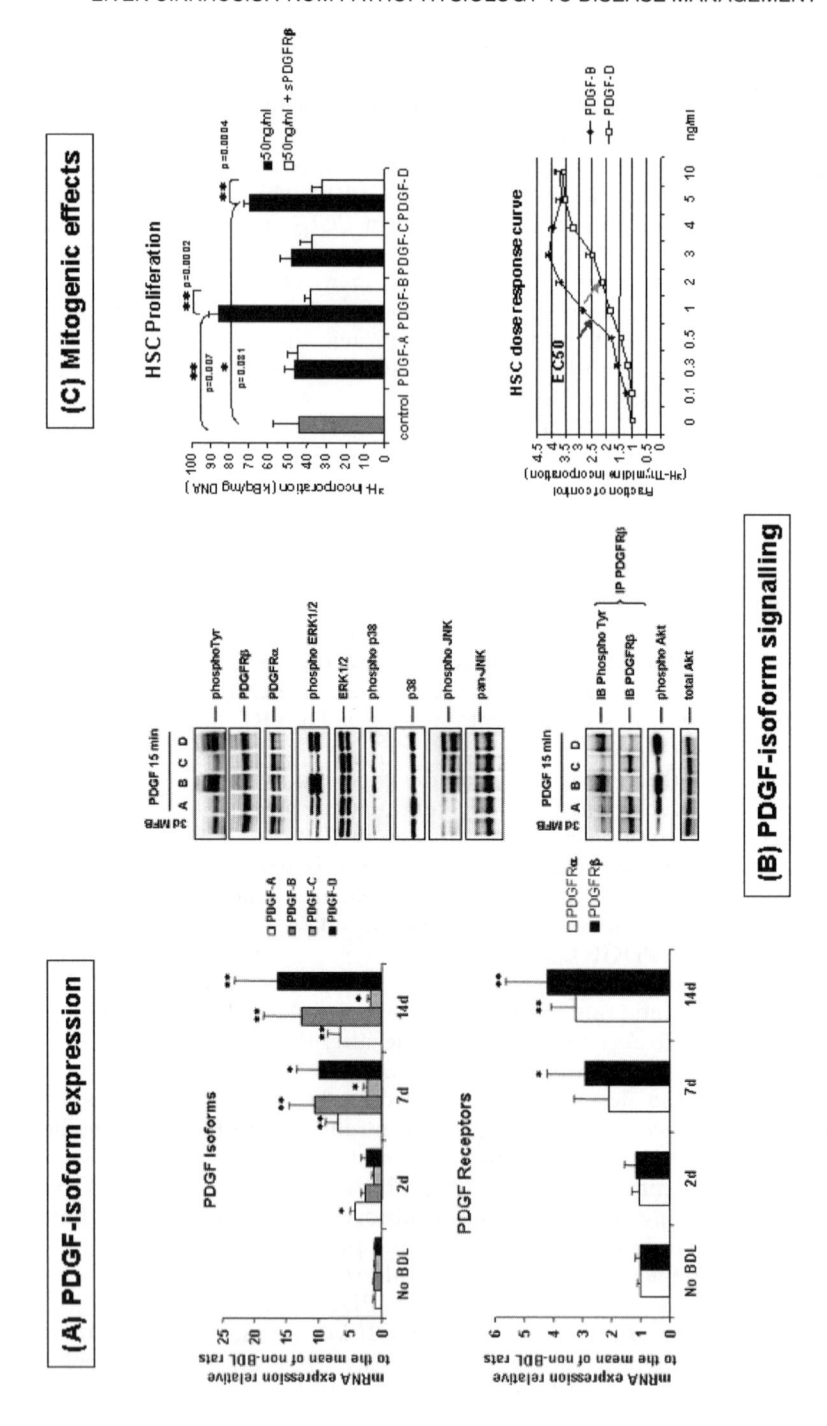

LIVER CIRRHOSIS: FROM PATHOPHYSIOLOGY TO DISEASE MANAGEMENT

and TGF-β with a combination of clinically comparable low doses of STI-571 and ACE-I exerted a significant inhibitory effect on ongoing liver fibrosis development[97].

In summary, the two PDGF-B and -D isoforms are significant contributors to HSC activation and matrix remodeling in *in vitro* and *in vivo* cholestatic liver fibrosis and are considered potential therapeutic targets.

NOVEL ASPECTS OF CELLULAR ACTIVATION AND TRANDIFFERENTIATION

Activated HSC are characterized not only by an increased ECM production but also by up-regulation of genes that are known as smooth muscle cell (SMC) differentiation markers, in particular α-SMA and SM22α, mediating contractility and cellular motility by cytoskeletal reorganization. In HSC the regulation of these genes is largely unknown, and only a few published observations provide an insight into the cellular players involved in the respective signalling cascades. Induction of α-SMA expression in HSC by TGF-β was shown in recent publications[98,99], which is in line with findings in SMC indicating that similar mechanisms mediate SMC marker gene regulation in this cell type. Intervention in the intracellular TGF-β signalling in activated HSC by blocking the classical profibrotic Smad2/3 pathway or inhibition of p38 MAPK resulted in impaired cytoskeletal organization or reduced α-SMA expression, respectively[3,100]. Another pathway of TGF-β signalling includes the activation of small GTP-binding proteins, e.g. RhoA. It has been demonstrated that the blockade of this pathway by trichostatin A or the Rho kinase inhibitor Y27632 was followed by an impaired organization of the cytoskeleton in HSC[101,102].

As known from SMC, a central mediator of TGF-β-induced SMC marker gene expression is the serum response factor (SRF), a ubiquitously expressed founding member of the MADS-box containing transcription factor family (reviewed in ref. 103). It is predominantly localized in the nucleus and binds to a specific sequence in the promoters of diverse target genes, called CArG-box. We looked for its expression in activated HSC and found an increase in protein level culminating in fully activated myofibroblast-like cells (MFB)[104]. Because SRF binds to a variety of diverse gene promoters, specific co-activators for

---

Figure 8 (opposite) PDGF isoform expression and functionality in HSC/MFB. **A**: Real-time quantitative PCR (Taqman) shows PDGF isoform and receptor mRNA expression in BDL rat livers. **B**: PDGF isoform signalling in HSC/MFB. SDS-PAGE and immunoblot HSC/MFB following PDGF isoforms stimulation, depicting autophosphorylation of the Tyr residues of PDGFR and the downstream signalling molecules phospho-ERK1/2, phospho-JNK, and phospho-p38 MAPK. Upon PDGFRβ immunoprecipitation only PDGF-B and -D stimulation show PDGFRβ Tyr phosphorylation. Following PDGF isoform stimulation, PI3K signalling is evidenced through phospho-Akt. **C**: Mitogenic effects of PDGF isoforms in HSC/MFB. (^{3}H)-incorporation proliferation assays of culture-activated HSC demonstrated that 50 ng/ml PDGF-D exerts significant mitogenic effects comparable to PDGF-B. The mitogenic effects of PDGF-B and PDGF-D were abolished in the presence of 1 µg/ml soluble PDGFRβ (sPDGFRβ). PDGF dose–response curve revealed that PDGF-B and -D posses EC_{50} values between 1 and 2.5 ng/ml respectively

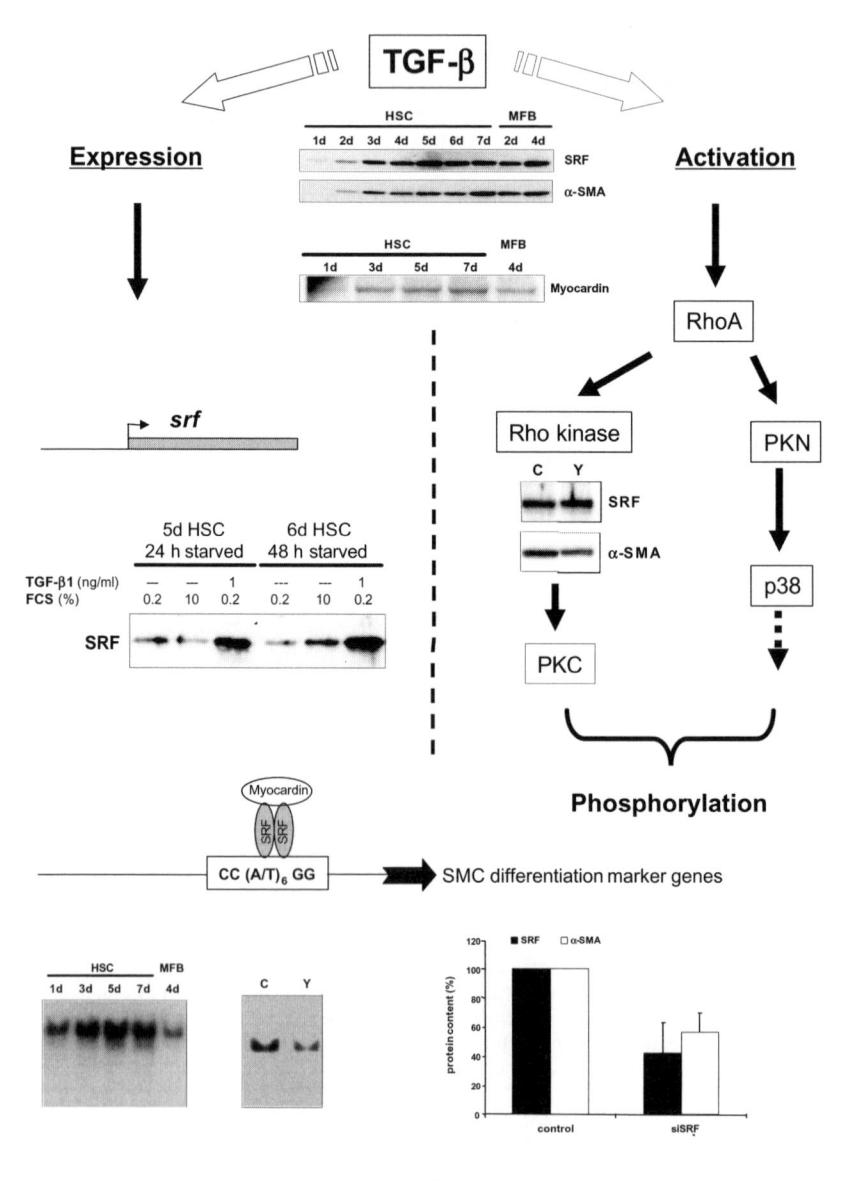

SMC marker gene regulation are necessary. The most important SRF co-factor in this relation is myocardin[105], which was also found increased in activated HSC, but in contrast to SRF the myocardin content was diminished in MFB. This expression pattern was also observable with other SMC marker gene-related SRF co-factors such as myocardin-related transcription factor-A (MRTF-A) or the cysteine- and glycine-rich protein 2 (CRP2)[106,107]. As phosphorylation at several serine or threonine residues of SRF is a prerequisite for its transcriptional activity we analysed the phosphorylation status of serine103 in HSC and observed that it indeed increased during transdifferentiation but declined in MFB. This reduced phosphorylation in MFB was accompanied by a smaller amount of nuclear SRF and a decreased DNA-binding potency of SRF. We also found that in HSC the expression of SRF itself was inducible by TGF-β and inhibition of Rho kinase, which is involved in activation of SRF, resulted in lowered DNA binding. Finally, direct antagonizing of SRF by specific siRNA repressed the contents of SMC markers in HSC.

All these findings indicate that the expression of contractile components of the cytoskeleton might be regulated by similar pathways converging to SRF as central player in activated HSC and differentiated SMC, as assumed in Figure 9. We conclude that, although TGF-β is the main effector of regulated gene expression during HSC transdifferentiation, the intracellular signalling resulting in expression of a multitude of target genes must be at least partially mediated by different pathways. Besides the classical TGF-β/Smad3 pathway that strictly participates in up-regulation of extracellular matrix proteins, we find alternative TGF-β signalling cascades which pass in parallel, but not independently, to regulate other sets of genes in activated HSC. It has been described that SRF and Smad3 are principally able to interact by physical contact via the MADS box and the MH2 domain, respectively, thereby modulating Smad3-mediated TGF-β signalling[108]. Vice-versa, it was found that TGF-β signalling by SRF was negatively influenced by overexpression of Smad7[109].

The presence of SRF and its relevant co-activators might also help to explain the role of PDGF in very early stages of HSC activation, because in SMC it has been demonstrated that PDGF-BB repressed binding of co-activators necessary for SMC marker gene expression to SRF, resulting in their decreased expression[110]. This finding is in line with the feature of SRF to regulate not only SMC marker genes but also genes relevant for cell growth and proliferation depending on specific co-activators which compete for SRF binding (reviewed in ref. 103).

Figure 9 (opposite) Scheme of the assumed TGF-β-dependent regulation of SRF activity in activated HSC. As shown in the upper Western blot analysis the up-regulation of α-SMA during transdifferentiation is accompanied by an increase in SRF and myocardin expression. In fully transdifferentiated MFB the myocardin expression is slightly decreased. The transcriptional activity of SRF correlates to its DNA-binding activity which was measured by EMSA (*bottom left side*). The expression of SRF in activated HSC is inducible by TGF-β (*left side*). The *srf* gene promoter contains a CArG-box. To shuttle into the nucleus, bind DNA, and become transcriptionally active, SRF must be phosphorylated at distinct serine or threonine residues. It is known from SMC that the RhoA/Rho kinase/protein kinase C (PKC) pathway plays a central role in SRF activation (*right side*). A parallel activation pathway using protein kinase N (PKN) and p38MAP was found in SMC. As shown by Western blot analysis, antagonism of the Rho kinase by the specific inhibitor Y27632 (Y) led to reduced α-SMA contents in activated HSC in comparison to untreated cells (C), while the SRF levels remained unaffected. This observation might be explained by a diminished DNA-binding capacity which was demonstrated in EMSA (*bottom left side*). The essential role of SRF in regulation of SMC differentiation marker genes in HSC was further evoked by usage of siRNA targeting SRF (siSRF) resulting in a down-regulation of SRF and α-SMA expression (*bottom right side*).

The knowledge that SRF is expressed in HSC and increased during transdifferentiation will extend our possibilities to explain and understand this highly dynamic process and additionally raise several new therapeutic targets for intervention in the process of liver fibrogenesis.

CONCLUSIONS

During recent decades the pathogenesis of liver fibrosis has been intensively investigated. Several growth factors and signalling pathways were identified that had critical impact on this fibroproliferative disease that is one of the leading causes of morbidity and mortality in humans. However, despite its enormous impact on human health, there are currently no approved curative treatments that directly target this disease. Surely, strategies targeting TGF-β and PDGF were effective in different animal models, but none of these 'therapeutics' was successfully translated into the clinics. The optimistic view that simple abrogation of TGF-β or PDGF signalling in HSC might be one ultimate strategy to medicate patients suffering from hepatic fibrosis must be potentially rethought. The different ligands and isoforms of both cytokine families are bound by many extracellular receptors that in turn activate different intracellular signalling cascades. The cellular effects that are induced and reflected in the different target genes that become activated or silenced are rather sophisticated. Moreover, the finding that some targets that become activated during the process of activation and transdifferentiation in the HSC/ MFB system are transcription factors (e.g. SRF) with a broad spectrum of activities suggests that HSC induce a tremendous change during ongoing fibrogenesis that might be irreversible when once initiated. The complexity of TGF-β and PDGF signalling is further increased by accessory receptors (e.g. endoglin), soluble factors (e.g. CTGF), or opposing cytokines (e.g. BMP-7) that modulate the overall activity of these cytokines with profibrogenic or mitogenic activities. In addition, the finding that several target molecules (e.g. ERK1/2, p38) are similarly triggered by TGF-β and PDGF suggests that the view 'one cytokine, some defined effects' is antiquated. Therefore, it is most likely that realistic future therapies will target special attributes of the fibrogenic response rather than targeting the process of fibrosis on the whole.

Acknowledgements

The authors are grateful to Sabine Weiskirchen for help in preparing figures. Relevant work incorporated in this chapter was supported by grants from the Deutsche Forschungsgemeinschaft (SFB-542 A9, WE2554/4-1, GR 463/14-1) and the BMBF financed German Network of Excellence for Viral Hepatitis (Kompetenznetz Hepatitis).

References

1. Winau F, Hegasy G, Weiskirchen R et al. Ito cells are liver-resident antigen-presenting cells for activating T cell responses. Immunity. 2007;26:117–29.

2. Gressner AM, Weiskirchen R. Modern pathogenetic concepts of liver fibrosis suggest stellate cells and TGF-β as major players and therapeutic targets. J Cell Mol Med. 2006;10:76–99.
3. Dooley S, Hamzavi J, Breitkopf K et al. Smad7 prevents activation of hepatic stellate cells and liver fibrosis in rats. Gastroenterology. 2003;125:178–91.
4. Bachem MG, Meyer D, Schafer W et al. The response of rat liver perisinusoidal lipocytes to polypeptide growth regulator changes with their transdifferentiation into myofibroblast-like cells in culture. J Hepatol. 1993;18:40–52.
5. Dooley S, Delvoux B, Lahme B, Mangasser-Stephan K, Gressner AM. Modulation of transforming growth factor β response and signaling during transdifferentiation of rat hepatic stellate cells to myofibroblasts. Hepatology. 2000;31:1094–106.
6. Dooley S, Delvoux B, Lahme B, Mangasser-Stephan K, Gressner AM. Modulation of transforming growth factor β response and signaling during transdifferentiation of rat hepatic stellate cells to myofibroblasts. Hepatology. 2000;31:1094–106.
7. Schnabl B, Kweon YO, Frederick JP, Wang XF, Rippe RA, Brenner DA. The role of Smad3 in mediating mouse hepatic stellate cell activation. Hepatology. 2001;34:89–100.
8. Furukawa F, Matsuzaki K, Mori S et al. p38 MAPK mediates fibrogenic signal through Smad3 phosphorylation in rat myofibroblasts. Hepatology. 2003;38:879–89.
9. Holmes A, Abraham DJ, Sa S, Shiwen X, Black CM, Leask A. CTGF and SMADs, maintenance of scleroderma phenotype is independent of SMAD signaling. J Biol Chem. 2001;276:10594–601.
10. Liu C, Gaca MD, Swenson ES, Vellucci VF, Reiss M, Wells RG. Smads 2 and 3 are differentially activated by transforming growth factor-β (TGF-β) in quiescent and activated hepatic stellate cells. Constitutive nuclear localization of Smads in activated cells is TGF-β-independent. J Biol Chem. 2003;278:11721–8.
11. Uemura M, Swenson ES, Gaca MD, Giordano FJ, Reiss M, Wells RG. Smad2 and Smad3 play different roles in rat hepatic stellate cell function and α-smooth muscle actin organization. Mol Biol Cell. 2005;16:4214–24.
12. Tahashi Y, Matsuzaki K, Date M et al. Differential regulation of TGF-β signal in hepatic stellate cells between acute and chronic rat liver injury. Hepatology. 2002;35:49–61.
13. Shen H, Huang G, Hadi M et al. Transforming growth factor-β1 downregulation of Smad1 gene expression in rat hepatic stellate cells. Am J Physiol Gastrointest Liver Physiol. 2003;285:G539–46.
14. Wiercinska E, Wickert L, Denecke B et al. Id1 is a critical mediator in TGF-β-induced transdifferentiation of rat hepatic stellate cells. Hepatology. 2006;43:1032–41.
15. Lebrin F, Deckers M, Bertolino P, Ten Dijke P. TGF-β receptor function in the endothelium. Cardiovasc Res. 2005;65:599–608.
16. Meurer SK, Tihaa L, Lahme B, Gressner AM, Weiskirchen R. Identification of endoglin in rat hepatic stellate cells: new insights into transforming growth factor β receptor signaling. J Biol Chem. 2005;280:3078–87.
17. Lebrin F, Goumans MJ, Jonker L et al. Endoglin promotes endothelial cell proliferation and TGF-β/ALK1 signal transduction. EMBO J. 2004;23:4018–28.
18. Hyytiäinen M, Penttinen C, Keski-Oja J. Latent TGF-β binding proteins: extracellular matrix association and roles in TGF-β activation. Crit Rev Clin Lab Sci. 2004;41:233–64.
19. Lyons RM, Keski-Oja J, Moses HL. Proteolytic activation of latent transforming growth factor-β from fibroblast-conditioned medium. J Cell Biol. 1988;106:1659–65.
20. Ribeiro SM, Poczatek M, Schultz-Cherry S, Villain M, Murphy-Ullrich JE. The activation sequence of thrombospondin-1 interacts with the latency-associated peptide to regulate activation of latent transforming growth factor-β. J Biol Chem. 1999;274:13586–93.
21. Saharinen J, Keski-Oja J. Specific sequence motif of 8-Cys repeats of TGF-β binding proteins, LTBPs, creates a hydrophobic interaction surface for binding of small latent TGF-β. Mol Biol Cell. 2000;11:2691–704.
22. Chen Y, Ali T, Todorovic V, O'Leary JM, Downing AK, Rifkin DB. Amino acid requirements for formation of the TGF-β-latent TGF-β binding protein complex. J Mol Biol. 2005;345:175–86.
23. Unsöld C, Hyytiäinen M, Bruckner-Tuderman L, Keski-Oja J. Latent TGF-β binding protein LTBP-1 contains potential extracellular matrix interacting domains. J Cell Sci. 2001;114:187–97.

24. Taipale J, Miyazono K. Heldin CH, Keski-Oja J. Latent transforming growth factor-β1 associates to fibroblast extracellular matrix via latent TGF-β binding protein. J Cell Biol. 1994;124:171–81.
25. Olofsson A, Ichijo H, Moren A, ten Dijke P, Miyazono K, Heldin CH. Efficient association of an amino-terminally extended form of human latent transforming growth factor-β binding protein with the extracellular matrix. J Biol Chem. 1995;270:31294–7.
26. Gong W, Roth S, Michel K, Gressner AM. Isoforms and splice variants of transforming growth factor β-binding protein in rat hepatic stellate cell. Gastroenterology. 1998;114:352–63.
27. Michel K, Roth S, Trautwein C, Gong W, Flemming P, Gressner, AM. Analysis of the expression pattern of the latent transforming growth factor β binding protein isoforms in normal and diseased human liver reveals a new splice variant missing the proteinase-sensitive hinge region. Hepatology. 1998;27:1592–9.
28. Öklu R, Metcalfe JC, Hesketh TR, Kemp PR. Loss of a consensus heparin binding site by alternative splicing of latent transforming growth factor-β binding protein-1. FEBS Lett. 1998;425:281–5.
29. Öklü R, Hesketh TR, Metcalfe JC, Kemp PR. Expression of alternatively spliced human latent transforming growth factor β binding protein-1. FEBS Lett. 1998;435:143–8.
30. Koski C, Saharinen J, Keski-Oja J. Independent promoters regulate the expression of two amino terminally distinct forms of latent transforming growth factor-β binding protein-1 (LTBP-1) in a cell type-specific manner. J Biol Chem. 1999;274:32619–30.
31. Noguera I, Obata H, Gualandris A, Cowin P, Rifkin DB. Molecular cloning of the mouse Ltbp-1 gene reveals tissue specific expression of alternatively spliced forms. Gene. 2003;308:31–41.
32. Weiskirchen R, Moser M, Günther K, Weiskirchen S, Gressner AM. The murine latent transforming growth factor-β binding protein (Ltbp-1) is alternatively spliced, and maps to a region syntenic to human chromosome 2p21-22. Gene. 2003;308:43–52.
33. Drews F, Knöbel S, Moser M et al. Disruption of the latent transforming growth factor-β binding protein-1 gene causes alteration in facial structure and influences TGF-β bioavailability. Biochim Biophys Acta. 2008;1783:34–48.
34. Bradham DM, Igarashi A, Potter RL, Grotendorst GR. Connective tissue growth factor: a cysteine-rich mitogen secreted by human vascular endothelial cells is related to the SRC-induced immediate early gene product CEF-10. J Cell Biol. 1991;114:1285–94.
35. Leask A, Abraham DJ. All in the CCN family: essential matricellular signaling modulators emerge from the bunker. J Cell Sci. 2006;119:4803–10.
36. Grotendorst GR, Okochi H, Hayashi N. A novel transforming growth factor β response element controls the expression of the connective tissue growth factor gene. Cell Growth Differ. 1996;7:469–80.
37. Rachfal AW, Brigstock DR. Structural and functional properties of CCN proteins. Vitam Horm. 2005;70:69–103.
38. Leivonen SK, Hakkinen L, Liu D, Kahari VM. Smad3 and extracellular signal-regulated kinase 1/2 coordinately mediate transforming growth factor-β-induced expression of connective tissue growth factor in human fibroblasts. J Invest Dermatol. 2005;124:1162–9.
39. Blom IE, Goldschmeding R, Leask A. Gene regulation of connective tissue growth factor: new targets for antifibrotic therapy? Matrix Biol. 2002;21:473–82.
40. Leask A, Holmes A, Black CM, Abraham DJ. Connective tissue growth factor gene regulation. Requirements for its induction by transforming growth factor-β2 in fibroblasts. J Biol Chem. 2003;278:13008–15.
41. Chen Y, Blom IE, Sa S, Goldschmeding R, Abraham DJ, Leask A. CTGF expression in mesangial cells: involvement of SMADs, MAP kinase, and PKC. Kidney Int. 2002;62:1149–59.
42. Van Beek JP, Kennedy L, Rockel JS, Bernier SM, Leask A. The induction of CCN2 by TGFβ1 involves Ets-1. Arthritis Res Ther. 2006;8:R36.
43. Holmes A, Abraham DJ, Chen Y et al. Constitutive connective tissue growth factor expression in scleroderma fibroblasts is dependent on Sp1. J Biol Chem. 2003;278:41728–33.
44. Li G, Xie Q, Shi Y et al. Inhibition of connective tissue growth factor by siRNA prevents liver fibrosis in rats. J Gene Med. 2006;8:889–900.

45. Mori T, Kawara S, Shinozaki M et al. Role and interaction of connective tissue growth factor with transforming growth factor-β in persistent fibrosis: a mouse fibrosis model. J Cell Physiol. 1999;181:153–9.
46. Leask A, Denton CP, Abraham DJ. Insights into the molecular mechanism of chronic fibrosis: the role of connective tissue growth factor in scleroderma. J Invest Dermatol. 2004;122:1–6.
47. Abreu JG, Ketpura NI, Reversade B, De Robertis EM. Connective-tissue growth factor (CTGF) modulates cell signalling by BMP and TGF-β. Nat Cell Biol. 2002;4:599–604.
48. Sicklick JK, Choi SS, Bustamante M et al. Evidence for epithelial–mesenchymal transitions in adult liver cells. Am J Physiol Gastrointest Liver Physiol. 2006;291:G575–83.
49. Zavadil J, Bottinger EP. TGF-β and epithelial-to-mesenchymal transitions. Oncogene. 2005;24:5764–74.
50. Gressner OA, Lahme B, Demirci I, Gressner AM, Weiskirchen R. Differential effects of TGF-β on connective tissue growth factor (CTGF/CCN2) expression in hepatic stellate cells and hepatocytes. J Hepatol. 2007;47:699–710.
51. Schmierer B, Schuster MK, Shkumatava A, Kuchler K. Activin A signaling induces Smad2, but not Smad3, requiring protein kinase A activity in granulosa cells from the avian ovary. J Biol Chem. 2003;278:21197–203.
52. Hoodless PA, Haerry T, Abdollah S et al. MADR1, a MAD-related protein that functions in BMP2 signaling pathways. Cell. 1996;85:489–500.
53. Reddi AH. Bone and cartilage differentiation. Curr Opin Genet Dev. 1994;4:737–44.
54. Wozney JM. The bone morphogenetic protein family and osteogenesis. Mol Reprod Dev. 1992;32:160–7.
55. Miller AF, Harvey SA, Thies RS, Olson MS. Bone morphogenetic protein-9. An autocrine/paracrine cytokine in the liver. J Biol Chem. 2000;275:17937–45.
56. Knittel T, Fellmer P, Muller L, Ramadori G. Bone morphogenetic protein-6 is expressed in nonparenchymal liver cells and upregulated by transforming growth factor-β1. Exp Cell Res. 1997;232:263–9.
57. Fan J, Shen H, Sun Y et al. Bone morphogenetic protein 4 mediates bile duct ligation induced liver fibrosis through activation of Smad1 and ERK1/2 in rat hepatic stellate cells. J Cell Physiol. 2006;207:499–505.
58. Koenig BB, Cook JS, Wolsing DH et al. Characterization and cloning of a receptor for BMP-2 and BMP-4 from NIH 3T3 cells. Mol Cell Biol. 1994;14:5961–74.
59. ten Dijke P, Yamashita H, Ichijo H et al. Characterization of type I receptors for transforming growth factor-β and activin. Science. 1994;264:101–4.
60. Macias-Silva M, Hoodless PA, Tang SJ, Buchwald M, Wrana JL. Specific activation of Smad1 signaling pathways by the BMP7 type I receptor, ALK2. J Biol Chem. 1998;273:25628–36.
61. Yamashita H, ten Dijke P, Huylebroeck D et al. Osteogenic protein-1 binds to activin type II receptors and induces certain activin-like effects. J Cell Biol. 1995;130:217–26.
62. Rosenzweig BL, Imamura T, Okadome T et al. Cloning and characterization of a human type II receptor for bone morphogenetic proteins. Proc Natl Acad Sci USA. 1995;92:7632–6.
63. Hu MC, Wasserman D, Hartwig S, Rosenblum ND. p38MAPK acts in the BMP7-dependent stimulatory pathway during epithelial cell morphogenesis and is regulated by Smad1. J Biol Chem. 2004;279:12051–9.
64. Wozney JM. The bone morphogenetic protein family: multifunctional cellular regulators in the embryo and adult. Eur J Oral Sci. 1998;106(Suppl. 1):160–6.
65. Kinoshita K, Iimuro Y, Otogawa K et al. Adenovirus-mediated expression of BMP-7 suppresses the development of liver fibrosis in rats. Gut. 2007;56:706–14.
66. Guo B, Slevin M, Li C et al. CD105 inhibits transforming growth factor-β-Smad3 signalling. Anticancer Res. 2004;24:1337–45.
67. Scherner O, Meurer SK, Tihaa L, Gressner AM, Weiskirchen R. Endoglin differentially modulates antagonistic transforming growth factor-β1 and BMP-7 signaling. J Biol Chem. 2007;282:13934–43.
68. Clement JH, Marr N, Meissner A et al. Bone morphogenetic protein 2 (BMP-2) induces sequential changes of Id gene expression in the breast cancer cell line MCF-7. J Cancer Res Clin Oncol. 2000;126:271–9.

69. Chambers RC, Leoni P, Kaminski N, Laurent GJ, Heller RA. Global expression profiling of fibroblast responses to transforming growth factor-β1 reveals the induction of inhibitor of differentiation-1 and provides evidence of smooth muscle cell phenotypic switching. Am J Pathol. 2003;162:533–46.
70. Miyazono K, Miyazawa K. Id: a target of BMP signaling. Sci STKE. 2002;2002:PE40.
71. Korchynskyi O, ten Dijke P. Identification and functional characterization of distinct critically important bone morphogenetic protein-specific response elements in the Id1 promoter. J Biol Chem. 2002;277:4883–91.
72. Vincent KJ, Jones E, Arthur MJ et al. Regulation of E-box DNA binding during *in vivo* and *in vitro* activation of rat and human hepatic stellate cells. Gut. 2001;49:713–19.
73. Heldin CH, Miyazono K, ten Dijke P. TGF-β signalling from cell membrane to nucleus through SMAD proteins. Nature. 1997;390:465–71.
74. Topper JN, Cai J, Qiu Y et al. Vascular MADs: two novel MAD-related genes selectively inducible by flow in human vascular endothelium. Proc Natl Acad Sci USA. 1997;94:9314–19.
75. Kavsak P, Rasmussen RK, Causing CG et al. Smad7 binds to Smurf2 to form an E3 ubiquitin ligase that targets the TGF β receptor for degradation. Mol Cell. 2000;6:1365–75.
76. Ebisawa T, Fukuchi M, Murakami G et al. Smurf1 interacts with transforming growth factor-β type I receptor through Smad7 and induces receptor degradation. J Biol Chem. 2001;276:12477–80.
77. Wang S, Chen Q, Simon TC et al. Bone morphogenic protein-7 (BMP-7), a novel therapy for diabetic nephropathy. Kidney Int. 2003;63:2037–49.
78. Nakatsuka R, Taniguchi M, Hirata M, Shiota G, Sato K. Transient expression of bone morphogenic protein-2 in acute liver injury by carbon tetrachloride. J Biochem (Tokyo). 2007;141:113–19.
79. Tacke F, Gabele E, Bataille F et al. Bone morphogenetic protein 7 is elevated in patients with chronic liver disease and exerts fibrogenic effects on human hepatic stellate cells. Dig Dis Sci. 2007;52:3404–15.
80. Pinzani M, Gesualdo L, Sabbah GM, Abboud HE. Effects of platelet-derived growth factor and other polypeptide mitogens on DNA synthesis and growth of cultured rat liver fat-storing cells. J Clin Invest. 1989;84:1786–93.
81. Li X, Ponten A, Aase K et al. PDGF-C is a new protease-activated ligand for the PDGF α-receptor. Nat Cell Biol. 2000;2:302–9.
82. LaRochelle WJ, Jeffers M, McDonald WF et al. PDGF-D, a new protease-activated growth factor. Nat Cell Biol. 2001;3:517–21.
83. Bergsten E, Uutela M, Li X et al. PDGF-D is a specific, protease-activated ligand for the PDGF β-receptor. Nat Cell Biol. 2001;3:512–16.
84. Heldin CH, Ostman A, Rönnstrand L. Signal transduction *via* platelet-derived growth factor receptors. Biochim Biophys Acta. 1998;1378:F79–113.
85. Marra F, Pinzani M, DeFranco R, Laffi G, Gentilini P. Involvement of phosphatidylinositol 3-kinase in the activation of extracellular signal-regulated kinase by PDGF in hepatic stellate cells. FEBS Lett. 1995;376:141–5.
86. Pagès G, Lenormand P, L'Allemain G, Chambard JC, Meloche S, Pouysségur J. Mitogen-activated protein kinases p42mapk and p44mapk are required for fibroblast proliferation. Proc Natl Acad Sci USA. 1993;90:8319–23.
87. Wong L, Yamasaki G, Johnson RJ, and Friedman SL. Induction of platelet-derived growth factor receptor in rat hepatic lipocytes during cellular activation *in vivo* and in culture. J Clin Invest. 1994;94:1563–9.
88. Borkham-Kamphorst E, van Roeyen CR, Ostendorf T, Floege J, Gressner AM, Weiskirchen R. Pro-fibrogenic potential of PDGF-D in liver fibrosis. J Hepatol. 2007;46:1064–74.
89. Borkham-Kamphorst E, Stoll D, Gressner AM, Weiskirchen R. Inhibitory effect of soluble PDGF-beta receptor in culture-activated hepatic stellate cells. Biochem Biophys Res Commun. 2004;317:451–62.
90. Borkham-Kamphorst E, Herrmann J, Stoll D, Treptau J, Gressner AM, Weiskirchen R. Dominant-negative soluble PDGF-beta receptor inhibits hepatic stellate cell activation and attenuates liver fibrosis. Lab Invest. 2004;84:766–77.

91. Campbell JS, Hughes SD, Gilbertson DG et al. Platelet-derived growth factor C induces liver fibrosis, steatosis, and hepatocellular carcinoma. Proc Natl Acad Sci USA. 2005;102:3389–94.
92. Kinnman N, Hultcrantz R, Barbu V et al. PDGF-mediated chemoattraction of hepatic stellate cells by bile duct segments in cholestatic liver injury. Lab Invest. 2000;80:697–707.
93. Czochra P, Klopcic B, Meyer E et al. Liver fibrosis induced by hepatic overexpression of PDGF-B in transgenic mice. J Hepatol. 2006;45:419–28.
94. Kinnman N, Francoz C, Barbu V et al. The myofibroblastic conversion of peribiliary fibrogenic cells distinct from hepatic stellate cells is stimulated by platelet-derived growth factor during liver fibrogenesis. Lab Invest. 2003;83:163–73.
95. Gonzalo T, Beljaars L, van de Bovenkamp M et al. Local inhibition of liver fibrosis by specific delivery of a platelet-derived growth factor kinase inhibitor to hepatic stellate cells. J Pharmacol Exp Ther. 2007;321:856–65.
96. Neef M, Ledermann M, Saegesser H et al. Oral imatinib treatment reduces early fibrogenesis but does not prevent progression in the long term. J Hepatol. 2006;44:167–75.
97. Yoshiji H, Kuriyama S, Noguchi R et al. Amelioration of liver fibrogenesis by dual inhibition of PDGF and TGF-β with a combination of imatinib mesylate and ACE inhibitor in rats. Int J Mol Med. 2006;17:899–904.
98. Cui X, Shimizu I, Lu G et al. Inhibitory effect of a soluble transforming growth factor β type II receptor on the activation of rat hepatic stellate cells in primary culture. J Hepatol. 2003;39:731–7.
99. Arias M, Lahme B, Van de Leur E, Gressner AM, Weiskirchen R. Adenoviral delivery of an antisense RNA complementary to the 3′ coding sequence of transforming growth factor-β1 inhibits fibrogenic activities of hepatic stellate cells. Cell Growth Differ. 2002;13:265–73.
100. Wang X, Tang X, Gong X, Albanis E, Friedman SL, Mao Z. Regulation of hepatic stellate cell activation and growth by transcription factor myocyte enhancer factor 2. Gastroenterology. 2004;127:1174–88.
101. Rombouts K, Knittel T, Machesky L et al. Actin filament formation, reorganization and migration are impaired in hepatic stellate cells under influence of trichostatin A, a histone deacetylase inhibitor. J Hepatol. 2002;37:788–96.
102. Kawada N, Seki S, Kuroki T, Kaneda K. ROCK inhibitor Y-27632 attenuates stellate cell contraction and portal pressure increase induced by endothelin-1. Biochem Biophys Res Commun. 1999;266:296–300.
103. Miano JM. Serum response factor: toggling between disparate programs of gene expression. J Mol Cell Cardiol. 2003;35:577–93.
104. Hermann J, Haas U, Gressner AM, Weiskirchen R. TGF-β up-regulates serum response factor in activated hepatic stellate cells. Biochim Biophys Acta. 2007;1772:1250–7.
105. Wang Z, Wang DZ, Pipes GCT, Olson EN. Myocardin is a master regulator of smooth muscle gene expression. Proc Natl Acad Sci USA. 2003;100:7129–34.
106. Selvaraj A, Prywes R. Expression profiling of serum inducible genes identifies a subset of SRF target genes that are MKL dependent. BMC Mol Biol. 2004;5:13.
107. Chang DF, Belaguli NS, Iyer D et al. Cysteine-rich LIM-only proteins CRP1 and CRP2 are potent smooth muscle differentiation cofactors. Dev Cell. 2003;4:107–18.
108. Lee HJ, Yun CH, Lim SH et al. SRF is a nuclear repressor of Smad3-mediated TGF-β signaling. Oncogene. 2007;26:173–85.
109. Camoretti-Mercado B, Fernandes DJ, Dewundara S et al. Inhibition of transforming growth factor β-enhanced serum response factor-dependent transcription by Smad7. J Biol Chem. 2006;281:20383–92.
110. Yoshida T, Gan Q, Shang Y, Owens GK. Platelet-derived growth factor-BB represses smooth muscle cell marker genes *via* changes in binding of MKL factors and histone deacetylases to their promoters. Am J Physiol Cell Physiol. 2007;292:C886–95.

6
Genetic determinants of liver fibrogenesis: a systems genetics approach in recombinant inbred mice

R. HALL and F. LAMMERT

Hepatic fibrosis is the result of chronic viral, toxic, autoimmune, or cholestatic liver injury. During the complex fibrotic response, distinct cell populations (e.g. activated hepatic stellate cells, portal myofibroblasts, bone-marrow-derived fibrocytes) might contribute to the excess deposition of abnormal extracellular matrix (ECM), and interactions between multiple cytokines, chemokines, receptors and ECM components modulate the fibrotic phenotypes[1,2]. Of note, course and extent of hepatic fibrosis display significant variability among individual patients. These well-known differences in progression of hepatic fibrosis have been attributed to age, gender, and exogenous factors, e.g. coinfections or alcohol consumption. However, host genetic factors are likely to modify liver fibrogenesis and to contribute to the overall variability in disease progression. In the past decade single variants of human genes encoding immunoregulatory proteins as well as pro- and anti-inflammatory cytokines were studied in association studies in patients with chronic hepatitis C virus infection, alcoholic liver disease, and autoimmune liver diseases, yielding inconsistent results[3]. Based on genome-wide association (GWA) analyses, a novel 'gene signature' consisting of seven variants has been proposed to identify patients at risk for progressive fibrosis during chronic hepatitis C virus infection[4].

Recently new and potent high-throughput methods for genome analysis have been implemented, in particular quantitative trait locus (QTL) analyses in experimental mouse crosses that allow the identification of genetic networks determining genetically complex diseases such as liver fibrosis[5,6], and systems genetics that offers the opportunity to define interacting clusters and networks of genes within a tissue or cell population[7]. Figure 1 illustrates that genetic networks controlling liver gene expression can be dissected through the combination of large-scale quantitative mRNA expression analysis in mapping populations such as BXD recombinant inbred mouse lines[8]. Recombinant inbred mouse lines are generated by crossing two inbred strains and inbreeding the progeny by brother–sister matings for at least 20

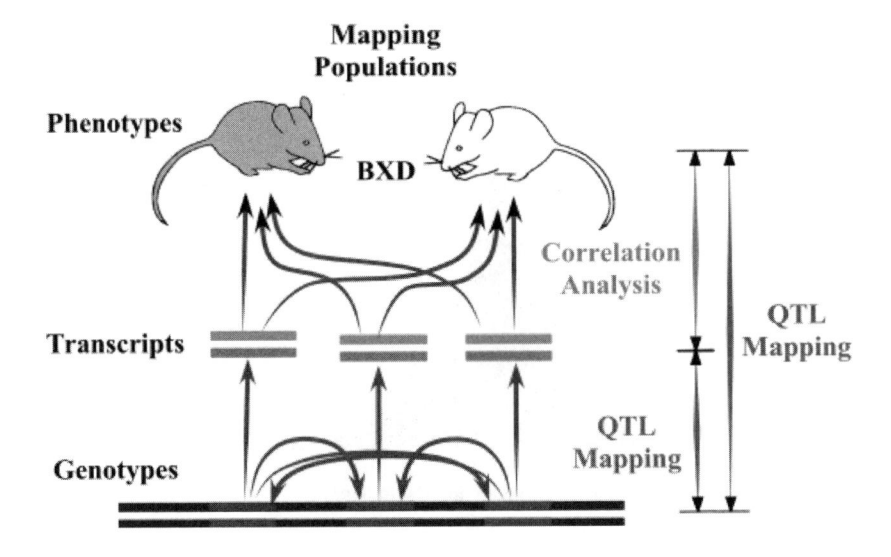

Figure 1 Systems genetics in the BXD mapping population. The BXD inbred lines can be used to map susceptibility loci that affect specific phenotypes (quantitative trait loci, QTL). Since each line serves as an infinite resource of genetically identical mice, replicated transcriptome profiling is possible. Therefore, all transcripts can be correlated with the phenotypes and QTL that regulate individual transcript levels can also be mapped. The experimental strategy to assess multiple phenotype × genotype correlations in reference populations is called 'systems genetics'

generations[9]. At this stage the progeny are inbred and each of the created lines shows a unique mosaic gene set of the two founder strains due to chromosomal recombination in every mating generation. The use of recombinant inbred mouse lines has several advantages compared to intercrosses. Most importantly, each mouse line serves as an infinite resource of genetically identical mice, allowing replicated analysis and mathematical modelling. The BXD recombinant inbred set with 80 lines is the largest panel available[10]. The lines have been generated by inbreeding progeny of a C57BL/6J and DBA/2J intercross. Furthermore, individual genotyping of BXD progeny is not required, as each inbred line has been genotyped for 13 377 single-nucleotide polymorphisms, and very soon >150 000 genotypes will provide dense genome coverage[11–14]. All genotype data are available at http://www.well.ox.ac.uk/mouse/INBREDS/RIL/BXD.shtml.

For characterization of liver fibrogenesis in BXD lines we employed a toxic model challenging the mice twice weekly with intraperitoneal injections of 0.7 mg/kg carbon tetrachloride (CCl_4) for 6 weeks[15,16]. Upon harvesting liver tissue we phenotyped the mice and determined histological stages of liver fibrosis after Sirius red staining[17] and hepatic collagen contents by colorimetric measurement of the collagen-specific amino acid hydroxyproline (Hyp)[18]. For the identification of profibrogenic QTL, whole genome-wide scans were performed with the dense map of previously genotyped SNP markers, as implemented in *WebQTL*[12,19] (http://genesys.helmholtz-hzi.de/).

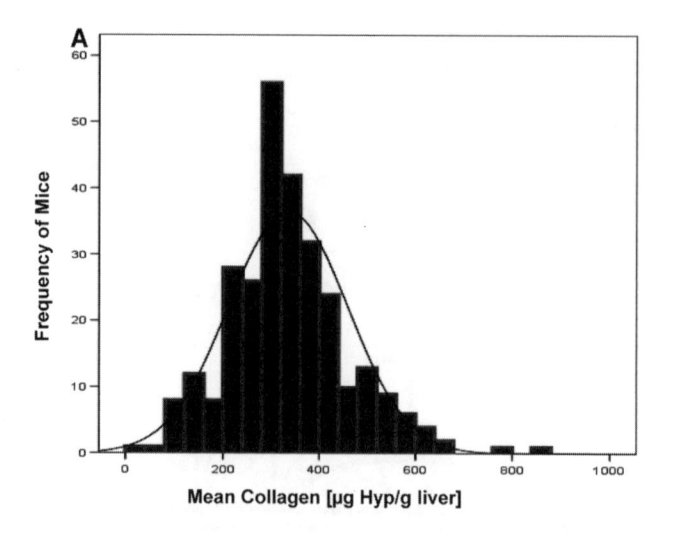

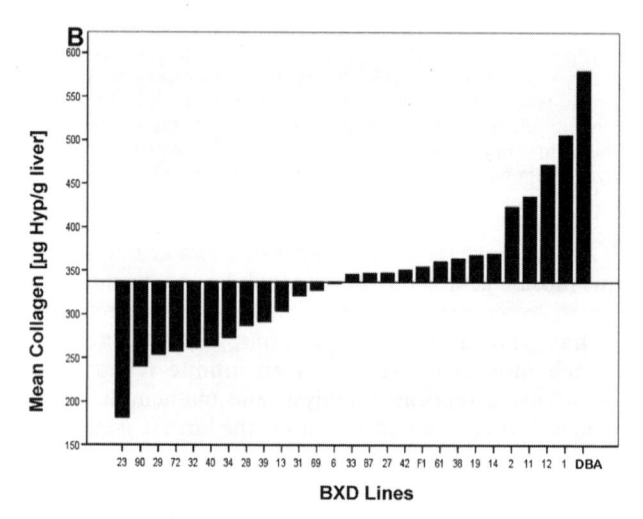

Figure 2 Phenotypic characterization of BXD recombinant inbred lines after fibrosis induction with CCl$_4$. **A**: Collagen contents show a normal distribution among BXD inbred mice, consistent with the polygenic inheritance of liver fibrosis in our model. Hepatic collagen contents were determined by measurement of the specific amino acid hydroxyproline (Hyp) ($n = 320$; mean collagen concentration 342 μg Hyp/g liver). **B**: Hepatic collagen contents of the BXD inbred lines ($n = 4$–20 per line). The vertical axis displays the mean collagen content of all BXD mice. Highest collagen levels are observed in line BXD1 (506 μg Hyp/g liver), whereas line BXD23 displays lowest concentrations (181 μg Hyp/g liver)

GENETIC DETERMINANTS OF LIVER FIBROGENESIS

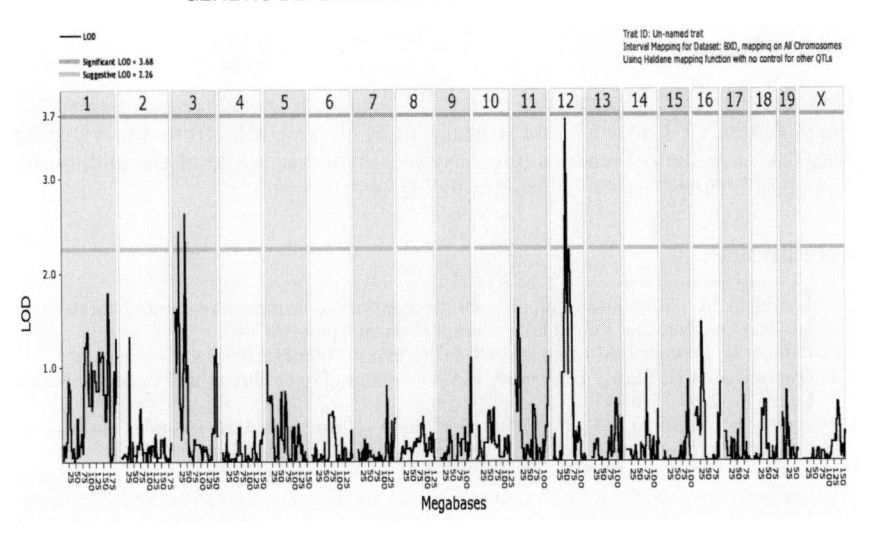

Figure 3 Whole genome QTL scan as implemented in WebQTL (http://genesys.helmholtz-hzi.de/). This scan was performed with 27 BXD lines ($n = 320$) to identify potential associations between variations in the quantitative trait (hepatic collagen contents after induction of liver fibrosis by CCl_4 challenge for 6 weeks) and the genetic variation across the chromosomes. The abscissa shows the genetic marker positions on the chromosomes. The LOD (logarithm of the odds ratio) score on the vertical axis and the black curve estimate the probability that a genetic locus influences the fibrosis phenotype. Vertical grey lines indicate empirical thresholds for suggestive and significant linkage. The scan identifies potential profibrogenic loci on chromosomes 3 and 12.

Analysis of the phenotypic data reveals that significant differences in susceptibility to fibrosis exist in the panel of BXD recombinant inbred lines. After 6 weeks of CCl_4 challenge the histological stages of fibrosis vary from F0 (normal liver) to F3 (septal fibrosis), and hepatic collagen contents range from 181 to 506 µg Hyp/g liver (Figure 2). Consistent with the polygenic inheritance of liver fibrosis in our model, collagen contents show a normal distribution among the BXD inbred lines. Figure 3 displays that preliminary genome-wide scans with *WebQTL* in 27 BXD lines identify suggestive susceptibility loci that predispose to more severe liver fibrosis.

The observed differences in susceptibility to fibrosis among the BXD lines demonstrate that this set qualifies as a genetic reference panel for the integrated analysis of profibrogenic susceptibility genes (Figure 1). We envisage that the use of such a panel, coupled with transcriptome profiling, will lead to novel insights into the complex genetic control of liver fibrogenesis and allow modelling of gene networks during chronic liver injury.

Acknowledgements

This work has been supported in part by Deutsche Forschungsgemeinschaft (grant LA997/4-1 to FL) and a grant to R.H. and F.L. from the German Network of Systems Genetics (GeNeSys), a Virtual Institute of the Helmholtz Association (http://www.helmholtz-hzi.de/de/genesys/).

References

1. Friedman SL. Mechanisms of disease: mechanisms of hepatic fibrosis and therapeutic implications. Nat Clin Pract Gastroenterol Hepatol. 2004;1:98–105.
2. Bataller R, Brenner DA. Liver fibrosis. J Clin Invest. 2005;115:209–18.
3. Österreicher CH, Stickel F, Brenner DA. Genomics of liver fibrosis and cirrhosis. Semin Liver Dis. 2007;27:28–43.
4. Huang H, Shiffman ML, Friedman S et al. A 7 gene signature identifies the risk of developing cirrhosis in patients with chronic hepatitis C. Hepatology. 2007;46:297–306.
5. Hillebrandt S, Wasmuth HE, Weiskirchen R et al. Complement factor 5 is a quantitative trait gene that modifies liver fibrogenesis in mice and humans. Nat Genet. 2005;37:835–43.
6. Lammert F. Genetic determinants of complex liver diseases: mouse models and quantitative trait locus analysis. In: Rodés J, Benhamou JP, Blei A, Reichen J, Rizzetto M, editors. Textbook of Hepatology: From Basic Science to Clinical Practice. Oxford: Blackwell, 2007:371–83.
7. Morahan G, Williams RW. Systems genetics: the next generation in genetics research. In: Bock G, Goode J, editors. Decoding the Genomic Control of Immune Reactions. Proceedings of Novartis Foundation Symposium 181. Chichester: Wiley, 2007:181–91.
8. Gatti D, Maki A, Chesler EJ et al. Genome-level analysis of genetic regulation of liver gene expression networks. Hepatology. 2007;46:548–57.
9. Peters LL, Robledo RF, Bult CJ, Churchill GA, Paigen BJ, Svenson KL. The mouse as a model for human biology: a resource guide for complex trait analysis. Nat Rev Genet. 2007;8:58–69.
10. Peirce JL, Lu L, Gu J, Silver LM, Williams RW. A new set of BXD recombinant inbred lines from advanced intercross populations in mice. BMC Genet. 2004;5:7.
11. Bystrykh L, Weersing E, Dontje B et al. Uncovering regulatory pathways that affect hematopoietic stem cell function using 'genetical genomics'. Nat Genet. 2005;37:225–32.
12. Chesler EJ, Lu L, Shou S et al. Complex trait analysis of gene expression uncovers polygenic and pleiotropic networks that modulate nervous system function. Nat Genet. 2005;37:233–42.
13. Broman KW. Mapping expression in randomized rodent genomes. Nat Genet. 2005;37:209–10.
14. Kempermann G, Chesler EJ, Lu L, Williams RW, Gage FH. Natural variation and genetic covariance in adult hippocampal neurogenesis. Proc Natl Acad Sci USA. 2006;103:780–5.
15. Tsukamoto H, Matsuoka M, French SW. Experimental models of hepatic fibrosis: a review. Semin Liver Dis. 1990;10:56–65.
16. Hillebrandt S, Goos C, Matern S, Lammert F. Genome-wide analysis of hepatic fibrosis in inbred mice identifies the susceptibility locus *Hfib1* on chromosome 15. Gastroenterology. 2002;123:2041–51.
17. Batts KP, Ludwig J. Chronic hepatitis. An update on terminology and reporting. Am J Surg Pathol. 1995;19:1409–17.
18. Jamall IS, Finelli VN, Que Hee SS. A simple method to determine nanogram levels of 4-hydroxyproline in biological tissues. Anal Biochem. 1981;112:70–5.
19. Chesler EJ, Lu L, Wang J, Williams RW, Manly KF. WebQTL: rapid exploratory analysis of gene expression and genetic networks for brain and behavior. Nat Neurosci. 2004;7:485–6.

7
Molecular mechanisms of fibrosis progression in non-alcoholic steatohepatitis (NASH)

C. HELLERBRAND

DEFINITION AND EPIDEMIOLOGY OF NON-ALCOHOLIC FATTY LIVER DISEASE (NAFLD)

NAFLD is a clinicopathological condition of emerging importance, now recognized as the most common cause of abnormal liver tests. NAFLD is associated with obesity, type 2 diabetes, dyslipidaemia and hypertension. These conditions have insulin resistance as the common factor and cluster to form the metabolic syndrome. Most patients with NAFLD have increased liver fat content alone (simple steatosis), but others develop increasing hepatic inflammation known as non-alcoholic steatohepatitis (NASH) and up to 20% of patients develop progressive hepatic fibrosis and may eventually develop cirrhosis or liver failure (Figure 1). In addition, the risk of development of hepatocellular carcinoma in NASH-related cirrhosis is comparable to hepatitis C infection. Considering the rising prevalence of obesity, NAFLD has to be considered as (one of) the most frequent chronic liver diseases in Western countries[1].

CURRENT MODEL OF DISEASE PROGRESSION IN NAFLD/NASH

A wealth of studies in animal models and humans with this disorder have increased our understanding of the pathogenesis of NASH; however, still the underlying mechanisms that influence that steatosis in progressing to steatohepatitis (i.e. the association of lipid overload and inflammation) and fibrosis are largely unknown. The 'two-hit' model summarizes important metabolic events leading to hepatocellular necrosis in NAFLD[2]. In addition to a 'first hit', namely steatosis characterized by an increase in lipid deposition in hepatocytes, a 'second hit' is required to induce inflammation (Figure 2). As one mechanism that promotes inflammation in NASH, lipid peroxidation has been identified, which induces increased DNA oxidative damage and cell

LIVER CIRRHOSIS: FROM PATHOPHYSIOLOGY TO DISEASE MANAGEMENT

NonAlcoholic Fatty Liver Disease (NAFLD)

Steatosis

Steato-Hepatitis (NASH)

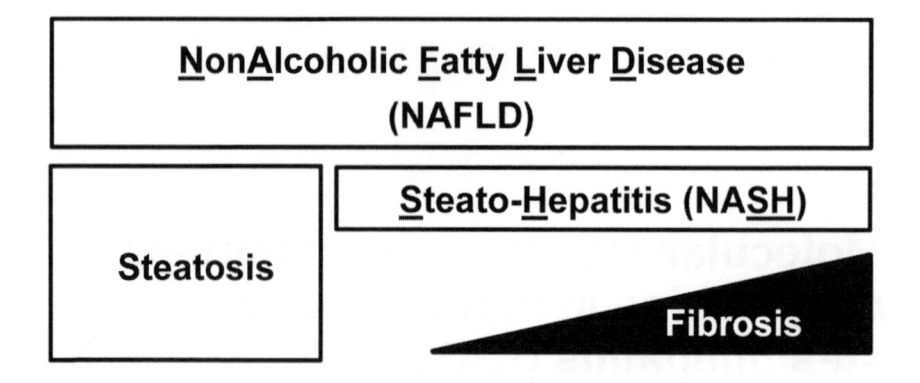

Fibrosis

Figure 1 The hallmark of NAFLD is hepatic steatosis, usually macrovascular fat. NAFLD may progress to NASH. NASH is characterized by an association between inflammation and other liver lesions such as fibrosis. In a subset of patients it may evolve to cirrhosis and hepatocellular carcinoma

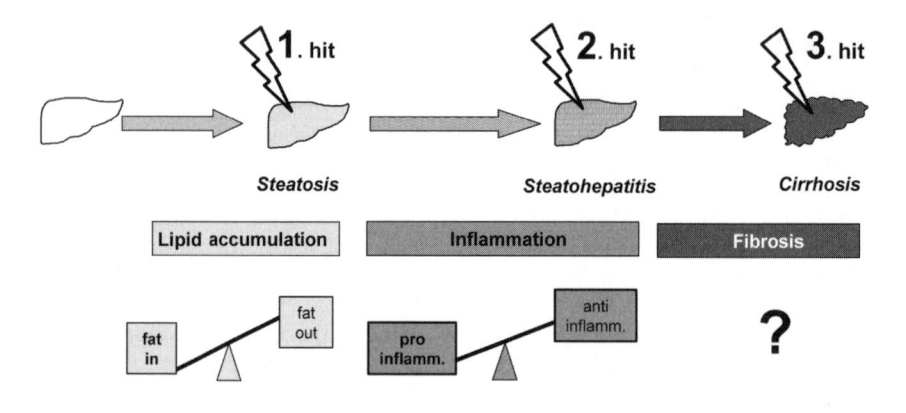

Figure 2 A three-step model for the pathogenesis of NAFLD. Initially, there is an imbalance between hepatic fat uptake and release resulting in hepatocellular lipid accumulation. In this model hepatic steatosis is considered as the 'first hit' of a pathophysiological cascade. Subsequently, there develops an imbalance between proinflammatory and anti-inflammatory mechanisms in the steatotic liver. The resulting inflammatory milieu is causing the 'second hit', leading to steatohepatitis. In only a subset of cases does NASH cause progressive hepatic fibrosis. This leads to the hypothesis that a 'third hit' is required to initiate the progression of NASH to fibrosis that may ultimately lead to cirrhosis and hepatocellular carcinoma

death. However, and interestingly, hepatic (necro)inflammation appears necessary but not sufficient for progression to severe fibrosis, since progression from NASH to cirrhosis develops only in a fraction of patients. This may reflect the requirement for additional factors, e.g. a 'third hit' or 'third hits', respectively, to initiate and perpetuate fibrogenesis.

Hepatic fibrosis is viewed as a relatively uniform response to different types of injury. It is characterized by an increased deposition of extracellular matrix (ECM) proteins as a result of increased fibrogenesis and decreased fibrolysis. Activated hepatic stellate cells (HSC) are the effector cells of hepatic fibrosis. After hepatic injury, HSC undergo an activation process and transform to an activated, myofibroblast-like phenotype. They are responsible for the excessive hepatic ECM deposition and their activity is recognized as a central event in the development of hepatic fibrosis[3,4]. Also in NAFLD HSC activation is the central pathophysiological mechanism underlying hepatic fibrosis, and this has to be kept in mind when searching for factors causing or enhancing the 'third hit'.

MOLECULAR MECHANISMS OF FIBROSIS IN NAFLD/NASH – LOOKING FOR THE 'THIRD HIT'

Lessons from alcohol-induced steatohepatitis (ASH)

Looking for such factors it appears that, in addition to histopathology of NASH, which resembles the picture of alcohol-induced steatohepatitis (ASH), common pathogenic mechanisms also exist.

As one example, tumour necrosis factor (TNF) has been shown to play an important role in the pathophysiology of alcoholic liver disease and its complications[5], and there is now a body of evidence showing that this proinflammatory cytokine is also critically involved in the progression of NASH. Thus, Tomita et al. applied the methionine-and-choline-deficient (MCD) diet, an established NASH animal model, to mice deficient in both TNF receptors 1 (TNFR1) and 2 (TNFR2)[6]. Notably, these mice had attenuated liver steatosis and fibrosis compared with control wild-type mice. In line with this observation, inhibition of TNF, using the monoclonal antibody infliximab, reduces inflammation and steatosis/fibrosis in Wistar rats fed a high-fat diet[7].

Further, similarly as in ASH, products of intestinal bacteria, particularly lipopolysaccharide (LPS), have been identified to promote disease progression in NASH. Thus, upon MCD dietary feeding both lipid accumulation and hepatic injury were significantly lower in toll-like receptor 4 (TLR-4) mutant mice as compared to wild-type mice[8]. Interestingly, intestinal bacterial overgrowth has been shown in diabetic subjects[9]. Further, a recent study by Brun et al. showed that genetically obese mice display enhanced intestinal permeability leading to increased portal endotoxaemia that makes HSC more sensitive to bacterial endotoxins[10]. Together these findings suggest that, also in obese and/or diabetic patients, intestinal mucosa permeability leads to increased endotoxin levels in portal blood that contribute to hepatic inflammation and fibrosis (Figure 3). Further, these results clearly show that, regarding progression of NAFLD, one has to consider that NASH is only one component of the metabolic syndrome. Thus, in addition to direct effects on the liver, indirect effects of other pathophysiologically altered organs such as the gut may indirectly influence NASH progression.

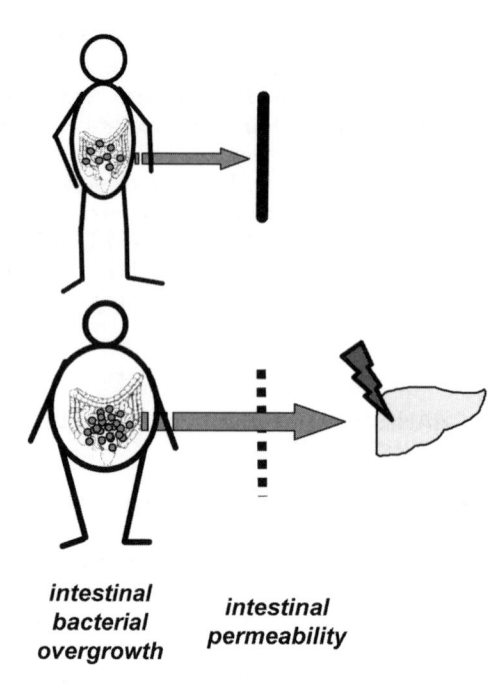

Figure 3 Model showing how gut-derived endotoxins may enhance progression of NASH in obese and/or diabetic patients. Both intestinal bacterial overgrowth and enhanced intestinal permeability cause portal endotoxaemia; thus promoting hepatic inflammation and fibrosis

Adipose tissue and adipokines expression

In parallel to increased levels of factors enhancing inflammation and fibrosis in NASH, the loss or reduced expression of (hepato)protective factors as adiponectin may also cause the 'third hit' promoting NASH progression. This adipokine is a main metabolic product of adipose tissue, and reduced adiponectin serum levels, which are usually observed in obese patients with or without metabolic syndrome, may result in fat accumulation in the liver and in the enhancement of liver inflammation and mostly fibrogenesis[11]. Conversely, obese patients frequently have increased levels of leptin, another adipokine mainly released by adipocytes, and associated leptin resistance[11]. Leptin is profibrogenic, and liver fibrosis is decreased in leptin- or leptin receptor-deficient mice[11,12]. Thus adipokines provide one further example of how other organs, e.g. adipose tissue, indirectly affect NASH progression. Obesity and mainly visceral fat accumulation impair adipocyte function and adipocytokine secretion, and the altered release of these proteins has a direct effect on hepatic inflammation and fibrosis (Figure 4).

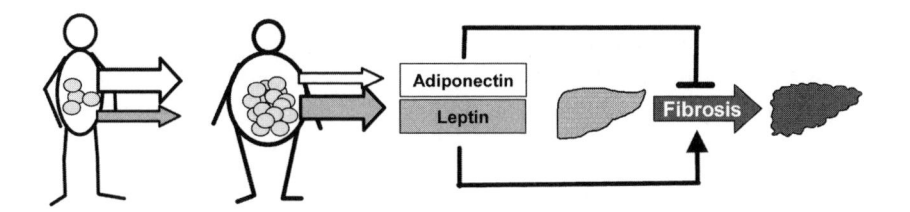

Figure 4 In obese patients adipose tissue often reveals increased release of the profibrogenic adipokine leptin, while there is decreased secretion of adiponectin that has antifibrotic potential

Obstructive sleep apnoea and chronic intermittent hypoxia

Another example of how the complexity of the metabolic syndrome or pathophysiological alterations associated with the metabolic syndrome, respectively, may affect the progression of NASH is obstructive sleep apnoea that causes chronic intermittent hypoxia during sleep. Obstructive sleep apnoea is frequent in obese individuals, and it has been shown that chronic intermittent hypoxia predisposes to liver injury[13]. Similarly, chronic intermittent hypoxia promotes the progression of NASH in animal models[14,15]. After exposure to chronic intermittent hypoxia mice with diet-induced hepatic steatosis developed lobular inflammation and fibrosis in the liver, which were not evident in control mice[14]. Moreover, in some patients severe obstructive sleep apnoea has also been identified as a risk factor for elevated liver enzymes and steatohepatitis independent of body weight in patients[16]. Interestingly, a recent study revealed that hypoxia may underlie the development of the inflammatory response in adipocytes[17]. This further indicates the complexity of the interaction of hepatic and extrahepatic pathophysiological mechanisms promoting the progression of NASH.

Amount and type of dietary fat affect progression of NAFLD

It has been shown that the amount of fatty infiltration of the liver, influenced by the dietary intake of both fat and protein, is related to the subsequent development of necrosis, inflammation, and fibrosis. However, in addition to the amount the type of dietary fat also has an influence on the pathogenesis of chronic liver disease. Thus, it has been shown in a rat model for alcoholic liver disease that dietary beef fat (tallow) prevented hepatocellular damage. In contrast, rats fed lard and ethanol developed minimal to moderate disease, while animals fed corn oil and the same amount of ethanol developed the most severe liver pathology[18]. Interestingly, systematic comparison of hepatic lipid accumulation in dietary high-fat models with varying fatty acid compositions revealed striking differences[19]. Thus, high-fat diets based on 42% (energy) lard or olive oil, respectively, showed the most pronounced hepatic steatosis. In contrast, after a fish oil diet, hepatic lipid accumulation was barely detectable. These findings indicate that the type of dietary fat directly affects the 'first hit'.

Furthermore, lipotoxic effects on hepatocytes also vary between different types of fatty acids. For example, palmitic and oleic acids are the most abundant fatty acids in liver triglycerides in both normal subjects and patients with NAFLD. However, both fatty acids exhibit a distinct toxic potential on hepatocytes[20]. Further, hepatocyte apoptosis is increased in patients with NASH and correlates with disease severity. Interestingly, long-chain saturated fatty acids, such as palmitate and stearate, induce apoptosis in liver cells, while oleate did not activate caspase-3 or induce DNA fragmentation in the same experimental setting. Together, these findings indicate that there is 'good fat' and 'bad fat' with regard to both development and progression of NAFLD.

The metabolic syndrome can bypass the first hit

Regardless of hepatic steatosis, obesity, high glucose levels and insulin resistance are major and independent risk factors for fibrosis progression in chronic liver disease of different aetiologies. For example, hepatic steatosis is an independent risk factor for the progression of fibrosis in patients with chronic hepatitis C infection, and weight reduction in these patients reduces fibrosis and hepatic stellate cell activation. Further, it has been shown that high glucose concentrations induce proliferation and collagen production by HSC[21]. Further again, high glucose and hyperinsulinaemia stimulate expression of further fibrogenic factors in HSC *in vitro* and *in vivo* in experimental models of obesity and type 2 diabetes[22]. Moreover, a recent study compared the effect of a high-fat diet on two strains of rats[11]. OLETF rats are prone to obesity, insulin resistance, hyperinsulinaemia and diabetes, while LETO rats are lean and insulin-sensitive. Interestingly, in OLETF rats the high-fat diet led to increased hepatic triglyceride accumulation and inflammation as well as HSC activation and fibrosis, while the hepatic response was significantly milder in LET rats. Together these results indicate that insulin resistance and/or diabetes may accelerate the entire pathological spectrum of NASH. Of note, the profibrotic action does not necessarily require hepatic lipid accumulation. Thus, the metabolic syndrome is independently associated with more severe fibrosis but not with the severity of steatosis both in chronic viral hepatitis and NASH[23]. Consequently, a recent study of livers of diabetics found activation of hepatic stellate cells and sinusoidal fibrosis without histologically detectable NASH and irrespective of the degree of steatosis[24]. Similarly, Abrams et al. found that a significant subset of morbidly obese individuals has portal fibrosis in the absence of NASH that is associated with glycaemic dysregulation[25].

SUMMARY

The 'hit model' is a valuable framework for understanding the molecular mechanisms of disease progression in NAFLD. However, as with every model, it is simplifying and it depicts only part of the (complexity of the) pathophysiological mechanisms promoting progression of hepatic steatosis to inflammation and fibrosis.

Thus, one has to consider that, in addition to the liver, the metabolic syndrome pathophysiologically affects several other organs. Such alterations as observed regarding adipokine release of adipose tissue, intestinal bacterial overgrowth or enhanced intestinal permeability additionally affect the progression of NAFLD. Further, it appears that the 'first hit', e.g. the amount and type of hepatic lipid accumulation, may already determine whether the liver will react with severe fibrosis in response to a 'second hit'. If true, this would have important prognostic, diagnostic and therapeutic implications for NAFLD and chronic liver disease in general.

References

1. Angulo P. Nonalcoholic fatty liver disease. N Engl J Med. 2002;346:1221–31.
2. Day CP, James OF. Steatohepatitis: a tale of two 'hits'? Gastroenterology. 1998;114:842–5.
3. Bataller R, Brenner DA. Liver fibrosis. J Clin Invest. 2005;115:209–18.
4. Friedman SL. Mechanisms of disease: mechanisms of hepatic fibrosis and therapeutic implications. Nat Clin Pract Gastroenterol Hepatol. 2004;1:98–105.
5. Terada T, Okada Y, Nakanuma Y. Expression of immunoreactive matrix metalloproteinases and tissue inhibitors of matrix metalloproteinases in human normal livers and primary liver tumors. Hepatology. 1996;23:1341–4.
6. Tomita K, Tamiya G, Ando S et al. Tumour necrosis factor alpha signalling through activation of Kupffer cells plays an essential role in liver fibrosis of non-alcoholic steatohepatitis in mice. Gut. 2006;55:415–24.
7. Barbuio R, Milanski M, Bertolo MB, Saad MJ, Velloso LA. Infliximab reverses steatosis and improves insulin signal transduction in liver of rats fed a high-fat diet. J Endocrinol. 2007;194:539–50.
8. Rivera CA, Adegboyega P, van Rooijen N, Tagalicud A, Allman M, Wallace M. Toll-like receptor-4 signaling and Kupffer cells play pivotal roles in the pathogenesis of non-alcoholic steatohepatitis. J Hepatol. 2007;47:571–9.
9. Zietz B, Lock G, Straub RH, Braun B, Scholmerich J, Palitzsch KD. Small-bowel bacterial overgrowth in diabetic subjects is associated with cardiovascular autonomic neuropathy. Diabetes Care. 2000;23:1200–1.
10. Brun P, Castagliuolo I, Di LV et al. Increased intestinal permeability in obese mice: new evidence in the pathogenesis of nonalcoholic steatohepatitis. Am J Physiol Gastrointest Liver Physiol. 2007;292:G518–25.
11. Tsochatzis E, Papatheodoridis GV, Archimandritis AJ. The evolving role of leptin and adiponectin in chronic liver diseases. Am J Gastroenterol. 2006;101:2629–40.
12. Marra F, Aleffi S, Bertolani C, Petrai I, Vizzutti F. Adipokines and liver fibrosis. Eur Rev Med Pharmacol Sci. 2005;9:279–84.
13. Savransky V, Nanayakkara A, Vivero A et al. Chronic intermittent hypoxia predisposes to liver injury. Hepatology. 2007;45:1007–13.
14. Savransky V, Bevans S, Nanayakkara A et al. Chronic intermittent hypoxia causes hepatitis in a mouse model of diet-induced fatty liver. Am J Physiol Gastrointest Liver Physiol. 2007;293:G871–7.
15. Zamora-Valdes D, Mendez-Sanchez N. Experimental evidence of obstructive sleep apnea syndrome as a second hit accomplice in nonalcoholic steatohepatitis pathogenesis. Ann Hepatol. 2007;6:281–3.
16. Tanne F, Gagnadoux F, Chazouilleres O et al. Chronic liver injury during obstructive sleep apnea. Hepatology. 2005;41:1290–6.
17. Wang B, Wood IS, Trayhurn P. Dysregulation of the expression and secretion of inflammation-related adipokines by hypoxia in human adipocytes. Pflugers Arch. 2007;455:479–92.
18. Nanji AA, Mendenhall CL, French SW. Beef fat prevents alcoholic liver disease in the rat. Alcohol Clin Exp Res. 1989;13:15–19.
19. Buettner R, Parhofer KG, Woenckhaus M et al. Defining high-fat-diet rat models: metabolic and molecular effects of different fat types. J Mol Endocrinol. 2006;36:485–501.

20. Gomez-Lechon MJ, Donato MT, Martinez-Romero A, Jimenez N, Castell JV, O'Connor JE. A human hepatocellular *in vitro* model to investigate steatosis. Chem Biol Interact. 2007;165:106–16.
21. Sugimoto R, Enjoji M, Kohjima M et al. High glucose stimulates hepatic stellate cells to proliferate and to produce collagen through free radical production and activation of mitogen-activated protein kinase. Liver Int. 2005;25:1018–26.
22. Paradis V, Perlemuter G, Bonvoust F et al. High glucose and hyperinsulinemia stimulate connective tissue growth factor expression: a potential mechanism involved in progression to fibrosis in nonalcoholic steatohepatitis. Hepatology. 2001;34:738–44.
23. Tsochatzis E, Papatheodoridis GV, Manesis EK, Kafiri G, Tiniakos DG, Archimandritis AJ. Metabolic syndrome is associated with severe fibrosis in chronic viral hepatitis and non-alcoholic steatohepatitis. Aliment Pharmacol Ther. 2007, Oct 6 [Epub ahead of print].
24. Jaskiewicz K, Rzepko R, Sledzinski Z. Fibrogenesis in fatty liver associated with obesity and diabetes mellitus type 2. Dig Dis Sci. 2007, Sep 12 [Epub ahead of print].
25. Abrams GA, Kunde SS, Lazenby AJ, Clements RH. Portal fibrosis and hepatic steatosis in morbidly obese subjects: a spectrum of nonalcoholic fatty liver disease. Hepatology. 2004;40:475–83.

8
New role of bile acid metabolism in intestinal bacteria translocation

M. PETRUZZELLI and A. MOSCHETTA

INTRODUCTION

Bile acids are endogenous molecules synthesized in the liver as endproducts of cholesterol catabolism. Secreted in bile, stored in the gallbladder in the interprandial period, bile acids are released in the intestine mainly in response to food intake. After active uptake in the ileum, bile acids return back to the liver through the portal vein, thus completing their enterohepatic circulation. Classical physiological functions of bile acids include promotion of hepatic homeostasis and bile flow, support of the smooth progression of lipid digestion and absorption, absorption of lipophilic vitamins, cholesterol solubilization and disposal[1]. Moreover, bile acids are directly involved in preserving the physiological commensal host–intestinal bacteria relationship. The gut microbiota hosted in the intestinal lumen is precious since it solves key metabolic roles for nutrient processing, as well as correct development and tuning of the immune system[2]. The delicate host–intestinal bacteria balance is regulated to maintain a fixed composition of microbial species, while preventing their excessive proliferation. In pathophysiological conditions the expansion of intestinal microflora leads to migration of bacteria through the intestinal mucosa, up to mesenteric lymph nodes and extra-intestinal tissues. Bacterial overgrowth and translocation play major pathophysiological roles, especially in cirrhotic patients, potentially leading to portal hypertension, ascites, spontaneous bacterial peritonitis, and hepatorenal syndrome[3].

BILE ACIDS AND INTESTINAL MICROFLORA

The bacteriostatic activity of bile acids has long being recognized. The first reports of the inhibitory effects of bile acids upon intestinal bacteria proliferation date back to 1970[4]. Both in experimental models and humans, interrupted bile flow results in hyperproliferation of intestinal microflora, leading to inflammation of intestinal epithelia, bacterial translocation, and systemic infection[5]. Since biliary bile acid output is markedly reduced in cirrhotic patients, the impairment of the gut microbiota observed during the course of the disease has been linked to bile acid depletion in the intestinal lumen[6]. Accordingly, therapeutic replenishment of bile acids by oral feeding in experimental cirrhotic rats resolves bacterial overgrowth and translocation, resulting in increased survival[7]. The mechanism whereby bile acids inhibit bacterial proliferation has been classically restricted to direct contact and detergency[8], a feature strictly related to bile acid hydrophobicity (Figure 1, left panel)[9]. In line with this hypothesis, conjugated bile acids which are resistant to intestinal absorption and last at higher concentration in the intestinal lumen would be best suited to exploit the antibacterial properties of bile acids. Indeed, the synthetic conjugated bile acid cholylsarcosine, which is resistant to biotransformation, is most effective in reducing bacterial counts in ascitic cirrhotic rats[7]. At variance, unconjugated bile acids are present at low concentration in the intestinal lumen because of fast uptake by the enterocyte, and should display little or no antibacterial activity. Unexpectedly, though,

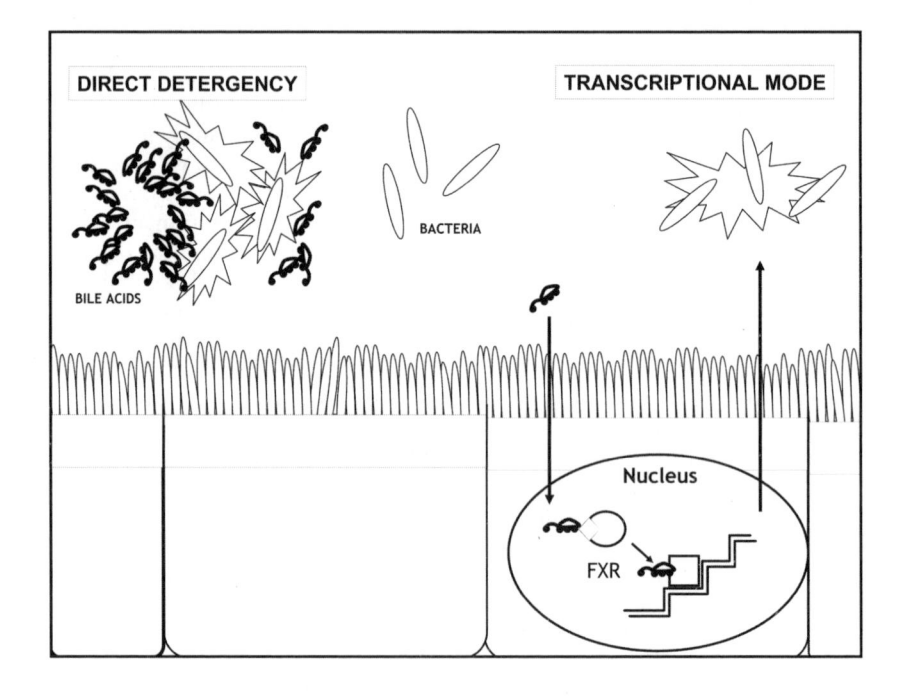

Figure 1 Molecular mechanisms involved in the antibacterial properties displayed by bile acids. In the upper segments of the intestinal tract, namely duodenum and jejunum, bile acids are not absorbed; therefore they are present at high concentration in the intestinal lumen. Intraluminal bile acids exert direct antibacterial activity, by means of their detergent properties (*left panel*). On the other hand, in the ileum, bile acids are actively absorbed and their intraluminal concentration falls dramatically (*right panel*). In these conditions intestinal mucosal defence is assured by FXR-mediated transcriptional activation of genes involved in antimicrobial defence, innate immune response and mucosal integrity

cholylglycine, which undergoes fast bacterial deconjugation and is rapidly absorbed, is only slightly less effective than cholylsarcosine[7]. The observation that unconjugated bile acids also display striking antibacterial properties suggests that mechanisms other than direct contact are implicated in the antibacterial activity of bile acids. Compelling new evidence links the bacteriostatic activity of bile acids to a transcriptional mode (Figure 1, right panel).

TRANSCRIPTIONAL PROPERTIES OF BILE ACIDS

The physiology of lipids has been revolutionized in recent years by the astonishing identification of their transcriptional properties. Some lipid molecules act as selective ligands for nuclear receptors, which are ligand-activated transcription factors. Through activation of nuclear receptors, lipids are able to switch genes on and off. Farnesoid X receptor (FXR) is the nuclear receptor bile acid sensor, responsible for the coherent transcriptional regulation of a series of genes directly involved in the maintenance of lipid homeostasis in the gut–liver axis[10]. FXR was cloned in 1995[11,12] and a few years later bile acids were identified as the natural ligands, giving this nuclear receptor the initial designation of bile acid receptor (BAR), which has now been abandoned[13,14]. At molecular level, nuclear receptors share a common modular organization: the ligand-binding domain (LBD) is located in the C-terminal part of the molecule and consists of a hydrophobic pocket where recognition and accommodation of the specific ligand take place. Following interaction of the ligand with the LBD, changes in the ternary structure of the nuclear receptor activate gene transcription at the DNA binding domain (DBD). Gene transcription occurs at precise sites, which are termed hormone response elements, and are unique for each nuclear receptor. In the case of FXR, the hormone response elements consist of inverted repeated sequences (the canonical AGGTCA repeats) separated by one nucleotide (IR-1). Gene transcription is additionally under control of co-regulatory proteins, which can either promote (co-activators) or restrain (co-repressors) the transcriptional activity of nuclear receptors. Interaction between co-regulatory proteins and nuclear receptors takes place at the N-terminal *trans*-activation domain (AF1) and the ligand-induced *trans*-activation domain (AF2). Some nuclear receptors exert their transcriptional activity as dimers, either homodimers or heterodimers with the retinoid X receptors (RXR), as it is the case for FXR.

Phenotyping of FXR knockout mice discloses the central role this nuclear receptor plays in bile acid metabolism[15,16]. FXR knockout mice display elevated serum bile acid with doubled bile acid pool size. Also, impairment of bile acid metabolism deeply affects the metabolism of other lipid species. FXR knockout mice also present elevated hepatic and serum levels of both cholesterol and triglycerides, plus a pro-atherogenic serum lipoprotein profile. The phenotype is the consequence of impaired activation of FXR target genes in the liver. FXR restrains bile acid synthesis by inhibiting gene transcription of cholesterol 7α-hydroxylase (CYP7α), the rate-limiting enzyme for bile acid synthesis[17,18]. Moreover, FXR promotes biliary secretion of bile acids, as a result of direct gene induction of canalicular bile acid transporter ATP binding cassette transporter B11 (ABC-B11; also known as bile salt export pump, BSEP)[19]. Of note, since bile acids are detergent molecules that could potentially be toxic for the hepatobiliary epithelia, FXR also promotes biliary secretion of phospholipids by direct gene induction of the canalicular phospholipid transporter ABC-B4 (also known as multi-drug resistance (mdr) 2 in mice, MDR3 in humans)[20]. Phospholipids prevent bile acid toxicity through the formation of mixed micelles with bile acid molecules[21,22]. The increased biliary secretion of bile acids and phospholipids induced by FXR activation has been exploited to reduce the saturation index of biliary cholesterol and prevent cholesterol gallstone disease in the mouse model[23].

FXR is also highly expressed in the intestine, where it chiefly promotes intracellular trafficking of bile acids from the apical to the basolateral membrane and ensuing basolateral efflux, through increased expression of ileal bile acid binding protein (IBABP)[13] and organic solute transporters (OST α and β)[24], respectively. Lastly, FXR drives the hormonal feedback response between the enterocyte and the hepatocyte, which results in reduced hepatic bile acid synthesis[25]. FXR stimulates in the intestine the expression of fibroblast growth factor (fgf) 15 in mice, or FGF19 in men, a hormone secreted in the portal vein and active in the liver after interaction with fibroblast growth factor receptor 4 (FGFR4), which in turn represses $CYP7\alpha$ expression through a mechanism that involves the orphan nuclear receptor small heterodimer partner (SHP). The bile acid–FXR–FGF15/19–FGFR4 metabolic cascade is also responsible for gallbladder filling in the postprandial period, as a result of inhibition of cholecystokinin-induced gallbladder contraction[26]. These reports highlight the role of FXR as the hub responsible for the synchronization of the gut–liver axis. Further investigations will in the near future disclose the relevance of this endocrine pathway for other physiological functions of the digestive tract.

Given the importance of FXR in bile acid physiology, and the high expression of this nuclear receptor in the intestine, it is plausible to hypothesize the involvement of FXR in the antibacterial properties of bile acids.

TRANSCRIPTIONAL PROTECTION OF INTESTINAL MUCOSA BY BILE ACIDS

To test the seminal hypothesis that FXR could be responsible, at least to some extent, for the antibacterial properties displayed by bile acids, the expression profile of FXR throughout the different sections of the intestine was investigated[27]. FXR is expressed in considerable amounts in duodenum and jejunum, at levels as high as the liver in the colon, while it peaks in the ileum, reaching values almost twice those in the liver. *In situ* hybridization analysis reveals that FXR is expressed in the intestinal epithelium which is most exposed to luminal content, namely the villi and the intervillus regions, while it is virtually absent in the crypts. Interestingly, microarray analysis shows that several genes involved in intestinal mucosal defence are activated by

Table 1 Genes involved in intestinal mucosal defence which are activated by administration of FXR synthetic ligand GW4064

Gene name	Acronym	Function	Reference
Inducible NO synthase	iNOS	Direct antimicrobial effects. Regulation of mucus secretion, vascular tone, and epithelial barrier function.	30, 31
Interleukin 18	IL18	Proinflammatory cytokine. Stimulation of resistance against intracellular and extracellular pathogens. Protective role during the early, acute phase of mucosal immune response.	32, 33
Angiogenin	ANG1	Involvement in the acute phase response to infection. Potent antibacterial and antimycotic actions.	34
RNase A family member 4	RNASE4	Exact function not yet established. Probably involved in the acute-phase response, since both RNASE4 and ANG1 arise by differential splicing from a common gene locus.	35
Carbonic anhydrase 12	CAR12	Maintenance of pH and ion balance.	36

administration of FXR synthetic ligand GW4064 (Table 1). At the molecular level, activation of FXR ignites transcription of genes involved in antimicrobial defence, innate immune response, mucosal health (mucus secretion, vascular tone, maintenance of the epithelial barrier). Such genes include inducible nitric oxide synthase, angiogenin, carbonic anhydrase 12, and interleukin 18. Definitive proof for the involvement of FXR in antibacterial properties of bile acids comes from bile duct ligation (BDL) experiments carried out in wild-type as well as FXR knockout mice. By abruptly interrupting bile flow, BDL determines the complete depletion of intestinal bile acids. The absence of intestinal bile acids is responsible for the increased colonization of aerobic and anaerobic bacteria in the ileum and caecum of BDL mice. Furthermore, BDL disrupts the barrier function which is assured by the integrity of the intestinal mucosa, as revealed by immunostaining for occludin, a structural component of the enterocyte tight junctions. Differently from sham-operated mice, in which occludin staining is continuous, in BDL mice the staining is severely interrupted. The breakdown of mucosal integrity after BDL is also confirmed by transmission electron microscopy, which reveals the ruptures in the mucosal surface and the penetration of bacteria in the intestinal epithelium. As a result of deteriorated epithelial integrity, bacteria translocation occurs from the intestinal mucosa to the mesenteric lymph node complexes. The pathological effects of BDL are largely prevented by FXR activation. Treatment with FXR agonists completely blocks bacterial overgrowth, restoring the presence of both aerobic and anaerobic bacteria at levels equal to those present in sham-operated mice. In addition, BDL wild-type mice treated with FXR agonists display a striking reduction in the pathological signs of intestinal mucosa damage, as evidenced by absence of oedema and dilated lymphatic vessels, and integrity of the epithelial barrier. Enteroprotection by synthetic FXR agonists is lost in FXR knockout mice. Most interestingly, even in sham-operated mice, the absence of FXR results in increased bacterial colonization. FXR knockout mice display increased levels of aerobic bacteria both in the ileum and intestine. At variance, the presence of anaerobic bacteria in FXR knockout sham-operated mice equals that of wild-type mice. The reason for the preferential protection against aerobic bacteria displayed by FXR is yet to be determined. FXR knockout mice also present a deteriorated epithelial barrier and greater bacterial population in mesenteric lymph nodes. Lastly, sham-operated FXR knockout mice host increased levels of neutrophils in the mucosa of the terminal ileum, at levels as high as those present in wild-type mice after BDL. One should remember that FXR knockout mice have a doubled bile acid pool size, so that the absence of protection in the gut points to the necessary importance of the transcriptional activity of bile acids to preserve the physiological host–intestinal bacteria balance. These findings extend the signalling competence of bile acids. Next to shielding the liver from the toxic effect of bile acid overload, FXR also promotes intestinal health.

FUTURE PERSPECTIVES

These recent major discoveries prompt the need for critical and systematic description of the FXR-mediated antibacterial activity of bile acids. A critical issue to address is the relative impact of direct bacteriostatic activity versus FXR-mediated transcriptional mode. One possibility is to determine the effect of bile acid supplementation in BDL FXR knockout mice. Theoretically, the two mechanisms may act in concert to protect the different segments of the intestinal tract against infectious threat[28]. In the upper parts of the intestine, i. e. duodenum and jejunum, where bile acids are not absorbed, the direct antibacterial properties of bile acids may prevail. On the contrary, in the ileum, where bile acids are actively absorbed, the FXR-mediated transcriptional mode may overcome. However, given the well-known sensitivity of FXR knockout mice to bile acid feeding, such experiments should be performed in intestinal-specific FXR knockout mice[29].

Regardless of these future experimental settings, FXR agonists stand as a potential new pharmacological tool to prevent or delay intestinal bacteria overgrowth and translocation. The pharmacological exploitation of FXR synthetic agonists is enormous, if one considers that the hydrophilic bile acid ursodeoxycholic acid is a very weak FXR agonist, while supplementation with hydrophobic bile acids would be extremely toxic, especially in conditions of intestinal bacterial overgrowth secondary to liver disease.

Would FXR agonists be helpful in the treatment and prevention of intestinal overgrowth in human conditions such as liver cirrhosis? The road is open, but a few obstacles are still there. One of the main questions is: how is FXR expression and function regulated in the intestinal villi?

Acknowledgements

The work described in this chapter has been generated with Takeshi Inagaki, Youn-Kyoung Lee, Li Peng, Guixiang Zhao, Michael Downes, Ruth T. Yu, John M. Shelton, James A. Richardson, and Joyce J. Repa, in the laboratories of David J. Mangelsdorf and Steven A. Kliewer. We thank members of the laboratory for critically reading the manuscript. This work was funded by the Italian Association for Cancer Research (AIRC, Milan, Italy), the University of Bari, Italy (ORBA07X7Q1, ORBA06BXVC), and the Fondazione Negri Sud, Santa Maria Imbaro, Italy. M.P. is a fellow of the Rosario Samanin Fund. We apologize to our distinguished colleagues that many primary references could not be included because of space limitation.

References

1. Hofmann AF. Biliary secretion and excretion in health and disease: current concepts. Ann Hepatol. 2007;6:15–27.
2. Xu J, Mahowald MA, Ley RE et al. Evolution of symbiotic bacteria in the distal human intestine. PLoS Biol. 2007;5:e156.
3. Wiest R, Garcia-Tsao G. Bacterial translocation (BT) in cirrhosis. Hepatology. 2005;41:422–33.
4. Floch MH, Gershengoren W, Elliott S, Spiro HM. Bile acid inhibition of the intestinal microflora – a function for simple bile acids? Gastroenterology. 1971;61:228–33.

5. Berg RD. Bacterial translocation from the gastrointestinal tract. Trends Microbiol. 1995;3:149–54.
6. Raedsch R, Stiehl A, Gundert-Remy U et al. Hepatic secretion of bilirubin and biliary lipids in patients with alcoholic cirrhosis of the liver. Digestion. 1983;26:80–8.
7. Lorenzo-Zuniga V, Bartoli R, Planas R et al. Oral bile acids reduce bacterial overgrowth, bacterial translocation, and endotoxemia in cirrhotic rats. Hepatology. 2003;37:551–7.
8. Binder HJ, Filburn B, Floch M. Bile acid inhibition of intestinal anaerobic organisms. Am J Clin Nutr. 1975;28:119–25.
9. Sung JY, Shaffer EA, Costerton JW. Antibacterial activity of bile salts against common biliary pathogens. Effects of hydrophobicity of the molecule and in the presence of phospholipids. Dig Dis Sci. 1993;38:2104–12.
10. Modica S, Moschetta A. Nuclear bile acid receptor FXR as pharmacological target: are we there yet? FEBS Lett. 2006;580:5492–9.
11. Forman BM, Goode E, Chen J et al. Identification of a nuclear receptor that is activated by farnesol metabolites. Cell. 1995;81:687–93.
12. Seol W, Choi HS, Moore DD. Isolation of proteins that interact specifically with the retinoid X receptor: two novel orphan receptors. Mol Endocrinol. 1995;9:72–85.
13. Makishima M, Okamoto AY, Repa JJ et al. Identification of a nuclear receptor for bile acids. Science. 1999;284:1362–5.
14. Parks DJ, Blanchard SG, Bledsoe RK et al. Bile acids: natural ligands for an orphan nuclear receptor. Science. 1999;284:1365–8.
15. Kok T, Hulzebos CV, Wolters H et al. Enterohepatic circulation of bile salts in farnesoid X receptor-deficient mice: efficient intestinal bile salt absorption in the absence of ileal bile acid-binding protein. J Biol Chem. 2003;278:41930–7.
16. Sinal CJ, Tohkin M, Miyata M, Ward JM, Lambert G, Gonzalez FJ. Targeted disruption of the nuclear receptor FXR/BAR impairs bile acid and lipid homeostasis. Cell. 2000;102:731–44.
17. Goodwin B, Jones SA, Price RR et al. A regulatory cascade of the nuclear receptors FXR, SHP-1, and LRH-1 represses bile acid biosynthesis. Mol Cell. 2000;6:517–26.
18. Lu TT, Makishima M, Repa JJ et al. Molecular basis for feedback regulation of bile acid synthesis by nuclear receptors. Mol Cell. 2000;6:507–15.
19. Ananthanarayanan M, Balasubramanian N, Makishima M, Mangelsdorf DJ, Suchy FJ. Human bile salt export pump promoter is transactivated by the farnesoid X receptor/bile acid receptor. J Biol Chem. 2001;276:28857–65.
20. Huang L, Zhao A, Lew JL et al. Farnesoid X receptor activates transcription of the phospholipid pump MDR3. J Biol Chem. 2003;278:51085–90.
21. Moschetta A, vanBerge-Henegouwen GP, Portincasa P, Palasciano G, Groen AK, van Erpecum KJ. Sphingomyelin exhibits greatly enhanced protection compared with egg yolk phosphatidylcholine against detergent bile salts. J Lipid Res. 2000;41:916–24.
22. Velardi AL, Groen AK, Elferink RP, van der MR, Palasciano G, Tytgat GN. Cell type-dependent effect of phospholipid and cholesterol on bile salt cytotoxicity. Gastroenterology. 1991;101:457–64.
23. Moschetta A, Bookout AL, Mangelsdorf DJ. Prevention of cholesterol gallstone disease by FXR agonists in a mouse model. Nat Med. 2004;10:1352–8.
24. Landrier JF, Eloranta JJ, Vavricka SR, Kullak-Ublick GA. The nuclear receptor for bile acids, FXR, transactivates human organic solute transporter-alpha and -beta genes. Am J Physiol Gastrointest Liver Physiol. 2006;290:G476–85.
25. Inagaki T, Choi M, Moschetta A et al. Fibroblast growth factor 15 functions as an enterohepatic signal to regulate bile acid homeostasis. Cell Metab. 2005;2:217–25.
26. Choi M, Moschetta A, Bookout AL et al. Identification of a hormonal basis for gallbladder filling. Nat Med. 2006;12:1253–5.
27. Inagaki T, Moschetta A, Lee YK et al. Regulation of antibacterial defense in the small intestine by the nuclear bile acid receptor. Proc Natl Acad Sci USA. 2006;103:3920–5.
28. Hofmann AF, Eckmann L. How bile acids confer gut mucosal protection against bacteria. Proc Natl Acad Sci USA. 2006;103:4333–4.
29. Kim I, Ahn SH, Inagaki T et al. Differential regulation of bile acid homeostasis by the farnesoid X receptor in liver and intestine. J Lipid Res. 2007;48:2664–72.
30. Nathan C. Inducible nitric oxide synthase: what difference does it make? J Clin Invest. 1997;100:2417–23.

31. Wallace JL, Miller MJ. Nitric oxide in mucosal defense: a little goes a long way. Gastroenterology. 2000;119:512–20.
32. Biet F, Locht C, Kremer L. Immunoregulatory functions of interleukin 18 and its role in defense against bacterial pathogens. J Mol Med. 2002;80:147–62.
33. Reuter BK, Pizarro TT. Commentary: The role of the IL-18 system and other members of the IL-1R/TLR superfamily in innate mucosal immunity and the pathogenesis of inflammatory bowel disease: friend or foe? Eur J Immunol. 2004;34:2347–55.
34. Hooper LV, Stappenbeck TS, Hong CV, Gordon JI. Angiogenins: a new class of microbicidal proteins involved in innate immunity. Nat Immunol. 2003;4:269–73.
35. Dyer KD, Rosenberg HF. The mouse RNase 4 and RNase 5/ang 1 locus utilizes dual promoters for tissue-specific expression. Nucl Acids Res. 2005;33:1077–86.
36. Halmi P, Lehtonen J, Waheed A, Sly WS, Parkkila S. Expression of hypoxia-inducible, membrane-bound carbonic anhydrase isozyme XII in mouse tissues. Anat Rec A Discov Mol Cell Evol Biol. 2004;277:171–7.

Section III
Cellular responses to chronic liver injury

Chair: D LEBREC and M PINZANI

9
The hepatic stellate cell: a progenitor cell

C. KORDES, I. SAWITZA and D. HÄUSSINGER

It is well known that isolated hepatic stellate cells (HSC) develop into myofibroblast-like cells during culture. These myofibroblast-like cells synthesize α-smooth muscle actin (α-SMA) and extracellular matrix proteins such as collagen type 1. Therefore, it is thought that HSC are involved in progression of liver fibrosis. Here we report that HSC are hitherto unrecognized progenitor cells of the liver. Freshly isolated HSC of rat liver displayed an active β-catenin-dependent Wnt signalling pathway and expressed the stem and progenitor cell marker CD133. This cell surface protein was used in the present study to select HSC by magnetic cell sorting after density gradient centrifugation. The selected CD133$^+$ HSC synthesized molecular markers of stem cells and displayed the expression pattern of endothelial progenitor cells as well as monocytes. CD133$^+$ HSC, which were cultured on plastic and treated with platelet-derived growth factor-BB (PDGF-BB), developed into α-SMA positive myofibroblast-like cells. However, if the CD133$^+$ HSC were cultured on collagen and treated with an appropriate cytokine cocktail, they differentiated into cells of hepatocyte or endothelial lineages. The cytokines fibroblast growth factor 4 (FGF$_4$), hepatocyte growth factor (HGF), basic fibroblast growth factor (bFGF), and interleukin-6 (IL-6) induced the hepatocyte markers α-fetoprotein (α-FP) and albumin in CD133$^+$ HSC. Endothelial cell markers such as endothelial nitric oxide synthase (eNOS) and vaso-endothelial cadherin (ve-CAD/CD144) were induced after treatment of CD133$^+$ HSC with vascular endothelial growth factor 164 (VEGF$_{164}$), bFGF, erythropoietin (EPO), and IL-6. In addition, these cytokines led to the formation of branched tube-like structures. Cells that formed these tubes synthesized numb similar to freshly isolated HSC. The presence of stem and progenitor cell markers, as well as β-catenin-dependent Wnt signalling in HSC, clearly indicates that stellate cells are undifferentiated cells of the vertebrate liver. These findings, in conjunction with the capability of HSC to differentiate into hepatocyte- or endothelial-like cells and to form tube-like structures, points towards an important function of stellate cells in liver regeneration.

HSC are vitamin A-storing cells of the liver[1,2], which are important for the hepatic wound-healing response. Following liver injury HSC become activated, lose their vitamin A stores, mainly consisting of retinyl palmitate, and develop a myofibroblast-like phenotype. These myofibroblasts produce α-SMA, become contractile, and synthesize extracellular matrix proteins such as collagens[3]. It is widely accepted that these properties of myofibroblast-like cells contribute to the pathogenesis of liver fibrosis and portal hypertension.

Stellate cells synthesize the filamentous proteins desmin[4] and glial fibrillary acidic protein (GFAP)[5], as well as several proteins typical for neuronal cells[6]. These proteins occur in cells of different embryonic germ layers, the mesoderm and ectoderm. The expression of ectodermal markers led to the hypothesis that stellate cells may originate from the neural crest. While this hypothesis was disproved recently[7], the gene expression of the endodermal protein cytokeratin 18 was also described for HSC[8]. The synthesis of elements of all three embryonic germ layers makes it difficult to give a final judgement about the origin of stellate cells. The finding that HSC can derive from the bone marrow[9,10] adds a new aspect to this topic. If HSC can originate from the bone marrow the question arises of whether HSC are already differentiated or still undifferentiated cells. An important feature of undifferentiated stem/progenitor cells is an active canonical Wnt signalling pathway via β-catenin. This signalling pathway is crucial for the maintenance of stem/progenitor cell characteristics. During investigation of the canonical Wnt signalling we observed a marked nuclear staining of β-catenin in freshly isolated HSC, indicating active canonical Wnt signalling (manuscript in preparation). Moreover, we detected the paired-like homeodomain transcription factor 2 isoform c (PITX2c)[11]. PITX2 is one of the target genes of β-catenin dependent Wnt signalling[12]. Interestingly, the PITX2c isoform appears in early haematopoietic stem/progenitor cells and its expression declines during their differentiation[13]. Both the active canonical Wnt signalling and the occurrence of PITX2c led us to test the hypothesis of whether HSC are stem or progenitor cells. To address this issue we searched for protein markers suitable to identify stem/progenitor cells and discovered that HSC express CD133 (AC133/prominin 1)[11]. The cellular function of the cell surface protein CD133 is unknown thus far, but it was found in somatic stem cells such as haematopoietic stem/progenitor cells[14,15].

The cell surface protein CD133 was detected by immunostaining in freshly isolated HSC after 1 day of culture (Figure 1A, B). The expression of CD133 was further verified by reverse transcriptase–polymerase chain reaction (RT-PCR; Figure 1C). The mature CD133 protein was identified by Western blot as a single band with approximately 120 kDa in cell membrane fractions obtained by the CNM Compartment Protein Isolation Kit (BioCat, Heidelberg, Germany) (Figure 1D). The unprocessed CD133 protein (about 99 kDa) was mainly detected in whole cell lysates of HSC[11]. CD133 was primarily synthesized by freshly isolated HSC, but its expression was also ascertained in cultured HSC that developed into myofibroblast-like cells (Figure 1C, D).

The occurrence of CD133 on the cell surface of HSC enabled us to further purify stellate cells by specific antibodies (2 µg/ml biotinylated CD133 antibody; Ancell, Bayport, MN, USA) and subsequent magnetic cell sorting

THE HEPATIC STELLATE CELL: A PROGENITOR CELL

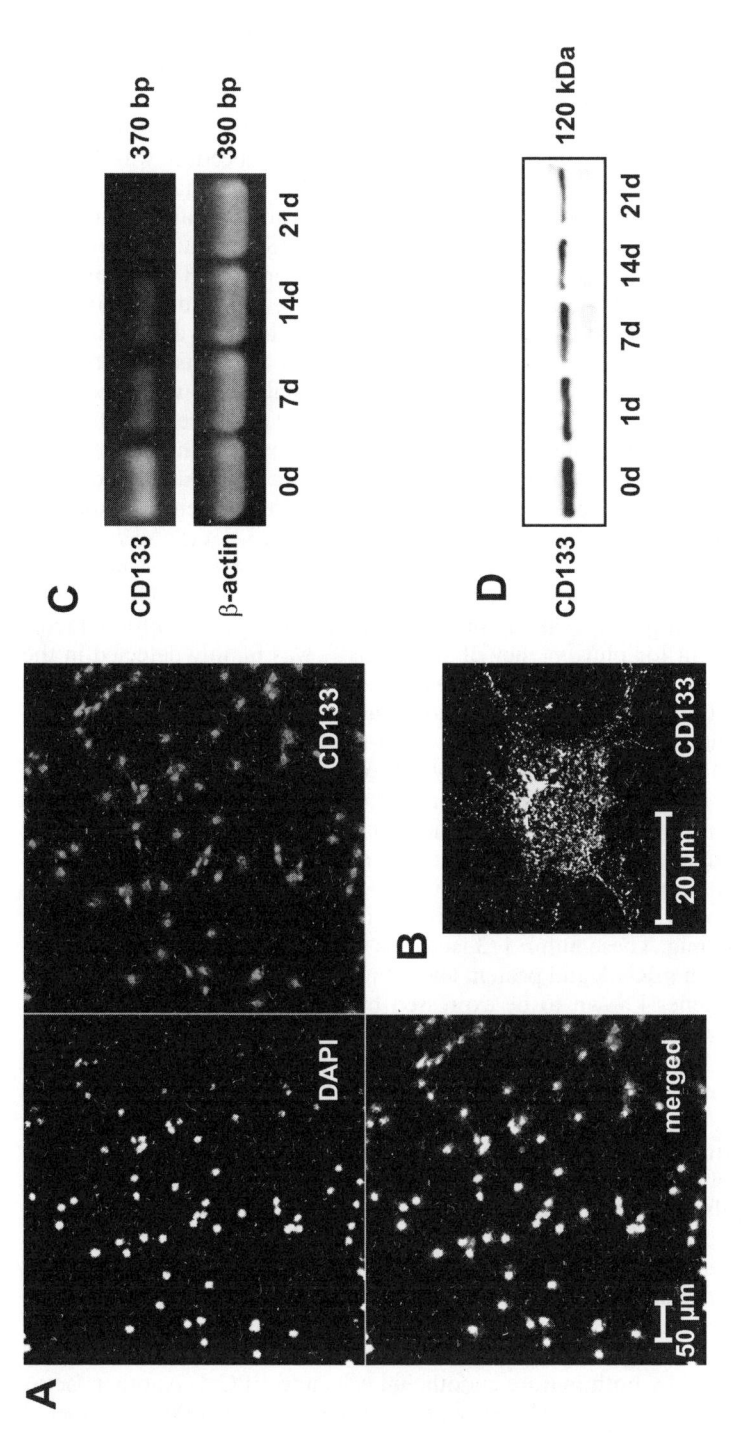

Figure 1 HSC express CD133 as investigated by immunofluorescence staining, RT-PCR, and Western blot. **A**: An overview of freshly isolated HSC cultured for 1 day. All HSC synthesized CD133 as indicated by simultaneous DAPI and CD133 labelling. **B**: A detailed fluorescence image of a single HSC, which was cultured for 1 day prior to staining with antibodies against CD133. **C**: The expression of CD133 was analysed by RT-PCR in a time-series of cultured HSC. **D**: The mature CD133 protein was detected by Western blot in cell membrane fractions of HSC during a culture period of 21 days

(EasySep cell separation kit, biotin; StemCell Technologies, Vancouver, Canada)[11]. Prior to cell sorting, HSC of male Wistar rats (500–600 g body weight) were enriched by density gradient centrifugation (8% Nycodenz, Axis-Shield, Oslo, Norway) essentially as described by Hendriks and colleagues[2]. About 60% of total HSC that survived the cell sorting procedure was selected by this method. The purity of the CD133$^+$ cells was analysed by cell morphology. The cells displayed stellate-shaped morphology and perinuclear lipid droplets typically observed in freshly isolated HSC of rats (Figure 2A). RT-PCR was also used to test the uniformity of selected HSC. Molecular markers such as α-SMA, elastin, eNOS, ve-CAD, stabilin 2, scavenger receptor F1 (SCARF1), C-type lectin 13, α-FP, albumin, and multidrug resistance protein 2 (MRP2), which are expressed by fibroblasts, endothelial cells, Kupffer cells, or hepatocytes (liver parenchymal cells), were absent in CD133$^+$ HSC (Figure 2B). This indicated a high purity of the cell selections.

The CD133$^+$ HSC exhibited lipid droplets that contained retinyl palmitate as measured by high-performance liquid chromatography (11). Furthermore, the selected CD133$^+$ HSC expressed the stellate cell marker proteins desmin and GFAP (Figure 3). These features proved that the CD133$^+$ cells were in fact stellate cells. In addition to CD133, the selected HSC expressed molecular markers of stem cells such as the octamer binding factor 4 (OCT4/POU domain class 5 transcription factor 1; Figure 3). The transcription factor OCT4, important for pluripotency of stem cells[16], was mainly detected in the cell nuclei of CD133$^+$ HSC that contained typical lipid droplets (Figure 4A, B). In contrast to this, the transcription factor nanog (Tir nan Og, land of the ever-young in Celtic mythology), also involved in sustaining pluripotency of stem cells[17,18], was found on protein level only without a distinct nuclear localization as expected[11]. Important for the maintenance of self-renewal and pluripotency of embryonic stem cells is the β-catenin-dependent canonical Wnt signalling pathway[19]. The nuclear staining of β-catenin in CD133$^+$ HSC indicated active canonical Wnt signalling (Figure 4C). Other factors involved in maintaining stem cell characteristics are the isoforms 1/3 of numb[20], which is an inhibitor of notch signalling. These numb 1/3 isoforms were detected in freshly isolated CD133$^+$ HSC on mRNA and protein level (Figures 3 and 4D).

Additional genes known to be expressed by stem/progenitor cells such as breast cancer resistance protein 1 (BCRP1/ATP-binding cassette transporter G2, ABCG2), PITX2c, and stem cell growth factor (SCGF) were also detected by RT-PCR analysis in freshly isolated CD133$^+$ HSC (Figure 3). Apart from CD133, the selected HSC exhibited the mRNA of bone morphogenetic protein-binding endothelial regulator (BMPER/crossveinless 2), CD31 (platelet endothelial cell adhesion molecule 1, PECAM1), fetal-like kinase 1 (FLK1/vascular endothelial growth factor receptor 2, VEGFR2), Lim only 2 (LMO2), runt-related transcription factor 1 (RUNX1), and angiopoietin receptor 1 precursor (TIE2; Figure 3). All these factors are known to occur in endothelial progenitor cells (EPC)[21–23]. EPC are negative for molecular markers of mature endothelial cells such as eNOS and ve-CAD, but their expression is induced during EPC differentiation[24]. An exception is CD31; this gene is expressed by both mature endothelial cells and EPC[23]. Another factor synthesized by undifferentiated cells with the potential to develop endothelial

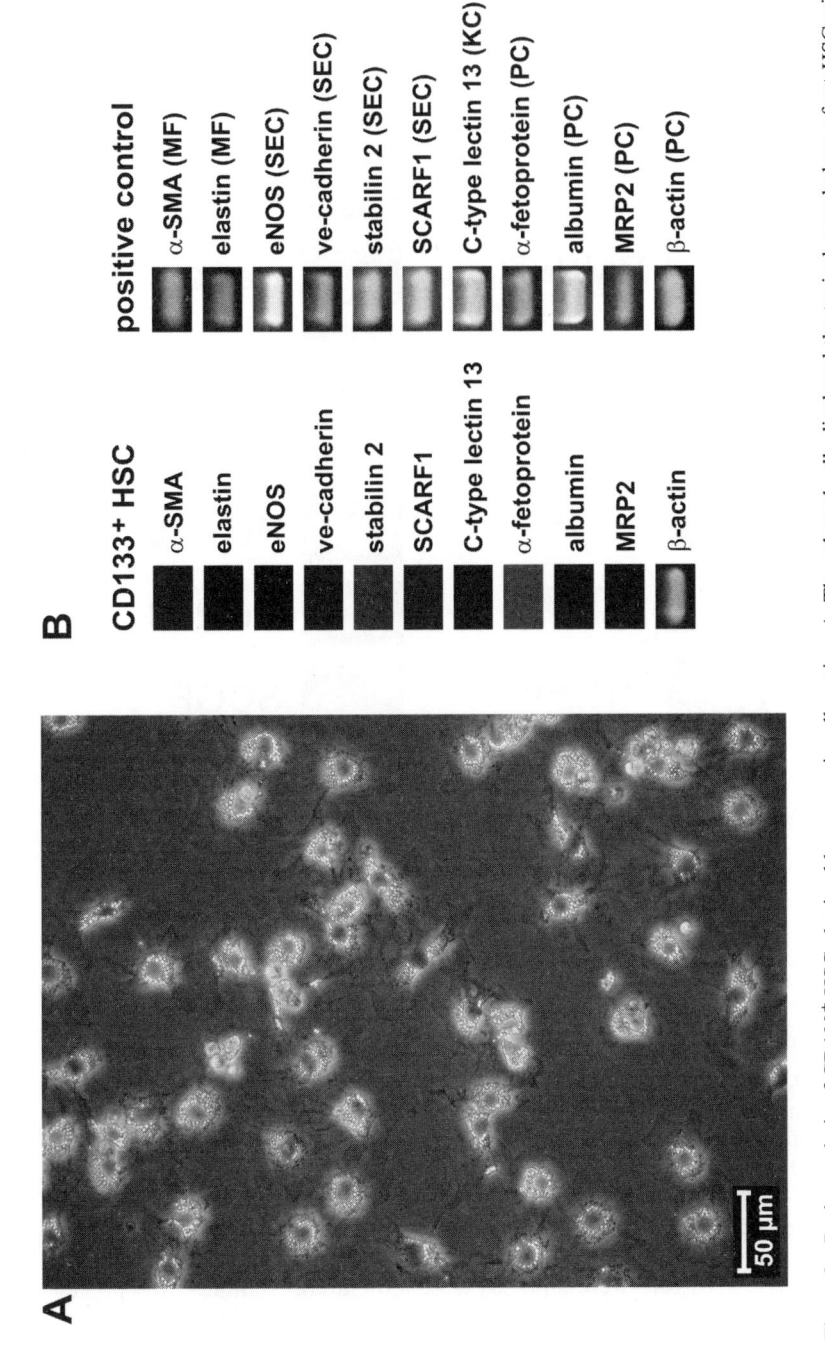

Figure 2 Purity analysis of CD133[+] HSC obtained by magnetic cell sorting. **A**: The selected cells displayed the typical morphology of rat HSC with perinuclear lipid droplets as documented by this phase contrast microscopic picture after 1 day of culture. **B**: RT-PCR analysis of freshly isolated CD133[+] HSC (0 days) was used to approve the cell purity. Differentiated cells such as muscle fibroblasts (MF), sinusoidal endothelial cells (SEC), Kupffer cells (KC), and hepatocytes (liver parenchymal cells, PC) served as a positive control for the molecular markers analysed

CD133+ HSC

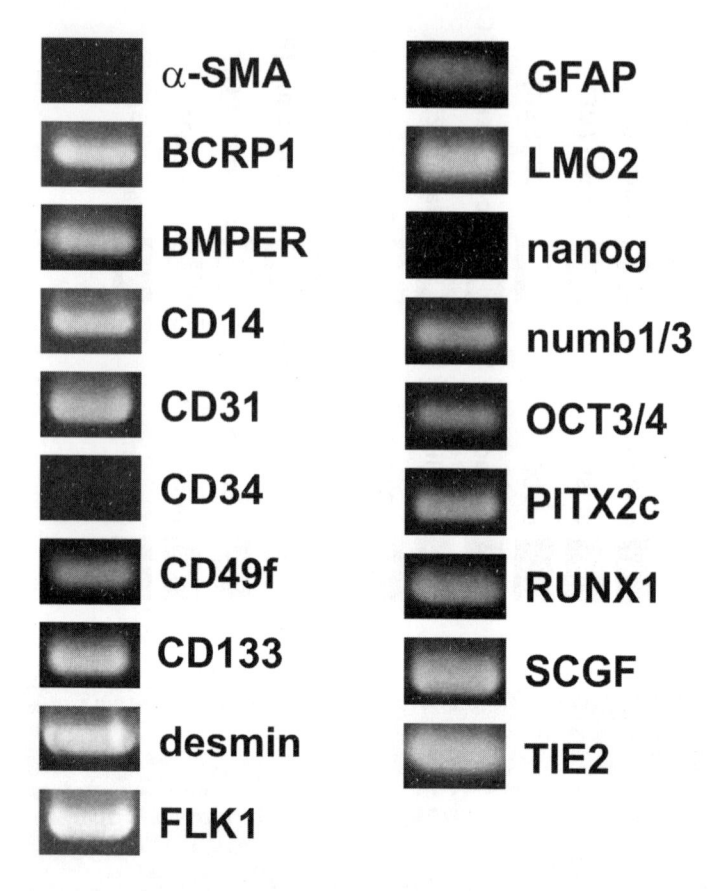

Figure 3 The expression pattern of freshly isolated CD133+ HSC. Molecular markers of HSC, stem/progenitor cells, and myeloid cells were investigated by RT-PCR immediately after magnetic cell sorting

cells is CD14[25,26]. The expression of the monocyte marker CD14 by HSC is already known[27]. CD14 was detected in CD133+ HSC (Figure 3), indicating a relation of HSC to cells of the haematopoietic system. This view was assured by the CD49f (integrin α6) synthesis of CD133+ HSC (Figure 3). CD49f is expressed by stem cells and cells of the myeloid lineage. Interestingly, the haematopoietic marker CD34, already described for HSC of the fetal liver[28], was not expressed by freshly selected CD133+ HSC. EPC characterized by CD34−/CD133+/FLK1+ were reported to be more undifferentiated and potent with respect to homing and vascular repair than their CD34+ counterpart[29].

The expression profile of CD133+ HSC, similar to stem and progenitor cells, indicated a high differentiation potential of stellate cells. Therefore, we tested whether they can give rise to other cell types after exposure to different cytokines known to initiate differentiation of stem cells. First, the CD133⁺ HSC were cultured with medium containing 10% fetal calf serum (FCS) and 20 ng/ml PDGF-BB (Sigma, Taufkirchen, Germany) on plastic for 7 days. The HSC developed into α-SMA-positive myofibroblast-like cells with decreased lipid stores and increased cell size (Figure 4E–G), a well-known behaviour of isolated HSC cultured on plastic. The expression of CD133 and FLK1 declined under these culture conditions and marker proteins of mature endothelial cells (i.e. eNOS, ve-CAD) or hepatocytes (i.e. α-FP, albumin) were detected neither in freshly isolated CD133⁺ HSC nor in myofibroblast-like cells. The expression of the haematopoietic cell marker CD34 increased during cultivation and myofibroblast formation (Figure 4F). At present the relevance of elevated CD34 expression in cultured stellate cells is unknown, but it might indicate first signs of cell maturation or differentiation.

CD133⁺ HSC were also cultured on thick self-made collagen from rat tail and treated with medium containing 10% FCS, 50 ng/ml FGF$_4$ (R&D Systems, Minneapolis, MN, USA), 40 ng/ml HGF (Abcam, Cambridge, UK), 50 ng/ml bFGF (Sigma), and 10 ng/ml interleukin 6 (IL-6) (Sigma) to investigate whether these cells can differentiate into hepatocytes. Selected cells reduced their lipid stores, started to proliferate, and within 4–7 days rotund cells appeared (Figure 4H). The cytokine treatment induced the mRNA synthesis of α-FP, albumin (Figure 4I), and MRP2[11]. The expression of these markers significantly increased after 14 days of cytokine treatment (not shown). The rotund cells synthesized α-FP as investigated by immunofluorescence staining (Figure 4J). These findings indicated that hepatocyte-like cells developed from CD133⁺ HSC. Under this culture condition, suitable to promote differentiation of stem cells into the hepatocyte lineage, the expression of CD133 and FLK1 decreased and molecular markers of endothelial cells (i.e. eNOS, ve-CAD) and myofibroblasts (i.e. α-SMA) remained undetectable.

In a third approach, CD133⁺ HSC were cultured on collagen and treated with medium containing 12% FCS (FCS for endothelial cell differentiation; StemCell Technologies), 50 ng/ml VEGF$_{164}$ (R&D Systems), 20 ng/ml bFGF, 10 ng/ml EPO (Sigma), and 10 ng/ml IL-6. These cytokines, known to promote differentiation of EPC into endothelial cells, caused a reduction of cellular lipid inclusions and subsequent cell proliferation. Between days 5 and 7 of cytokine treatment the HSC started to migrate and finally formed branched tube-like structures (Figure 4K). The expression of CD133 remained detectable after tube formation. The FLK1 mRNA synthesis was sustained and the gene expression of eNOS, ve-CAD (Figure 4L), stabilin 2, and SCARF1[11] was induced under these culture conditions. Stabilin 2 and SCARF1 are both involved in cellular uptake of macromolecules and are typical elements of endothelial cells also present in sinusoidal endothelial cells[30,31]. The induction of these endothelial cell markers indicated that endothelial-like cells developed from CD133⁺ HSC. Moreover, cells that surrounded tubular structures were able to take up fluorescent acetylated low-density lipoprotein (DIL-AC-LDL; 2.5 μg/ml, Biogenesis, Poole, UK; Figure 4M), a typical feature of endothelial cells. In contrast to this, DIL-AC-LDL was not incorporated by freshly isolated CD133⁺ HSC and myofibroblast-like cells (not shown). The myofibroblast

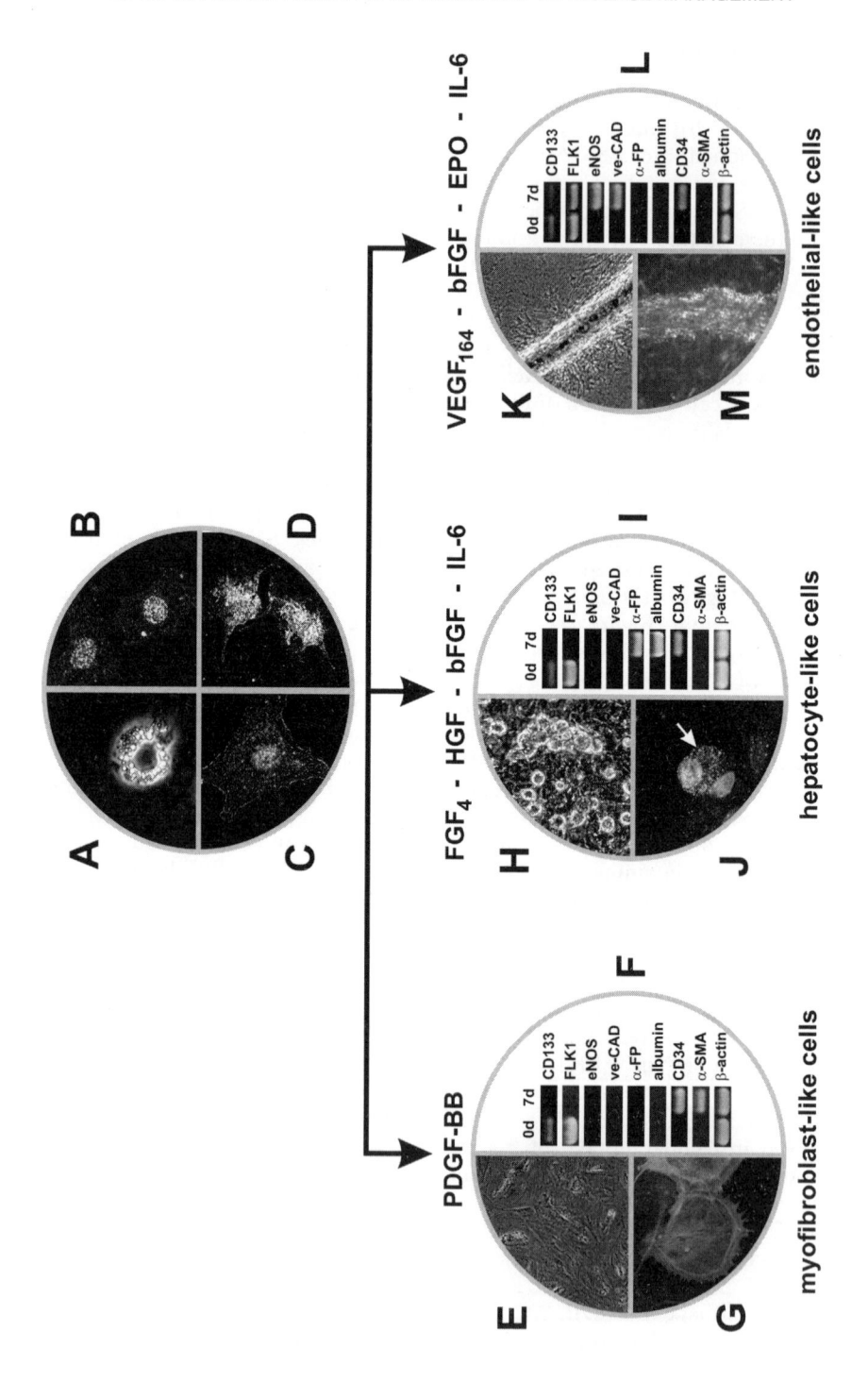

LIVER CIRRHOSIS: FROM PATHOPHYSIOLOGY TO DISEASE MANAGEMENT

Figure 4 The differentiation potential of CD133+ HSC. Selected CD133+ HSC displayed **A**: the typical cell morphology of stellate cells as well as a nuclear localization of **B**: OCT4 and **C**: β-catenin as investigated by immunofluorescence staining after 1 day of culture. **D**: These freshly isolated CD133+ HSC were also positively stained with antibodies against numb. The selected HSC were treated with three experimental media designed to facilitate their development into myofibroblast-, hepatocyte-, or enothelial-like cells. **E-G**: The culture medium was supplemented with PDGF-BB to promote the formation of myofibroblast-like cells in plastic culture dishes. **E**: Phase contrast microscopic image of myofibroblast-like cells derived from CD133+ HSC after 7 days of culture. **F**: CD133+ HSC were lysed for RT-PCR analysis directly after cell selection (0 days) and 7 days of culture (7d). **G**: The synthesis of α-SMA by myofibroblast-like cells that derived from CD133+ HSC was verified by immunofluorescence staining after 7 days of culture. **H-J**: The selected CD133+ HSC were cultured on collagen and treated with FGF$_4$, bFGF, HGF, and IL-6. **(H)** Phase contrast microscopic image of rotund cells that appeared after 7 days. **I**: The gene expression was analysed by RT-PCR in freshly isolated CD133+ HSC and after treatment with FGF$_4$, bFGF, HGF, and IL-6 for 7 days. **J**: The hepatocyte marker α-FP (spotted grey) was detected by immunofluorescence staining in rotund cells (white arrow). The cell nuclei were labelled by DAPI staining (pale grey). **K-M**: CD133+ HSC were also cultured with medium containing VEGF$_{164}$, bFGF, EPO, and IL-6 on collagen. **K**: These cytokines led to the formation of tube-like structures within 7 days of culture as documented by this phase contrast microscopic image. **L**: RT-PCR analysis of freshly isolated and cultured CD133+ HSC. The selected HSC were treated with VEGF$_{164}$, bFGF, EPO, and IL-6 for 7 days. **M**: Cells that surrounded tube-like structures were able to take up fluorescent DiI-Ac-LDL

marker α-SMA and the hepatocyte markers α-FP and albumin remained undetectable during tube formation (Figure 4L). However, the tubular structures that initially displayed discontinuous cavities were unstable and developed into islet-like structures when the cytokines were applied for 14 days (not shown). The tubes were formed by cells that synthesized numb-like freshly isolated CD133$^+$ HSC as investigated by immunofluorescence staining. The islet-like structures were covered by numb-positive cells and harboured numb-negative cells inside (not shown). The expression of numb and the transient appearance of tubes indicate that the tube formation is rather a feature of immature or undifferentiated cells. Similar tubular structures were described in regenerating liver tissue. This so-called ductular reaction is thought to represent a stem cell response[32]. The tube formation by CD133$^+$ HSC and their potential to differentiate into endothelial- and hepatocyte-like cells suggest an important function of stellate cells in liver regeneration. However, the expression of pluripotency-sustaining factors by HSC, such as OCT4 and nanog, indicate an even higher differentiation potential of stellate cells. On the other hand CD133$^+$ HSC possess properties of determined cells, because they exhibited the typical expression pattern of EPC and haematopoietic cells. Indeed, EPC and haematopoietic cells are related cell types, because they both derive from common precursor cells, the haemangioblasts, during early embryogenesis of vertebrates.

As shown in this study, HSC express the stem cell marker CD133 and exhibit a gene expression pattern of EPC and of cells that derived from the haematopoietic system. Our findings demonstrate that CD133$^+$ HSC are obviously undifferentiated cells with the potential to develop into myofibroblast-, hepatocyte-, or endothelial-like cells *in vitro*. Thus CD133$^+$ HSC represent not-yet-recognized progenitor cells of the vertebrate liver, and obviously fulfil functions beyond participation in liver fibrogenesis.

Acknowledgements

We are grateful to Claudia Rupprecht for her excellent technical assistance. This work was supported by the Collaborative Research Center 575 'Experimental Hepatology' (Deutsche Forschungsgemeinschaft SFB575) and the Research Commission of the Medical Faculty of the Heinrich–Heine University Düsseldorf.

References

1. Wake K. Sternzellen in the liver: perisinusoidal cells with special reference to storage of vitamin A. Am J Anat. 1971;132:429–62.
2. Hendriks HFJ, Verhoofstad WA, Brouwer A, DeLeeuw AM, Knook DL. Perisinusoidal fat-storing cells are the main vitamin A storage sites in rat liver. Exp Cell Res. 1985;160:138–49.
3. Friedman SL. Molecular regulation of hepatic fibrosis, an integrated cellular response to tissue injury. J Biol Chem. 2000;275:2247–50.
4. Yokoi Y, Namihisa T, Kuroda H et al. Immunocytochemical detection of desmin in fat-storing cells (Ito cells). Hepatology 1984;4:709-14.

5. Gard A, White F, Dutton G. Extra-neural glial fibrillary acidic protein (GFAP) immunoreactivity in perisinusoidal stellate cells of rat liver. J Neuroimmunol. 1985;8:359–75.
6. Geerts A. History, heterogeneity, developmental biology, and functions of quiescent hepatic stellate cells. Semin Liver Dis. 2001;21:311–35.
7. Cassiman D, Barlow A, Borght SV, Libbrecht L, Pachnis V. Hepatic stellate cells do not derive from the neural crest. J Hepatol. 2006;44:1098–104.
8. Lim Y-S, Kim K-A, Jung J-O et al. Modulation of cytokeratin expression during in vitro cultivation of human hepatic stellate cells: evidence of transdifferentiation from epithelial to mesenchymal phenotype. Histochem Cell Biol. 2002;118:127–36.
9. Baba S, Fujii H, Hirose T et al. Commitment of bone marrow cells to hepatic stellate cells in mouse. J Hepatol. 2004;40:255–60.
10. Russo FP, Alison MR, Bigger BW et al. The bone marrow functionally contributes to liver fibrosis. Gastroenterology. 2006;130:1807–21.
11. Kordes C, Sawitza I, Müller-Marbach A et al. CD133+ hepatic stellate cells are progenitor cells. Biochem Biophys Res Commun. 2007;352:410–17.
12. Kioussi C, Briata P, Baek SH et al. Identification of a Wnt/Dvl/beta-catenin–Pitx2 pathway mediating cell-type-specific proliferation during development. Cell. 2002;111:673–85.
13. Degar BA, Baskaran N, Hulspas R, Quesenberry PJ, Weissman SM, Forget BG. The homeodomain gene Pitx2 is expressed in primitive hematopoietic stem/progenitor cells but not in their differentiated progeny. Exp Hematol. 2001;29:894–.902.
14. Yin AH, Miraglia S, Zanjani ED et al. AC133, a novel marker for human hematopoietic stem and progenitor cells. Blood. 1997;90:5002–12.
15. Kania G, Corbeil D, Fuchs J et al. Somatic stem cell marker prominin-1/CD133 is expressed in embryonic stem cell-derived progenitors. Stem Cells. 2005;23:791–804.
16. Niwa H. Molecular mechanism to maintain stem cell renewal of ES cells. Cell Struct Funct. 2001;26:137–48.
17. Chambers I, Colby D, Robertson M et al. Functional expression cloning of Nanog, a pluripotency sustaining factor in embryonic stem cells. Cell. 2003;113;643–55.
18. Chambers I. The molecular basis of pluripotency in mouse embryonic stem cells. Cloning Stem Cells. 2004;6:386–91.
19. Sato N, Meijer L, Skaltsounis L, Greengard P, Brivanlou AH. Maintenance of pluripotency in human and mouse embryonic stem cells through activation of Wnt signaling by a pharmacological GSK-3-specific inhibitor. Nat Med. 2004;10:55–63.
20. Bani-Yaghoub M, Kubu CJ, Cowling R et al. A switch in numb isoforms is a critical step in cortical development. Dev Dyn. 2007;236:696–705.
21. Moser M, Binder O, Wu Y et al. BMPER, a novel endothelial cell precursor-derived protein antagonizes bone morphogenetic protein signaling and endothelial cell differentiation. Mol Cell Biol. 2003;23:5664–79.
22. Asahara T, Murohara T, Sullivan AK et al. Isolation of putative progenitor endothelial cells for angiogenesis. Science. 1997;275:964–7.
23. Urbich C, Heeschen C, Aicher A, Dernbach E, Zeiher AM, Dimmeler S. Relevance of monocytic features for neovascularization capacity of circulating endothelial progenitor cells. Circulation. 2003;108:2511–16.
24. Hristov M, Weber C. Endothelial progenitor cells: characterization, pathophysiology, and possible clinical relevance. J Cell Mol Med. 2004;8:498–508.
25. Harraz M, Jiao C, Hanlon HD, Hartley RS, Schatteman GC. CD34− blood-derived human endothelial cell progenitors. Stem Cells. 2001;19:304–12.
26. Romagnani P, Annunziato F, Liotta F et al. CD14+CD34^{low} cells with stem cell phenotypic and functional features are the major source of circulating endothelial progenitors. Circ Res. 2005;97:314–22.
27. Paik YH, Schwabe RF, Bataller R, Russo MP, Jobin C, Brenner DA. Toll-like receptor 4 mediates inflammatory signaling by bacterial lipopolysaccharide in human hepatic stellate cells. Hepatology. 2003;37:1043–55.
28. Suskind DL, Muench MO. Searching for common stem cells of the hepatic and hematopoietic systems in the human fetal liver: CD34+ cytokeratin 7/8+ cells express markers for stellate cells. J Hepatol. 2004;40:261–8.

29. Friedrich EB, Walenta K, Scharlau J, Nickenig G, Werner N. CD34$^-$/CD133$^+$/VEGFR-2$^+$ endothelial progenitor cell subpopulation with potent vasoregenerative capacities. Circ Res. 2006;98:e20–5.
30. Adachi H, Tsujimoto M, Arai H, Inoue K. Expression and cloning of novel scavenger receptor from human endothelial cells. J Biol Chem. 1997;272:31217–20.
31. Enomoto K, Nishikawa Y, Omori Y et al. Cell biology and pathology of liver sinusoidal endothelial cells. Med Electron Microsc. 2004;37:208–15.
32. Forbes SJ, Vig P, Poulsom R, Thomas H, Alison MR. Hepatic stem cells. J Pathol. 2002;197:510–18.

10
Role of non-parenchymal cells in portal hypertension

R. C. HUEBERT and V. H. SHAH

PORTAL HYPERTENSION

Chronic liver disease and its associated complications are increasing in frequency, due in large part to rising rates of obesity and the hepatitis C epidemic. Cirrhosis is the final common pathway in chronic liver disease and a syndrome of increased portal pressure is the final common pathway in all aetiologies of cirrhosis. Ohm's law (pressure = flow × resistance) describes portal pressure mathematically as a function of the portal inflow and the resistance across the portal vasculature. The pathophysiology of portal hypertension is complex, involving alterations in both flow and resistance. Increases in portal inflow are largely the result of systemic vasodilation, decreased systemic vascular resistance, and a resultant hyperdynamic circulation. Changes in intrahepatic resistance occur via mechanical changes involving not only fibrosis of the parenchyma, but also vascular factors including altered vasoreactivity and pathological vascular remodelling. Importantly, while fibrosis may be a dynamic process, vascular factors are thought to be more reversible, are attractive targets for pharmacological intervention, and may be responsible for 25% or more of the increases in resistance. This chapter addresses the specific roles of, and interplay between liver sinusoidal endothelial cells (LEC) and hepatic stellate cells (HSC) in the development of portal hypertension, and identifies several key signalling pathways and mechanisms thought to contribute. Specifically discussed are the roles of nitric oxide (NO) and endothelin (ET) signalling in altering hepatic vasoreactivity, and the role of platelet-derived growth factor (PDGF) signalling in pericyte recruitment and vascular remodelling.

NON-PARENCHYMAL LIVER CELLS

The hepatic parenchyma consists of hepatocytes and cholangiocytes, the epithelial cells that line the intrahepatic bile ducts. The remaining cell types within the liver are considered non-parenchymal. Two particularly important cell types are discussed here: LEC and HSC.

Liver sinusoidal endothelial cells

The hepatic sinusoids are situated between the hepatocyte plates and separated from them by the perisinusoidal space of Disse. They carry a mixture of portal venous and hepatic arterial blood from their origin at the portal tracts to their termination at the central vein. LEC are a distinct subpopulation of cells lining these sinusoids. They are morphologically unique in their multiple fenestrae and the lack of a basement membrane. Their anatomical location makes them the first intrahepatic cells to contact portal blood flow and thus LEC are uniquely situated to interact quickly with vasoregulatory mediators. Additionally, LEC are in intimate contact with other cell types including HSC, allowing complex paracrine signalling mechanisms.

Hepatic stellate cells

HSC are liver-specific pericytes that are well established as vitamin A-storing cells in the quiescent state and collagen-producing cells following activation. However, they are being increasingly recognized in diverse hepatic vascular processes, both normal and pathological, including roles in vascular development, vessel stability, vasoregulation, pathological vascular remodelling, and the pathogenesis of portal hypertension and tumour angiogenesis. In the normal liver HSC are vascular mural cells in intimate contact with the endothelium that are important for retinoid storage and vascular development and stabilization. In chronic liver disease HSC acquire an 'activated' phenotype, which includes increased contractility, migration, proliferation, and fibrogenesis. Increases in contractility are of key importance in the pathogenesis of portal hypertension and are discussed in detail below. HSC locomotion and proliferation are of fundamental importance in several disease processes, including portal hypertension, tumour angiogenesis, and hepatic fibrogenesis, and these topics are discussed here as well as in other chapters.

NITRIC OXIDE

One of the major phenotypic changes in LEC during portal hypertension includes alteration of the NO generation system that results in a regional NO deficiency. Deficient NO generation, coupled with other changes that reduce its local effect, results in a myriad of downstream alterations in both LEC and HSC. NO is a hydrophobic gas that diffuses freely across cellular membranes and can have both autocrine and paracrine signalling effects on LEC and HSC, respectively. It is generated by the enzyme nitric oxide sythase (NOS) during the conversion of arginine to citrulline. Three isoforms exist: the endothelial (eNOS), inducible (iNOS), and neuronal (nNOS) forms. eNOS is constitutively expressed by LEC and is thought to be chiefly responsible for regulating sinusoidal vascular tone. In the normal liver, increased portal inflow creates a shear stress to the LEC and a subsequent increase in production of NO. The NO generated within LEC acts in a paracrine fashion upon adjacent HSC via activation of soluble guanylyl cyclase, cGMP accumulation, activation of protein kinase G, and ultimately results in HSC relaxation. This process results in a local vasodilation effect which serves to autoregulate hepatic resistance and portal pressure. In cirrhotic states, changes at multiple levels within LEC disrupt this system and reduce the amount of eNOS-derived NO. While eNOS protein levels appear to be unchanged, there is an increase in eNOS binding by the inhibitory protein caveolin. Additionally, Akt phosphorylation and activation of eNOS is impaired in cirrhosis. In animal models of cirrhosis there is significantly less phosphorylated eNOS in the liver, but transduction of a constitutively active Akt can restore eNOS activity and reduce portal pressures. In addition to reduced local levels of NO, defects in the guanylyl cyclase system appear to make HSC resistant to NO-mediated relaxation in cirrhosis. HSC in cirrhotic states thus become more contractile, having important consequences on total hepatic vascular resistance and contributing to the development of portal hypertension. NO is an attractive therapeutic target in the treatment of portal hypertension and the study of several experimental approaches is ongoing, including strategies for the activation of hepatic eNOS, liver-specific NO donors, and others.

ENDOTHELIN-1

The endothelin family of proteins are potent vasoconstrictors that have been implicated in vasoregulatory phenomena in both myocardial and cerebral vascular tissues. These proteins are synthesized and released from endothelial cells and act via receptor–ligand interactions with G-protein-coupled receptors on multiple cell types, including pericytes. As with NOS, three endothelin isoforms are known, but one isoform (ET-1) appears to play a prominent role in the liver. Luminal ET-1 release gives detectable serum levels of the protein, whereas abluminal release towards the contractile cell types allows for a local, paracrine, contractile effect. ET-1 binds to two endothelin receptor subtypes (ET-A and ET-B). Binding of the ET-1 ligand to the ET-A receptor results in the intracellular release of calcium stores, activation of protein kinase C (PKC) and, ultimately, a contractile effect. Signalling mediated by the ET-B receptor is more complex, affecting LEC in an autocrine fashion with a paradoxical increase in eNOS activation, but is also capable of mediating the traditional contractile response in HSC. The role of ET-1-mediated vasoconstriction in portal hypertension is supported by multiple lines of evidence. In human serum there is an increase in the detectable levels of ET-1 in patients with portal hypertension. Furthermore, in animal models of hepatic fibrosis, such as carbon tetrachloride (CCl_4) feeding and bile duct ligation (BDL), LEC have increased levels of ET-1. An increase in ET-1 mRNA within HSC also suggests an autocrine effect within these cells. Blocking the ET-A receptor with the antagonist BQ-123 prevents the increase in intrahepatic resistance in BDL rats. However, administration of the combined ET-A/ET-B antagonist, RO 48-5695, does not improve portal haemodynamics in portal hypertensive rats. As such, further study of the binding kinetics and downstream effects of these receptor subtypes is needed before modulation of this pathway can result in effective therapies.

PLATELET-DERIVED GROWTH FACTOR

PDGF is a mitogen and chemotactic factor for many cell types including fibroblasts, vascular smooth muscle cells, mesangial cells, and glial cells. It is, in fact, the single most potent stellate cell mitogen currently identified, and also appears to be the most critical growth factor in pericyte recruitment during vascular remodelling. PDGF exists as a dimeric protein that can form homodimers or heterodimers. Two PDGF polypeptide subunits, A and B, have been most extensively studied and can form homodimers or heterodimers. The recently identified C and D polypeptides form only homodimers. Five distinct ligand isoforms can thus form (PDGF-AA, PDGF-BB, PDGF-CC, PDGF-DD, and PDGF-AB). The PDGF receptors (PDGFR) exist as homodimers or heterodimers of two ~ 180 kDa, transmembrane, receptor tyrosine kinases, α and β. Thus three distinct receptor complexes can form (PDGFR-$\alpha\alpha$, PDGRF-$\beta\beta$, and PDGFR-$\alpha\beta$). The interactions and biological effects of the various PDGF and PDGFR isoforms are complex and variable among different cell types. A pathophysiological role for PDGFR signalling has been demonstrated in several fibrogenic disorders including pulmonary fibrosis, glomerulonephritis, atherosclerosis, and liver fibrosis. In cirrhotic liver, and in animal models of liver fibrosis, the expression of PDGF and its receptors is markedly up-regulated. In the non-activated phonotype HSC express PDGFR-α, but not PDGFR-β. Upon activation they dramatically increase the expression of PDGFR-β. This is consistent with the observation that PDGF-BB is a more potent mitogen to cultured HSC than PDGF-AA. These findings suggest an important role for PDGF signalling in the HSC-mediated fibrogenesis that ultimately leads to portal hypertension. HSC are also thought to contribute to angiogenesis and pathological vascular remodelling in portal hypertension. HSC density and coverage of the sinusoids are increased in cirrhosis. This process involves recruitment and proliferation of HSC to sites of vascular development via LEC-derived factors. There is significant evidence to support the theory that LEC-derived PDGF signals control pericyte recruitment to angiogenic vessels via chemotactic gradients. The increase in contractile HSC leads to a constricted, high-resistance vessel and contributes importantly to increased portal pressure. In mice, while knockout of PDGF or PDGFR is lethal, the developing vasculature is devoid of pericytes and displays abnormal vessel diameter, endothelial hyperplasia, and vascular leak. Interference of PDGF signalling pathways with tyrosine kinase inhibitors such as imatinib can limit vascular remodelling in other tissues such as the lung, and are also attractive therapeutic considerations in portal hypertension.

SUMMARY

Non-parenchymal cells in the liver contribute importantly to the development of portal hypertension. In addition to classic parenchymal fibrosis, alterations in the hepatic vasculature may contribute 25% or more of the increases in intrahepatic resistance. These changes involve the related concepts of vasoreactivity and pathological vascular remodelling. LEC and HSC represent two particularly important populations of non-parenchymal liver cells that function together in complex autocrine and paracrine signalling mechanisms to affect these changes. Recent work has elucidated a detailed molecular understanding of several key signalling pathways in these cells, including NO, ET-1, and PDGF signalling. These pathways constitute important potential therapeutic targets in the treatment of portal hypertension.

Literature

1. Alvarez RH, Kantarjian HM, Cortes JE. Biology of platelet-derived growth factor and its involvement in disease. Mayo Clin Proc. 2006;81:1241–57.
2. Blei AT. Portal hypertension and its complications. Curr Opin Gastroenterol. 2007;23:275–82.
3. Langer DA, Shah VH. Nitric oxide and portal hypertension: interface of vasoreactivity and angiogenesis. J Hepatol. 2006;44:209–16.
4. Lee JS, Semela D, Iredale J, Shah VH. Sinusoidal remodeling and angiogenesis: a new function for the liver-specific pericyte? Hepatology. 2007;45:817–25.
5. Pinzani M. PDGF and signal transduction in hepatic stellate cells. Front Biosci. 2002;7:d1720–6.
6. Reeves HL, Friedman SL. Activation of hepatic stellate cells – a key issue in liver fibrosis. Front Biosci. 2002;7:d808–26.
7. Shah V. Cellular and molecular basis of portal hypertension. Clin Liver Dis. 2001;5:629–44.

11
Role of angiogenesis in portal hypertension

M. FERNANDEZ, M. MEJIAS, E. GARCIA-PRAS and J. BOSCH

INTRODUCTION

Portal hypertension is a frequent syndrome caused by diseases interfering with portal blood flow, and is a major complication of chronic liver diseases including cirrhosis of the liver, chronic hepatitis and alcoholic liver disease, or portal vein thrombosis, which are leading causes of death and liver transplantation all over the world[1,2]. As resistance to portal vein blood flow increases, the portal venous system becomes hypertensive. In an attempt to get portal blood back to the systemic circulation and decompress the portal system, portosystemic collateral vessels develop. In the areas where portal and systemic systems anastomose, the collateral vessels are engorged, creating gastro-oesophageal varicosities. These varices are particularly prone to rupture, causing a massive gastro-oesophageal bleeding that is usually torrential and difficult to arrest, and that is associated with a high mortality rate[1,2]. In addition, collateral vessels result in shunting of portal blood into the systemic circulation, causing high systemic concentrations of several substances normally metabolized by the liver, such as drugs, toxins, hormones and bacteria. These in turn contribute to major complications of chronic liver disease, including portosystemic encephalopathy and sepsis[1,2].

Successful design of medical treatment for portal hypertension requires a better understanding of the mechanisms underlying the formation of portosystemic collateral vessels, an issue that has remained largely unexplored. Traditionally, formation of collaterals was considered to be a mechanical consequence of the increased portal pressure that will result in the opening of these vascular channels. Accordingly, all therapeutic strategies aimed at decreasing portal pressure[1,2]. We hypothesized that the development of these collateral vessels could also involve active angiogenesis.

Another characteristic feature of the portal hypertensive syndrome is the development of a hyperdynamic splanchnic circulatory state, with an increase in blood flow in splanchnic organs draining into the portal vein and a subsequent increase in portal venous inflow[1,2]. Such an increased portal venous inflow represents a significant factor maintaining and worsening the portal pressure elevation[1,2]. The mechanisms underlying this splanchnic hyperaemia are not fully understood, but it has been shown that it is associated with an overproduction of endogenous vasodilators and decreased vascular reactivity to vasoconstrictors[1,2]. An intriguing possibility is that an increased formation of splanchnic blood vessels through an angiogenic process could also be involved in the maintenance of a hyperdynamic splanchnic circulation in portal hypertension.

In the past few years we have attempted to address these possibilities by studying the effects of different anti-angiogenic strategies aimed at inhibiting the vascular endothelial growth factor (VEGF) and the platelet-derived growth factor (PDGF) signalling pathways, which are essential mediators of angiogenesis[3–5], on the development and maintenance of hyperdynamic splanchnic circulation and portosystemic collateralization in experimental models of portal hypertension.

OVEREXPRESSION OF ANGIOGENESIS MEDIATORS AND INCREASED SPLANCHNIC NEOVASCULARIZATION IN PORTAL HYPERTENSION

First, we have demonstrated the presence of increased angiogenesis in the splanchnic territory of portal hypertensive animals (mice and rats), evidenced by overexpression of VEGF, VEGF receptor-2 and CD31 (Figures 1 and 2)[3,6–8]. Up-regulation of VEGF receptor-2 and CD31 reflects an increase in the amount of splanchnic blood vessels in portal hypertensive animals, since these molecules are exclusively expressed on vascular endothelial cells and are up-regulated once these cells proliferate during angiogenesis. These results indicate that a VEGF-stimulated splanchnic neovascularization occurs in portal hypertensive animals.

Other studies also found evidence of increased angiogenesis and VEGF overexpression in the abdominal cavity of portal hypertensive rats and cirrhotic patients[9–14]. The precise mechanism triggering VEGF-dependent angiogenesis in portal hypertension remains speculative, but it is likely to be multifactorial. Indeed, several factors relevant to the pathogenesis of portal hypertension, such as tissue hypoxia, cytokines, and mechanical stress, have been shown to promote VEGF expression in various cell types and tissues[1–3].

Prevention of the formation of portosystemic collateral vessels and hyperdynamic splanchnic circulation by vascular endothelial growth factor blockade in portal hypertension

We have also determined the effects of several angiogenesis inhibitors, with different modes of action, in experimental models of portal hypertension during the development of the portal hypertensive syndrome. In these studies, treatment with the angioinhibitors started immediately after induction of portal hypertension by partial portal vein ligation and continued for 5 or 7 days. The idea was to assess whether blockade of angiogenesis could prevent the circulatory abnormalities observed in portal hypertension.

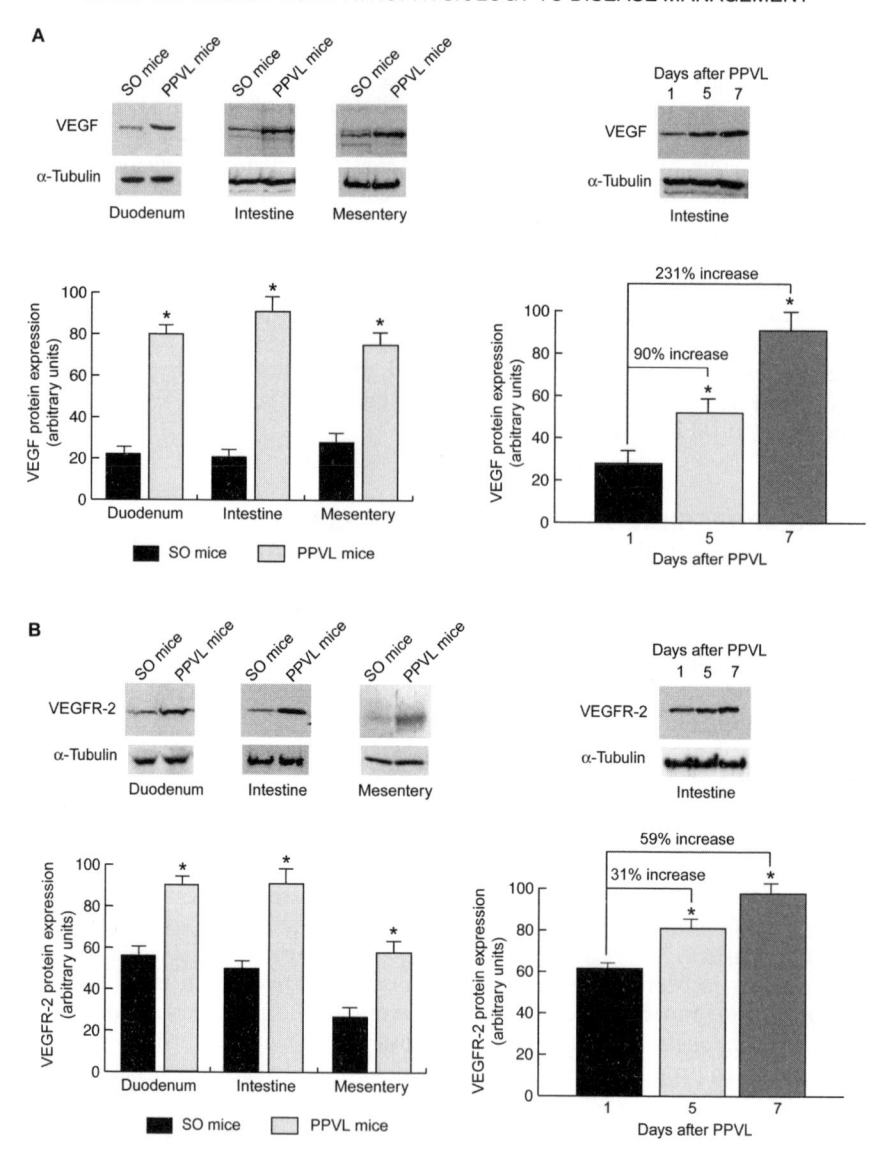

First, we used in portal hypertensive mice a function-blocking neutralizing monoclonal antibody directed against the receptor-2 of VEGF as anti-angiogenic strategy. This monoclonal antibody, known as DC101, binds to VEGF receptor-2 with high affinity, potently blocks VEGF-induced signalling, and strongly inhibits angiogenesis[15]. We found a marked and significant inhibition in the formation of portosystemic collateral vessels in portal hypertensive mice treated with DC101[6]. This inhibitory effect of DC101 was

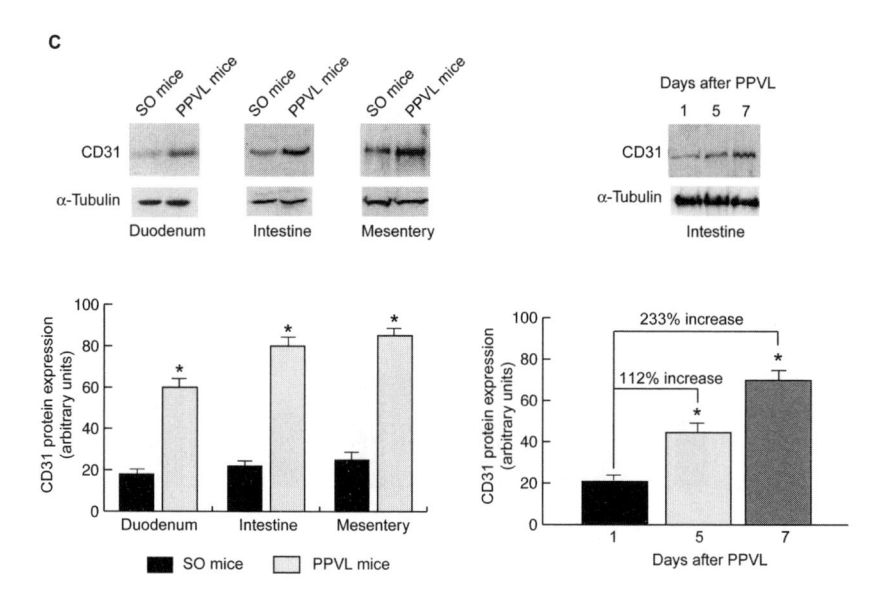

Figure 1 (and opposite) Overexpression of VEGF (**A**), VEGF receptor-2 (**B**) and CD31 (**C**) in portal hypertensive mice. *Left*: Protein expressions in splanchnic organs from partial portal vein-ligated (PPVL) mice and sham-operated (SO) control animals, 7 days after the initial surgery. *Right*: Protein expressions at days 1, 5 and 7 after the induction of portal hypertension in mice. Representative Western blots are shown at the top and densitometric quantification normalized to α-tubulin is shown at the bottom of each panel. *$p < 0.05$ vs SO mice (left) or vs day 1 (right)

consistent and effective after treatment for 5 days (40% inhibition) and 7 days (68% inhibition)[6]. These results indicate that VEGF-dependent angiogenesis plays a crucial role in the formation of portosystemic collateral vessels. The administration of anti-VEGF receptor-2 monoclonal antibodies also effectively decreased the intestinal neovascularization observed in portal hypertensive mice, demonstrating that the effects of the DC101 therapy on the formation of collateral vessels were mediated through inhibition of VEGF-induced angiogenesis[6].

Second, we used, in portal hypertensive rats, a potent anti-angiogenic agent (known as SU5416) that selectively and specifically inhibits VEGF-stimulated VEGF receptor-2 autophosphorylation, by interfering with the tyrosine kinase domain of the VEGF receptor-2[8,16]. Interestingly, findings in these additional experiments were almost superimposable to those observed with DC101 in portal hypertensive mice[6]. Indeed, we found a significant decrease (52% inhibition) in the extent of collateral vessels in portal hypertensive rats treated with SU5416, compared with those receiving vehicle[8]. In addition, blockade of VEGF receptor-2 by SU5416 markedly attenuated the splanchnic hyperdynamic circulation observed in portal hypertensive rats. Thus, portal

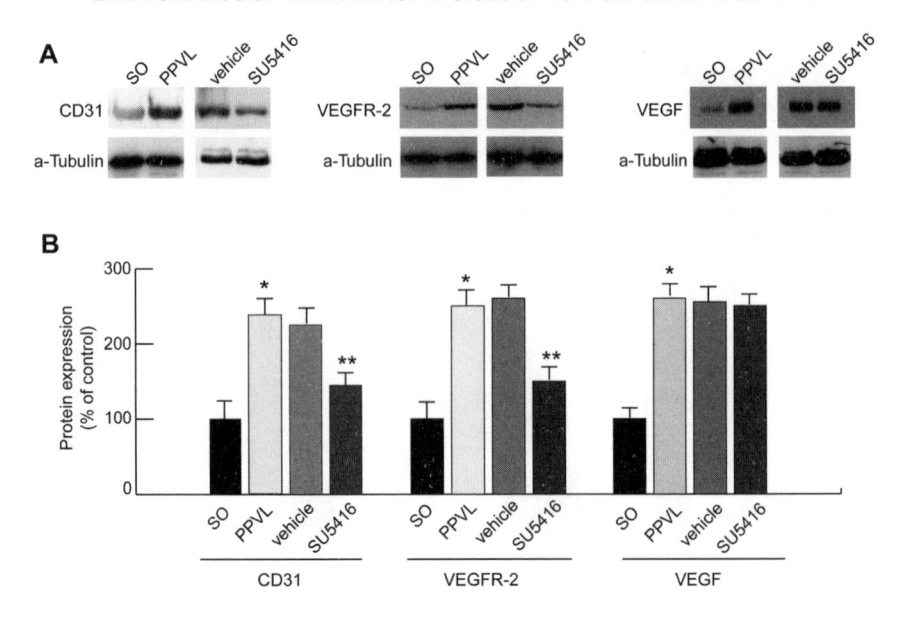

Figure 2 Overexpression of CD31, VEGF receptor-2 and VEGF in the mesentery from portal hypertensive (PPVL) rats compared with sham-operated (SO) controls, 5 days after the initial surgery. Effects of SU5416 treatment on the expression of these proteins in PPVL rats compared with vehicle-treated PPVL rats. **A**: Representative western blots. **B**: Densitometric quantification of protein expression normalized to α-tubulin. *$p < 0.05$ vs SO rats; **$p < 0.05$ vs PPVL–vehicle

venous inflow was significantly decreased (by 44%) and splanchnic arteriolar resistance increased (by 68%) in portal hypertensive rats treated with SU5416, compared with those receiving vehicle[8]. These splanchnic effects were predominantly located in the mesentery and intestine, organs where we found a significant decrease in blood flow[8]. These results indicate that an increase in the splanchnic vascular bed size mediated by a VEGF-dependent angiogenic process significantly contributes to increase overall blood flow in splanchnic tissues of portal hypertensive animals. Despite the reduction in portal venous inflow after SU5416 treatment, portal pressure did not decrease; most probably because of the concomitant inhibition in the formation of portosystemic collateral vessels[8]. The net effect of diminished extent of the collateral network is an increase in overall portocollateral resistance. In addition, the increased splanchnic neovascularization (i.e. CD31 and VEGF receptor-2 overexpressions) observed in portal hypertensive rats was significantly reduced after SU5416 treatment (Figure 2), indicating that the effects of SU5416 on splanchnic hyperaemia were mediated through inhibition of VEGF-induced angiogenesis in portal hypertensive rats[8].

Finally, we determined the effects of rapamycin, which inhibits VEGF production[17,18], in portal hypertensive rats. Rapamycin effectively prevented the increase in VEGF expression and the formation of new blood vessels in the splanchnic territory of portal hypertensive rats as reflected by a significant inhibition in the intestinal expression of the vascular endothelial cell markers

CD31 and VEGF receptor-2 (Figure 3)[18]. The rapamycin-induced inhibition of splanchnic neovascularization was paralleled by a significant prevention of the hyperdynamic splanchnic circulation of portal hypertensive rats, as indicated by a significant 24% decrease in superior mesenteric artery blood flow and a 66% increase in superior mesenteric artery resistance compared with vehicle-treated portal hypertensive rats, reaching values not significantly different to those observed in rapamycin-treated sham-operated rats (Figure 4)[18]. Despite the decrease in superior mesenteric artery blood flow, portal pressure was not reduced by rapamycin in portal hypertensive animals (Figure 4)[18]. That was most probably due to the marked 67% reduction in portosystemic collateral vessel formation observed in portal hypertensive rats after VEGF signalling inhibition (Figure 4)[18].

Taken together, these data indicate that the development of hyperdynamic splanchnic circulation and splanchnic neovasculature, as well as the formation of portosystemic collateral vessels in portal hypertensive animals, are in part VEGF-dependent angiogenic processes that can be significantly prevented by administration of inhibitors of the VEGF/VEGF receptor-2 signalling pathway, starting at the time of portal hypertension initiation[6,8,18].

REVERSAL OF PORTAL HYPERTENSION AND HYPERDYNAMIC SPLANCHNIC CIRCULATION BY COMBINED VASCULAR ENDOTHELIAL GROWTH FACTOR AND PLATELET-DERIVED GROWTH FACTOR BLOCKADE IN PORTAL HYPERTENSION

The studies described so far in this chapter highlight the importance of angiogenesis in the pathogenesis of portal hypertension, and suggest that anti-angiogenic treatment might be a promising therapeutic strategy to prevent the progression of the portal hypertensive syndrome[6,8,18]. In clinical practice, however, an anti-angiogenic drug would have to be given to a patient who is usually diagnosed, and eventually treated, when portal hypertension is already advanced and has caused clinical manifestations. Thus, it was imperative to confirm our previous prophylactic studies by therapeutic models that most closely mirror advanced human portal hypertension, and to determine whether anti-angiogenic agents could not only prevent but also revert the circulatory abnormalities associated with portal hypertension once these are fully developed. Therefore, we evaluated long-term anti-angiogenic treatment in an animal model of established portal hypertension[18].

Recent studies indicate that, in the process of neovascularization, VEGF plays a predominant role in the formation of new blood vessels by activating the proliferation of endothelial cells and the subsequent formation of an endothelial tubule, while maturation of the newly formed vessels is mainly modulated by the proangiogenic growth factor platelet-derived growth factor (PDGF), which regulates the investiture of the endothelial tubule with mural cell and pericyte populations, thereby stabilizing the vascular architecture of the nascent vessel[19–21]. It thus seems reasonable to hypothesize that established portal hypertension should be associated with overexpression not only of VEGF, but also of PDGF on splanchnic tissues, and that reversal of

A

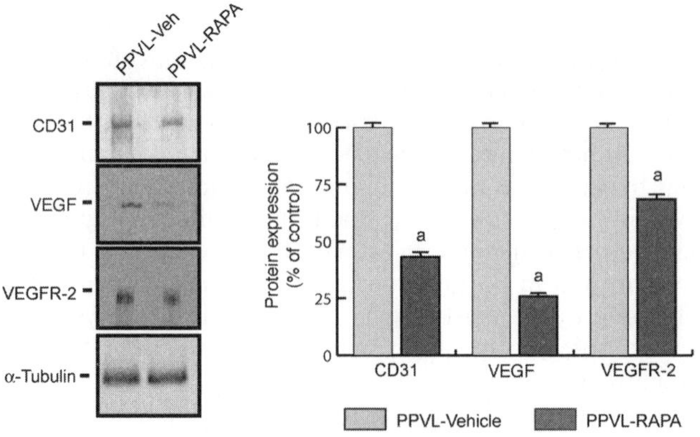
PPVL-Veh
PPVL-RAPA
CD31
VEGF
VEGFR-2
α-Tubulin
Protein expression
(% of control)
100
75
50
25
0
a
a
a
CD31
VEGF
VEGFR-2
PPVL-Vehicle
PPVL-RAPA

C

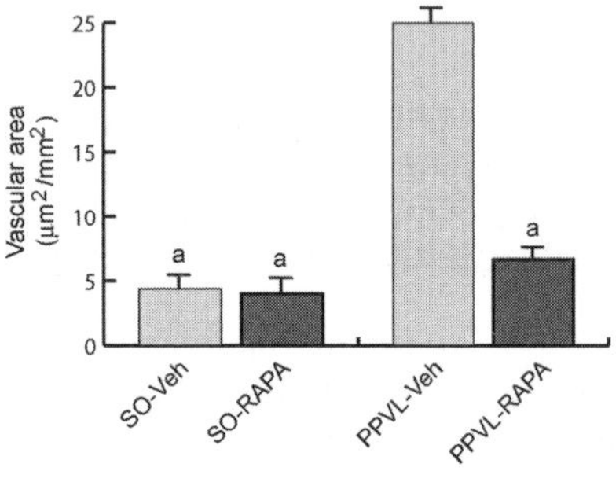
Vascular area
(μm²/mm²)
25
20
15
10
5
0
a
a
a
SO-Veh
SO-RAPA
PPVL-Veh
PPVL-RAPA

D

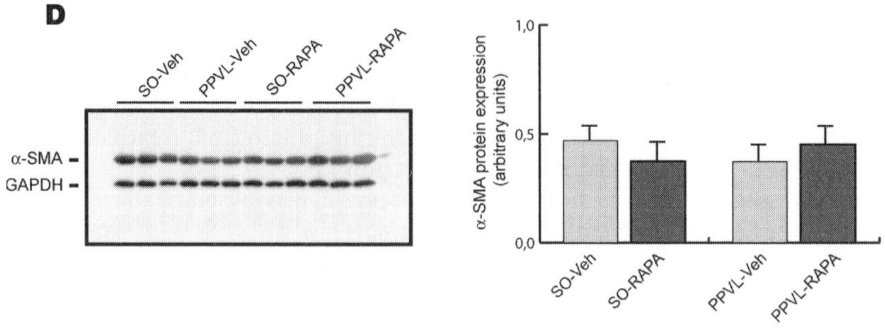
SO-Veh
PPVL-Veh
SO-RAPA
PPVL-RAPA
α-SMA
GAPDH
α-SMA protein expression
(arbitrary units)
1,0
0,5
0,0
SO-Veh
SO-RAPA
PPVL-Veh
PPVL-RAPA

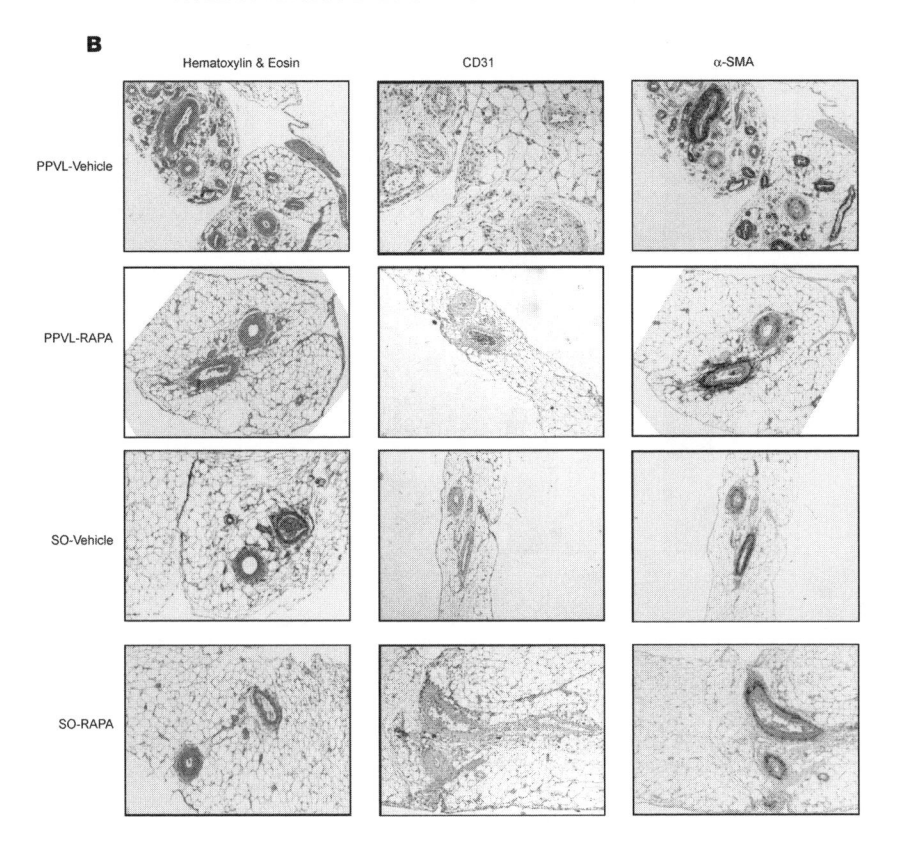

Figure 3 (and opposite) Effects of rapamycin (RAPA) on angiogenesis mediators when portal hypertension was actively developing. **A**: Expression of CD31, VEGF and VEGF receptor-2 in the intestine of partial portal vein-ligated (PPVL) rats treated with RAPA or vehicle. Representative Western blots are shown at the left and quantification of protein expression normalized to α-tubulin is shown at the right. **B**: Representative histological images of mesentery tissues, stained with H&E, or immunostained for CD31 and α-smooth muscle actin (α-SMA) from PPVL and SO rats treated with RAPA or vehicle. Original magnification ×40 (×100 magnification in CD31 staining of PPVL-vehicle). **C**: Quantitative analysis of neovascularization in the mesentery from RAPA or vehicle-treated PPVL and SO rats. (a) $p<0.05$ vs PPVL–vehicle. **D**: Expression of α-SMA in the mesentery of PPVL and SO rats treated with RAPA or vehicle showing lack of effect of RAPA on α-SMA expression. Representative Western blot is shown at the left and quantification of protein expression normalized to GAPDH is shown at the right

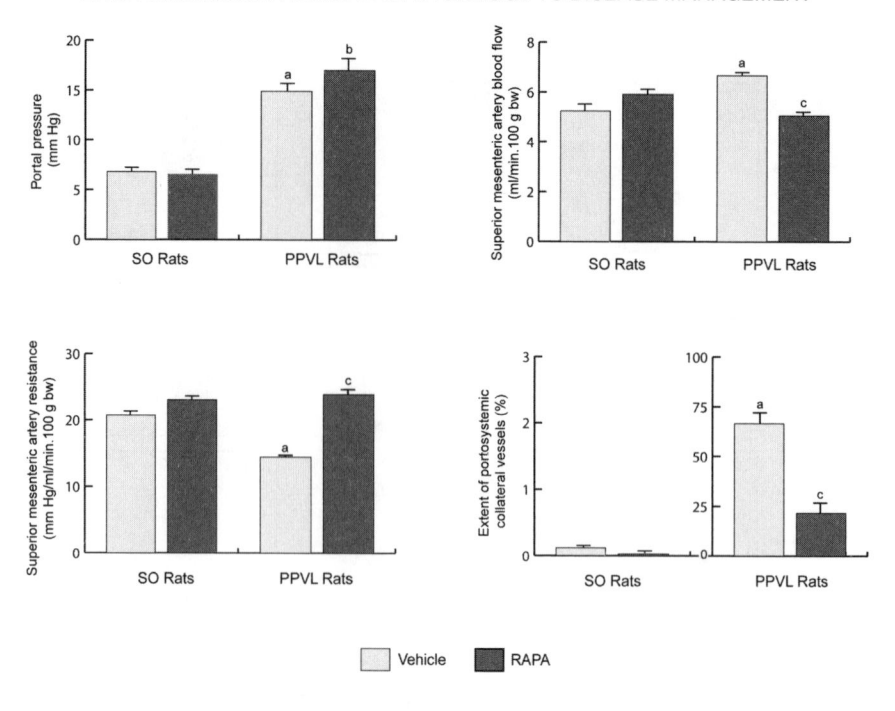

Figure 4 Effects of rapamycin (RAPA) on splanchnic haemodynamics and the extent of portosystemic collateral vessels when portal hypertension was actively developing. (a) $p<0.05$ vs SO–vehicle; (b) $p<0.05$ vs SO–RAPA; (c) $p<0.05$ vs PPVL–vehicle

splanchnic circulatory changes associated with portal hypertension might be greater after the combined blockade of VEGF and PDGF (i.e. after simultaneous targeting of endothelial cells and pericytes) than after either alone. Indeed, we demonstrated that, besides VEGF, portal hypertension development is associated with a progressive overexpression of PDGF, which reached its peak later in the course of portal hypertension than VEGF overexpression (Figure 5)[18].

We used rapamycin and Gleevec as strategies to inhibit VEGF and PDGF signalling pathways, respectively[17,22,23]. We chose these drugs because, in addition to their well-known effects as inhibitors of VEGF and PDGF pathways, they are already broadly used in the treatment of several human malignancies, and proved to be well tolerated in these indications[17,22,23]. Rats were treated with rapamycin, Gleevec or a combination of rapamycin plus Gleevec over a 2-week period, beginning 1 week after partial portal vein ligation, when portal hypertension is already fully established[18].

Therapy with rapamycin alone induced a significant decrease in VEGF expression, which was associated with a substantial attenuation of the increased splanchnic neovascularity (i.e. attenuation of the overexpression of the endothelial cell markers CD31 and VEGF receptor-2 and decrease in vascular area) (Figure 6) and a marked reduction in portal pressure (by 17%)

and splanchnic hyperaemia (17% decrease in superior mesenteric artery blood flow and a 38% increase in superior mesenteric artery resistance) (Figure 7)[18]. These effects were specific for the neovasculature of portal hypertensive rats since they were not observed in sham-operated control animals. We therefore concluded that VEGF signalling is required not only for development but also for maintenance of the portal hypertensive syndrome, and that inhibition of the VEGF pathway results in significant attenuation of the increased portal pressure and the hyperdynamic splanchnic circulation in rats with advanced portal hypertension. However, despite the significant decreases in portal pressure, superior mesenteric artery blood flow and splanchnic neovascularization, the extent of collateralization was unchanged (Figure 7)[18]. This finding is discussed later.

Treatment with the PDGF inhibitor Gleevec alone had no major effects other than a reduction in PDGF expression as well as a decrease in the perivascular cell coverage of splanchnic neovessels, as indicated by a significant decrease in the expression of the pericyte-specific markers α-smooth muscle actin and PDGF receptor-β (Figure 6). However, the combined treatment with rapamycin and Gleevec, on top of the expected

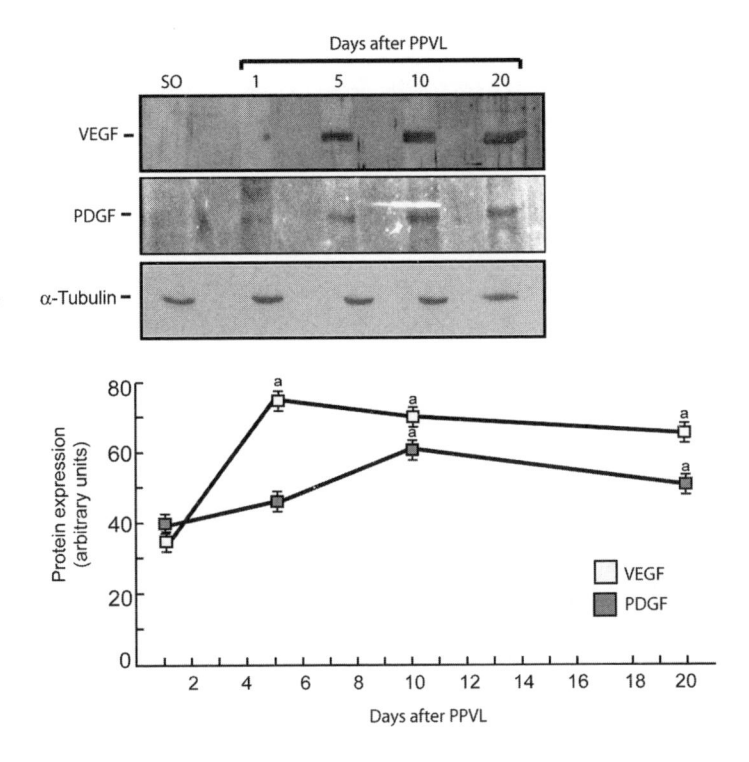

Figure 5 Expression of VEGF and PDGF at days 1, 5, 10 and 20 after PPVL and also in SO rats. Representative blots are shown above, and quantification of expression normalized to α-tubulin is shown below. (a) $p < 0.05$ vs SO rats

significant decrease in the expression of VEGF, VEGF receptor-2, CD31, PDGF, PDGF receptor-β and α-smooth muscle actin (Figure 6), also resulted in a virtually complete reversal of the increased portal pressure (40% reduction) and the increased splanchnic hyperaemia (30% decrease in superior mesenteric artery blood flow and 63% increase in superior mesenteric artery resistance) (Figure 7). Notably, the magnitude of the effects of the combination treatment was superior to the addition of the effects of either drug alone, suggesting the existence of a synergistic regulatory interaction between the VEGF and PDGF signalling pathways in mediating the maintenance of the vascular and circulatory abnormalities observed in portal hypertensive rats[18]. These findings also have important clinical implications: in the absence of perivascular cells (i.e. after PDGF signalling inhibition), the endothelium is more vulnerable to anti-angiogenic therapies targeting endothelial cells, such as VEGF signalling blockade[24].

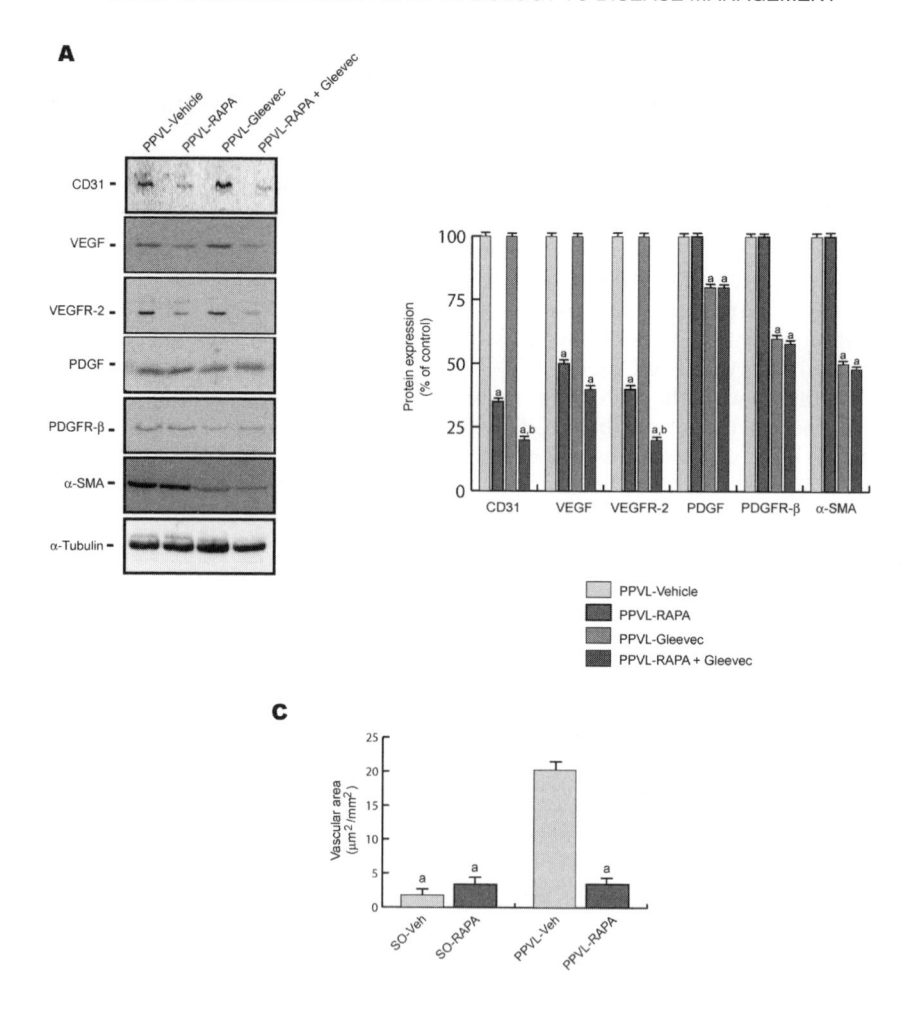

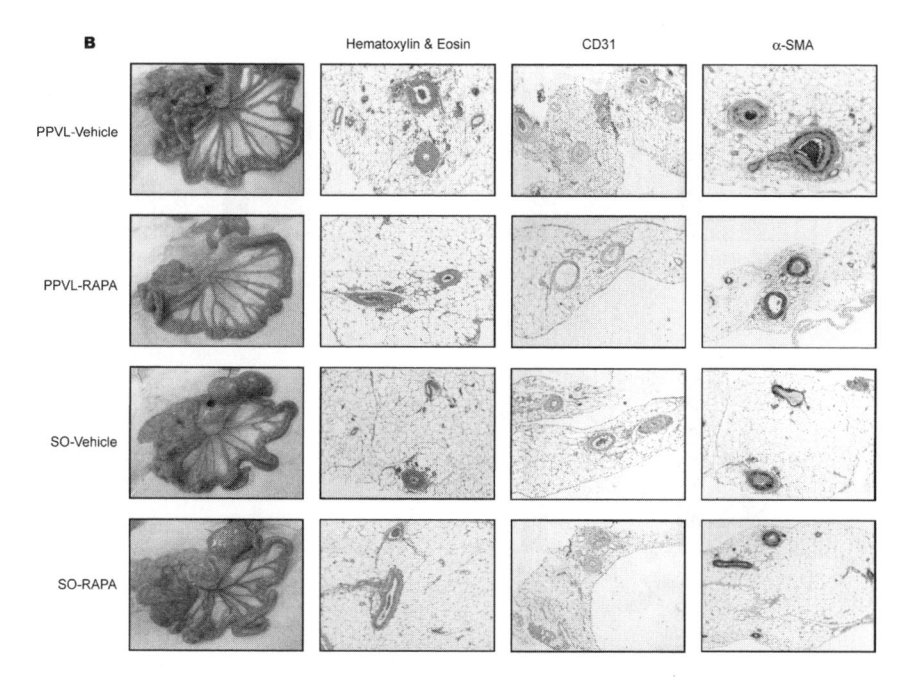

	Hematoxylin & Eosin	CD31	α-SMA
PPVL-Vehicle			
PPVL-RAPA			
SO-Vehicle			
SO-RAPA			

Figure 6 (and opposite) Effects of rapamycin (RAPA), Gleevec or RAPA + Gleevec on angiogenesis mediators when portal hypertension was completely established. A: Expression of CD31, VEGF, VEGFR-2, PDGF, PDGFR-β and α-SMA in the intestine of PPVL rats after treatment with RAPA, Gleevec, RAPA + Gleevec or vehicle. Representative blots are shown at the left and quantification of expression normalized to α-tubulin is shown at the right. (a) $p < 0.05$ vs PPVL–vehicle; (b) $p < 0.05$ vs PPVL–RAPA. B: Representative mesentery photographs, and representative histological images of mesentery sections stained with H&E, or immunostained for CD31 and α-SMA from PPVL and SO rats treated with RAPA or vehicle. Original magnification × 40. C: Quantitative analysis of neovascularization in the mesentery from PPVL and SO rats treated with RAPA or vehicle. (a) $p < 0.05$ vs PPVL–vehicle

As remarked earlier, although VEGF inhibition suppressed the development of new portosystemic collateral vessels, selective VEGF signalling blockade had no significant effects on the extent of already-established collateral vessels, and the simultaneous inhibition of VEGF plus PDGF signalling, despite much greater effects on portal pressure and superior mesenteric artery blood flow, caused a significant but slight reduction in the extent of portosystemic collaterals. Why did the anti-angiogenic therapy markedly reduce the formation of collaterals when these vessels began to develop but not when collateralization was already established? A likely explanation is that a measurable decrease in collateralization may take longer than the 2-week course of treatment evaluated in this study. It should be noted in this regard that patients with cirrhosis receiving an orthotopic liver transplant maintain an increased portocollateral blood flow for months[25]. The extent of portosystemic collaterals decreased slightly (9% decrease) but significantly ($p < 0.05$) after the

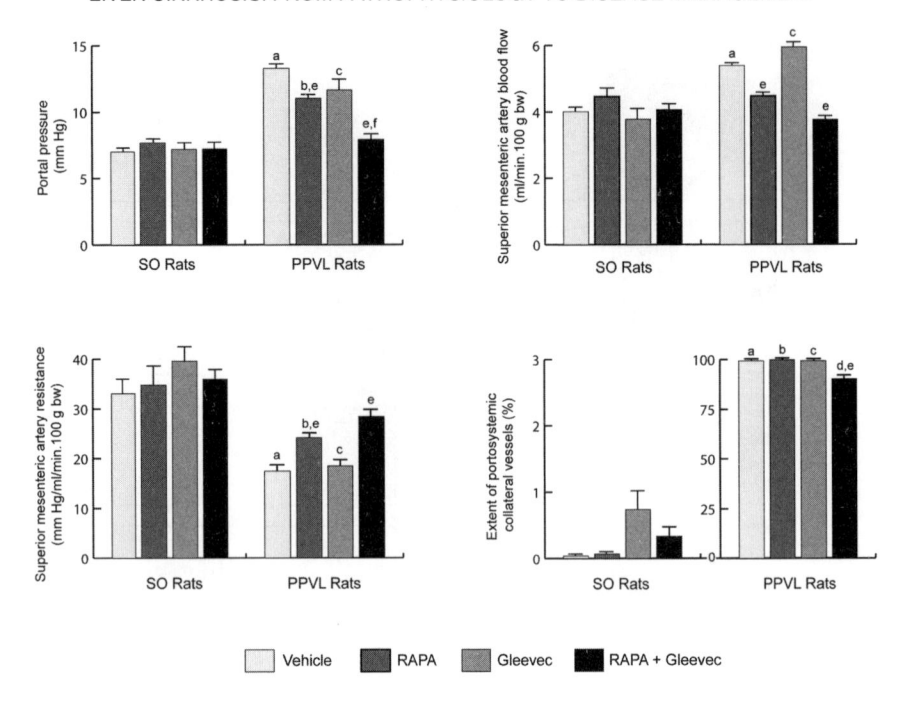

Figure 7 Effects of RAPA, Gleevec or RAPA + Gleevec on splanchnic haemodynamics and the extent of portosystemic collaterals when portal hypertension was completely established. (a) $p<0.05$ vs SO–vehicle; (b) $p<0.05$ vs SO–RAPA; (c) $p<0.05$ vs SO–Gleevec; (d) $p<0.05$ vs SO–RAPA + Gleevec; (e) $p<0.05$ vs PPVL–vehicle; (f) $p<0.01$ vs PPVL–RAPA

combined inhibition of VEGF plus PDGF signalling (Figure 7). On the other hand, it is also possible that there are either intrinsic differences in the sensitivity of vessels to the lack of growth factors, or differences in the extent of vessel maturation[19,20,26,27]. In this regard it is important to point out that collaterals frequently become large vessels, suggesting a high degree of vessel maturation[28]. Therefore, it could be that the dependence on VEGF and PDGF for collateral vessel growth and maintenance changes over time and, upon their maturation, portosystemic collateral dependence from VEGF and PDGF is less accentuated. Nevertheless, the marked decrease in portal pressure and splanchnic hyperaemia in response to the combined VEGF and PDGF signalling inhibition suggests that, even if collaterals are still present, their potential to result in clinical complications could be substantially reduced[28–30]. Importantly, the use of rapamycin and Gleevec as inhibitors of the VEGF and PDGF signalling pathways, respectively, has the additional advantage that their efficacy and safety in the treatment of several human malignancies has already been broadly documented[17,22,23].

Overall, these results provide new and important biological insights into the role of growth factors and angiogenesis in portal hypertension by suggesting the existence of a regulatory interaction between VEGF and PDGF pathways to maintain the haemodynamic and vascular changes provoked by portal hypertension in the partial portal vein ligated rat model. This study is also the first to our knowledge to describe the successful therapeutic use of the combination of rapamycin and Gleevec in an animal model of portal hypertension. Taking into account the limitations of experimental studies, we still believe that these findings will be stimulating for consideration of this novel therapeutic approach in patients suffering from advanced portal hypertension, in which VEGF and PDGF signalling pathways may be up-regulated, as suggested by the findings in the currently investigated portal hypertensive animals[18].

ANGIOGENESIS, HAEM OXYGENASE AND OXIDATIVE STRESS IN PORTAL HYPERTENSION

Haem oxygenase (HO) is the enzyme catalysing the degradation of haem and produces carbon monoxide, iron, and biliverdin[31]. Biliverdin is converted to bilirubin by biliverdin reductase[31]. In mammals, three isoforms of HO have been described: the inducible HO-1, and the constitutives HO-2 and HO-3. In the past few years evidence has accumulated showing that the HO enzymes and their by-products are important players in the pathophysiology of portal hypertension. For example, increased HO activity and/or expression of HO-1 have been described in experimental models of portal hypertension and cirrhosis[31–37], as well as in patients with cirrhosis of the liver[38–40]. It has been suggested that this HO-1 induction plays a role in mediating the hyperdynamic splanchnic circulation in portal hypertension[33,41]. More recently we have determined the potential role of endogenous HO on oxidative stress and angiogenesis in portal hypertensive rats[41]. The rationale and specific hypotheses for these studies are discussed below.

First, HO-1 is a stress-responsive protein induced by various oxidative agents, and HO-1 induction is considered to be an adaptive cellular response to survive exposure to enviromental stresses[31]. The cytoprotective function of HO-1 is derived from its ability to eliminate the pro-oxidant haem[31], the release of biliverdin and subsequent conversion to bilirubin, both of which are potent antioxidants[42], and the generation of carbon monoxide, which has vasodilatory and anti-inflammatory properties[43]. We have recently demonstrated the presence of enhanced oxidative stress in the splanchnic territory of portal hypertensive rats[41]. Therefore, it was reasonable to hypothesize that HO-1 induction in portal hypertension would be part of a defensive response against stress. We found that chronic HO inhibition further exacerbated oxidative stress, and resulted in a marked inflammatory response in splanchnic organs of portal hypertensive rats[41]. These results strongly suggest that HO-1 up-regulation constitutes an important antioxidant mechanism in portal hypertension that attenuates oxidative stress and inflammation.

Second, emerging evidence indicates the participation of HO-1 in angiogenesis. Thus, HO-1 activity has been shown to induce the expression of VEGF in vascular cells, stimulating endothelial cell proliferation and capillary formation[44-46]. Since we have demonstrated that the expression of VEGF is increased in experimental models of portal hypertension, and that the formation of portosystemic collaterals is, in part, a VEGF-dependent angiogenic process[6,8], it could be possible that HO-1 was involved in the modulation of VEGF expression and/or angiogenesis in portal hypertensive rats. Interestingly, we found that chronic HO inhibition markedly and significantly decreased (by 74%) VEGF protein expression in the mesentery of portal hypertensive rats, suggesting that HO enzymatic activity is an important stimulus for VEGF production in portal hypertension[41]. In this regard recent *in vitro* studies have shown that carbon monoxide, derived from HO-1, increases VEGF synthesis in vascular cells[45,46]. In addition, we and other authors have previously demonstrated that VEGF is also able to induce HO-1 expression *in vivo* and *in vitro*[47,48], further suggesting the existence of a reciprocal relationship between VEGF and the HO-1 system. Despite the decrease in VEGF expression observed after HO blockade in portal hypertensive rats, neither the formation of portosystemic collaterals nor the increased splanchnic vascularization was significantly modified[41]. This was unexpected, since we have recently demonstrated that both the development of collaterals and the increased splanchnic vascularity in portal hypertension are, in part, VEGF-dependent angiogenic processes[6,8]. It is interesting to note that HO inhibition also led to a significant increase in VEGF receptor-2 expression in the mesentery of portal hypertensive rats. This VEGFR-2 up-regulation could be a compensatory mechanism to maintain VEGF angiogenic activity in a situation in which VEGF expression is markedly suppressed. This could partly explain why neither the splanchnic neovascularization nor the formation of portosystemic collaterals decreased after HO blockade in portal hypertensive rats[41]. An additional explanation could be related to our finding that HO inhibition potentiated oxidative stress in portal hypertensive rats[41]. This increased oxidative stress can lead to angiogenesis by activating the VEGF signalling pathway, even in the presence of decreased VEGF, as has been previously observed *in vitro*[49]. The molecular mechanism(s) underlying this effect are incompletely understood, but it has been suggested that reactive oxygen species could directly activate VEGF receptor-2, as well as other signalling pathways, such as ERK1/2 and Akt kinase, which have been implicated in VEGF-induced angiogenesis[49]. Therefore, although HO inhibition in portal hypertensive rats decreased VEGF expression, angiogenesis was maintained, probably by means of both a compensatory increase in VEGF receptor-2 expression, and by the activation of the VEGF signalling pathway through enhanced oxidative stress.

Interestingly, recent data derived from our studies indicate that NAD(P)H oxidase, a major source of reactive oxygen species in the vasculature[50,51], plays an important role modulating VEGF-induced angiogenesis in portal hypertension[52]. Thus, chronic NAD(P)H oxidase inhibition not only significantly reduced the excessive splanchnic production of reactive oxygen species observed in portal hypertensive rats, but also markedly decreased VEGF expression and splanchnic neovascularization, as well as the portosystemic collateralization and the splanchnic hyperaemia in this animal model[52]. The underlying molecular mechanisms by which activation of NAD

(P)H oxidase stimulates angiogenesis are incompletely understood[53]. As described above, reactive oxygen species produced by NAD(P)H oxidases can activate multiple signalling pathways, such as mitogen-activated protein kinases, tyrosine kinases and transcription factors, which have been implicated in VEGF-induced neovascularization[49].

Collectively taken, these findings suggest that oxidative stress modulates angiogenesis in portal hypertension, directly by activating the VEGF signalling pathway, and indirectly by stimulating the induction of haem oxygenase-1, which, in turn, increases the expression of VEGF.

References

1. Bosch J, Pizcueta P, Feu F, Fernandez M, Garcia-Pagan JC. Pathophysiology of portal hypertension. Gastroenterol Clin N Am. 1992;21:1–13.
2. Bosch J, Garcia-Pagan JC. The splanchnic circulation in cirrhosis. In: Gines P, Arroyo V, Rodes J, Schrier RW, editors. Ascites and Renal Dysfunction in Liver Disease. Pathogenesis, Diagnosis, and Treatment. Oxford: Blackwell, 2005:125–36.
3. Ferrara N, Gerber H-P, LeCouter J. The biology of VEGF and its receptors. Nat Med. 2003;9:669–76.
4. Folkman J, D'Amore PA. Blood vessel formation: what is its molecular basis? Cell. 1996;87:1153–5.
5. Carmeliet P. Mechanisms of angiogenesis and arteriogenesis. Nat Med. 2000;6:389–95.
6. Fernandez M, Vizzutti F, Garcia-Pagan JC, Rodes J, Bosch J. Anti-VEGF receptor-2 monoclonal antibody prevents portal-systemic collateral vessel formation in portal hypertensive mice. Gastroenterology. 2004;126:886–94.
7. Newman PJ, Berndt MC, Gorski J et al. PECAM-1 (CD31) cloning and relation to adhesion molecules of the immunoglobulin gene superfamily. Science. 1990;247:1219–22.
8. Fernandez M, Mejias M, Angermayr B, Garcia-Pagan JC, Rodes J, Bosch J. Inhibition of VEGF receptor-2 decreases the development of hyperdynamic splanchnic circulation and portal-systemic collateral vessels in portal hypertensive rats. J Hepatol. 2005;43:98–103.
9. Sumanovski LT, Battegay E, Stumm M, van der Kooij M, Sieber CC. Increased angiogenesis in portal hypertensive rats: role of nitric oxide. Hepatology. 1999;29:1044–9.
10. Sieber CC, Sumanovski LT, Stumm M, van der Kooij M, Battegay E. *In vivo* angiogenesis in normal and portal hypertensive rats: role of basic fibroblast growth factor and nitric oxide. J Hepatol. 2001;34:644–50.
11. Tsugawa K, Hashizume M, Tomikawa M et al. Immunohistochemical localization of vascular endothelial growth factor in the rat portal hypertensive gastropathy. J Gastroenterol Hepatol. 2001;16:429–37.
12. Tsugawa K, Hashizume M, Migou S et al. Role of vascular endothelial growth factor in portal hypertensive gastropathy. Digestion. 2000;61:98–106.
13. Cejudo-Martin P, Ros J, Navasa M et al. Increased production of vascular endothelial growth factor in peritoneal macrophages of cirrhotic patients with spontaneous bacterial peritonitis. Hepatology. 2001;34:487–93.
14. Perez-Ruiz M, Ros J, Morales-Ruiz M et al. Vascular endothelial growth factor production in peritoneal macrophages of cirrhotic patients: regulation by cytokines and bacterial lipopolysaccharide. Hepatology. 1999;29:1057–63.
15. Witte L, Hicklin DJ, Zhu Z et al. Monoclonal antibodies targeting the VEGF receptor-2 (Flk-1/KDR) as an anti-angiogenic therapeutic strategy. Cancer Metastasis Rev. 1998;17:155–61.
16. Fong TAT, Shawver LK, Sun L et al. SU5416 is a potent and selective inhibitor of the vascular endothelial growth factor receptor (Flk-1/KDR) that inhibits tyrosine kinase catalysis, tumor vascularization, and growth of multiple tumor types. Cancer Res. 1999;59:99–106.
17. Guba M, von Breitenbuch P, Steinbauer M et al. Rapamycin inhibits primary and metastatic tumor growth by antiangiogenesis: involvement of vascular endothelial growth factor. Nat Med. 2002;8:128–35.

18. Fernandez M, Mejias M, Garcia-Pras E, Mendez R, Garcia-Pagan JC, Bosch J. Reversal of portal hypertension and hyperdynamic splanchnic circulation by combined vascular endothelial growth factor and platelet-derived growth factor blockade in rats. Hepatology. 2007;46:1208–18.
19. Carmeliet P. Mechanisms of angiogenesis and arteriogenesis. Nat Med. 2000;6:389–95.
20. Jain RK. Molecular regulation of vessel maturation. Nat Med. 2003;9:685–93.
21. Heldin CH, Westermark B. Mechanism of action and *in vivo* role of platelet-derived growth factor. Physiol Rev. 1999;79:1283–316.
22. Capdeville R, Buchdunger E, Zimmermann J, Matter A. Glivec (STI571, imatinib), a rationally developed, targeted anticancer drug. Nat Rev Drug Discov. 2002;1:493–502.
23. Pietras K, Sjöblom T, Rubin K, Heldin CH, Ostman A. PDGF receptors as cancer drug targets. Cancer Cell. 2003;3:439–43.
24. Bergers G, Song S, Meyer-Morse N, Bergsland E, Hanahan D. Benefits of targeting both pericytes and endothelial cells in the tumor vasculature with kinase inhibitors. J Clin Invest. 2003;111:1287–95.
25. Navasa M, Forns X, Sanchez V et al. Quality of life, major medical complications and hospital service utilization in patients with primary biliary cirrosis after liver transplantation. J Hepatol. 1996;25:129–34.
26. Eberhard A, Kahlert S, Goede V, Hemmerlein B, Plate KH, Augustin HG. Heterogeneity of angiogenesis and blood vessel maturation in human tumors: implications for antiangiogenic tumor therapies. Cancer Res. 2000;60:1388–93.
27. Gee MS, Procopio WN, Makonnen S, Feldman MD, Yeilding NM, Lee WM. Tumor vessel development and maturation impose limits on the effectiveness of anti-vascular therapy. Am J Pathol. 2003;162:183–93.
28. Escorsell A, Bosch J. Pathophysiology of variceal bleeding. In: Groszmann RJ, Bosch J, editors. Portal Hypertension in the 21st Century. Dordrecht: Kluwer Academic Publishers, 2004:155–66.
29. Abraldes JG, Tarantino I, Turnes J, Garcia-Pagan JC, Rodes J, Bosch J. Hemodynamic response to pharamcological treatment of portal hypertension and long-term prognosis of cirrhosis. Hepatology. 2003;37:902–8.
30. D'Amico G, Garcia-Pagan JC, Luca A, Bosch J. Hepatic vein pressure gradient reduction and prevention of varicela bleeding in cirrosis: a systematic review. Gastroenterology. 2006;131:1611–24.
31. Lambrecht RW, Fernandez M, Shan Y, Bonkovsky HL. Heme oxygenase in portal hypertension and liver disease. In: Gines P, Arroyo V, Rodes J, Schrier RW, editors. Ascites and Renal Dysfunction in Liver Disease. Pathogenesis, Diagnosis, and Treatment. Oxford: Blackwell, 2005:125–36.
32. Fernandez M, Bonkovsky HL. Increased heme oxygenase-1 gene expression in liver cells and splanchnic organs from portal hypertensive rats. Hepatology. 1999;29:1672–79.
33. Fernandez M, Lambrecht RW, Bonkovsky HL. Increased heme oxygenase activity in splanchnic organs from portal hypertensive rats: role in modulating mesenteric vascular reactivity. J Hepatol. 2001;34:812–17.
34. Schroeder RA, Ewing CA, Sitzmann JV, Kuo PC. Pulmonary expression of iNOS and HO-1 protein is upregulated in a rat model of prehepatic portal hypertension. Dig Dis Sci. 2000;45:2405–10.
35. Liu H, Song D, Lee SS. Role of heme oxygenase–carbon monoxide pathway in pathogenesis of cirrhotic cardiomyopathy in the rat. Am J Physiol. 2001;280:G68–74.
36. Chen YC, Gines P, Yang J et al. Increased vascular heme oxygenase-1 expression contributes to arterial vasodilation in experimental cirrhosis in rats. Hepatology. 2004;39:1075–87.
37. Wei CL, Lee KH, Khoo HE, Hon WM. Expression of haem oxygenase in cirrhotic rat liver. J Pathol. 2003;199:324–34.
38. Makino N, Suematsu M, Sugiura Y et al. Altered expression of heme oxygenase-1 in the livers of patients with portal hypertensive diseases. Hepatology. 2001;33:32–42.
39. Matsumi M, Takahashi T, Fujii H et al. Increased heme oxygenase-1 gene expression in the livers of patients with portal hypertension due to severe hepatic cirrhosis. J Int Med Res. 2002;30:282–8.

40. De las Heras D, Fernandez J, Gines P et al. Increased carbon monoxide production in patients with cirrhosis with and without spontaneous bacterial peritonitis. Hepatology. 2003;38:452-9.
41. Angermayr B, Mejias M, Gracia-Sancho J, Garcia-Pagan JC, Bosch J, Fernandez M. Heme oxygenase attenuates oxidative stress and inflammation, and increases VEGF expression in portal hypertensive rats. J Hepatol. 2006;44:1033-9.
42. Stocker R, Yamamoto Y, McDonagh AF, Glazer AN, Ames BN. Bilirubin is an antioxidant of possible physiological importance. Science. 1987;235:1043-6.
43. Otterbein LE, Bach FH, Alam J et al. Carbon monoxide has anti-inflammatory effects involving the mitogen-activated protein kinase pathway. Nat Med. 2000;6:422-8.
44. Deramaudt BM, Braunstein S, Remy P, Abraham NG. Gene transfer of human heme oxygenase into coronary endothelial cells potentially promotes angiogenesis. J Cell Biochem. 1998;68:121-7.
45. Dulak J, Jozkowicz A, Foresti R et al. Heme oxygenase activity modulates vascular endothelial growth factor synthesis in vascular smooth muscle cells. Antioxid Redox Signal. 2002;4:229-40.
46. Jozkowicz A, Huk I, Nigisch A et al. Heme oxygenase and angiogenic activity of endothelial cells: stimulation by carbon monoxide and inhibition by tin protoporphyrin-IX. Antioxid Redox Signal. 2003;5:155-62.
47. Fernandez M, Bonkovsky HL. Vascular endothelial growth factor increases heme oxygenase-1 protein expression in the chick embryo chorioallantoic membrane. Br J Pharmacol. 2003;139:634-40.
48. Bussolati B, Ahmed A, Pemberton H et al. Bifunctional role for VEGF-induced heme oxygenase-1 *in vivo*: induction of angiogenesis and inhibition of leukocytic infiltration. Blood. 2004;103:761-6.
49. Maulik N. Redox signaling of angiogenesis. Antioxid Redox Signal. 2002;4:805-15.
50. Cai H, Griendling KK, Harrison DG. The vascular NAD(P)H oxidases as therapeutic targets in cardiovascular diseases. Trends Pharmacol Sci. 2003;24:471-8.
51. Griendling KK, Sorescu D, Ushio-Fukai M. NAD(P)H oxidase: role in cardiovascular biology and disease. Circ Res. 2000;86:494-501.
52. Angermayr B, Fernandez M, Mejias M, Gracia-Sancho J, Garcia-Pagan JC, Bosch J. NAD(P)H oxidase modulates angiogenesis and the development of portosystemic collaterals and splanchnic hyperemia in portal hypertensive rats. Gut. 2007;56:560-4.
53. Ushio-Fukai M, Alexander RW. Reactive oxygen species as mediators of angiogenesis signaling. Role of NAD(P)H oxidase. Mol Cell Biochem. 2004;264:85-97.

12
Current concept of hepatic fibrogenesis in mouse models of liver fibrosis

D. SCHOLTEN and D. BRENNER

INTRODUCTION

Hepatic fibrosis is an outcome of many liver diseases. It can progress to liver cirrhosis which often results in liver failure, portal hypertension and the development of hepatocellular cancer[1]. During this process the composition of the hepatic extracellular matrix (ECM) in fibrotic liver changes dramatically. Pathological stimuli such as viral infections and toxic, autoimmune or metabolic injury induce recruitment of inflammatory cells to the liver. Further on, collagen-producing cells such as hepatic stellate cells (HSC) contribute to the deposition of ECM, especially collagen α_1 in the liver tissue. Low-density collagen type IV is replaced with high-density collagen types I and III[2]. HSC are the major source of collagen type I in the liver. In the normal liver they reside in the space of Disse in a quiescent state. In response to liver injury HSC undergo a phenotypic transformation into activated myofibroblasts which produce collagen and interact with other cells contributing to liver fibrosis (Figure 1)[3]. Beside HSC, other fibrogenic cells contribute to liver fibrosis. Portal fibroblasts and bone marrow-derived fibrocytes can transform to collagen-producing myofibroblasts[4,5]. Furthermore, similar to organs such as lung or kidney, hepatocytes and cholangiocytes may undergo a process called epithelial–mesenchymal transition and differentiate into myofibroblasts[6]. Changes which lead to liver fibrosis are regulated by a complex crosstalk between hepatic and non-parenchymal cells. Damaged or apoptotic hepatocytes release reactive oxygen species (ROS) as well as many different cytokines and chemokines. This leads to the recruitment of inflammatory cells, such as lymphocytes and macrophages, to the damaged liver, and activation of hepatic stellate cells. Upon activation quiescent HSC activate into collagen expressing myofibroblasts. HSC play a major role in modulating the signalling cascade leading to the deposition of collagen. HSC have a significant impact on recruitment of inflammatory cells. Bone marrow-derived macrophages recruited into the injured liver and Kupffer cells, liver resident macrophages,

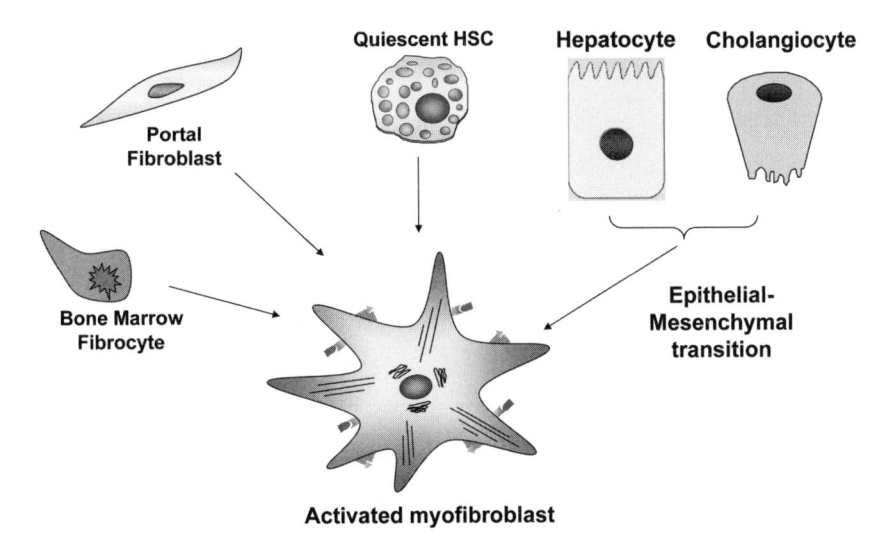

Figure 1 Cells contributing to liver fibrosis derive from several sources. Besides HSC, portal fibroblasts and bone marrow-derived fibrocytes can transform to collagen-producing myofibroblasts. Furthermore, similar to organs such as lung or kidney, hepatocytes and cholangiocytes are believed to undergo a process called epithelial–mesenchymal transition and also change into myofibroblasts

upon activation also secrete ROS and produce profibrogenic cytokines such as transforming growth factor β_1 (TGF-β_1) and tumour necrosis factor α (TNF-α) and stimulate T cells and HSC directly. Finally the recruitment of T cells to the injured liver tissue shifts the local cytokine production towards a Th2 (T helper 2) type response which is associated with fibrosis.

ANIMAL MODELS OF LIVER INJURY

Several rodent models have been developed to study pathogenesis of liver fibrosis and to characterize the key steps of fibrogenesis to find new therapeutic targets to prevent or reverse the fibrogenic process[7]. In this regard the bile duct ligation model can be used to study chronic cholestatic disorders (Table 1)[8]. Carbon tetrachloride (CCl$_4$), thioacetamide (TAA) and dimethylnitrosamine (DMN) induce acute liver injury by massive apoptosis of hepatocytes, and mimic toxic liver injury[9]. Intragastric ethanol administration, a model developed by Dr French and Dr Tsukamoto, and referred to as Tsukamoto–French model, provides a new strategy to study alcohol-induced liver injury in mice[10]. A model of metabolically induced liver injury specifically designed to induce a non-alcoholic steatohepatitis (NASH), can be induced by administration of a methionine choline-deficient diet in mice[11]. In addition, some infectious and parasitic diseases cause liver fibrosis, which is associated

Table 1 Rodent models of liver fibrosis and the diseases they mimic

Rodent models of liver fibrosis	Comparable human disease
Bile duct ligand (BDL)	Cholestatic diseases
Carbon tetrachloride (CCl$_4$), thioacetamide, dimethylnitrosamine (DMN)	Toxic liver injury
Intragastric ethanol feeding	Chronic alcohol abuse
Methionine choline-deficient diet, high sucrose diet	Metabolically induced liver injury, NAFLD, NASH
Schistosomiasis-induced liver fibrosis	Immunological and inflammatory diseases

Within limitations the bile duct ligation model induces cholestatic injury, application of CCl$_4$, thioacetamide and DMN mimics toxic liver injury; feeding with ethanol resembles liver injury after chronic alcohol abuse in humans. Histological changes as seen in human NAFLD (non-alcoholic liver disease) and NASH (non-alcoholic steatohepatitis) are induced in rodents by feeding with a methionine choline-deficient or high-sucrose diet, and immunological or inflammatory changes can be seen after infection of mice with schistosomiasis.

with the release of Th2 cytokines and mediation of acquired immunity. Thus, infection of mice with schistosomiasis causes release of Th2-type cytokines, interleukins IL-4 and IL-5, subsequent secretion of IL-13 and TGF-β_1 and development of liver fibrosis[12]. These models were successfully used to study the pathophysiology of liver fibrosis in wild-type mice. They were also exploited in different knockout mice to determine the role of single genes in progression of fibrosis. Although experimental models of liver fibrosis in mice have been particularly useful in elucidating the molecular mechanisms of fibrosis, all of these approaches have limitations.

The major problem remains to duplicate chronic injury in long-standing progressive liver diseases in patients. However, experimental models of liver fibrosis provide new insights into cellular and molecular processes of regulation of fibrogenesis. Data obtained from mouse models of liver fibrosis contributed to the current understanding of fibrogenesis. In addition, experimental fibrosis serves as a useful tool to test antifibrotic strategies and to investigate mechanisms of their action at the preclinical stage.

CYTOKINES AND CHEMOKINES CONTRIBUTING TO LIVER FIBROSIS

The event which triggers the development of liver fibrosis is damage to hepatocytes and chronic inflammation. Upon chronic liver injury, inflammation is characterized by the infiltration of mononuclear cells, i.e. macrophages, lymphocytes, eosinophils and plasma cells. Recruitment of inflammatory cells to the injured liver induces a complex cascade of signalling events and interactions between bone marrow cells, liver resident macrophages, Kupffer cells, and HSC, regulated by lymphokines, cytokines and chemokines.

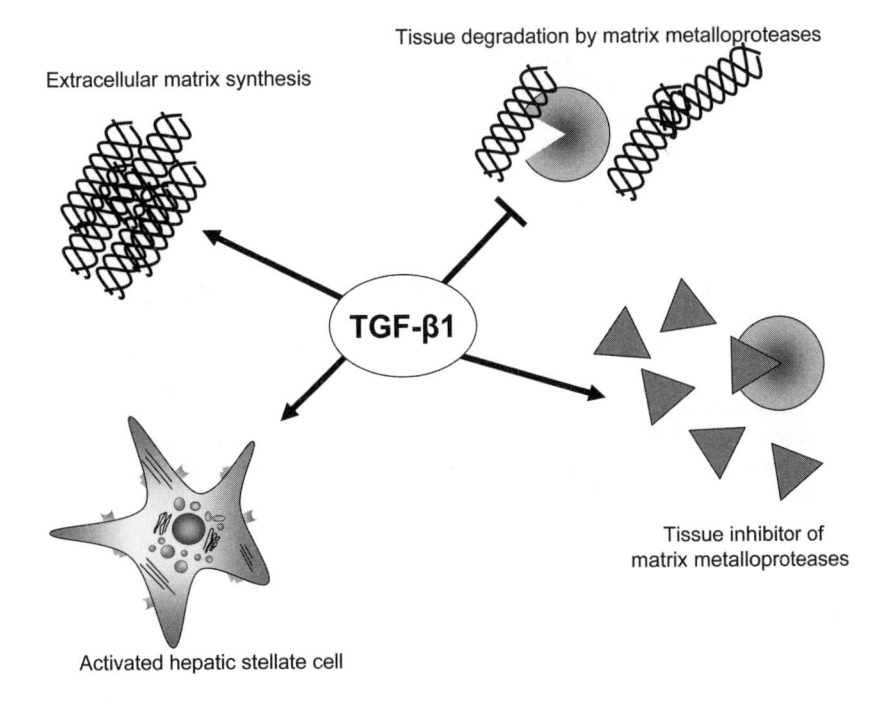

Figure 2 TGF-β_1 plays a major role in the development of liver fibrosis. Not only is the activation of HSC triggered by this cytokine, but it leads to increased production of ECM (extracellular matrix), it inhibits tissue degradation by MMP and it induces the production of TIMP

TGF-β_1 is the major profibrotic cytokine and is secreted mostly by cells of myelo-monocytic lineage during inflammation (Figure 2). Therefore, depletion of macrophages in the early stages of liver fibrosis leads to the attenuation of liver fibrosis[13]. Mice deficient in TGF-β_1 are less susceptible to liver fibrosis than wild-type mice. Consistent with this, Smad3$^{-/-}$ mice which lack Smad3 transcription factor show less fibrosis after liver injury than wild-type mice, since TGF-β_1 mediates its fibrogenic function through Smad3 signalling.

CD4$^+$ cells play an important role in the regulation of the complex crosstalk of liver fibrosis. In particular the type of response CD4$^+$ cells develop is very important for fibrogenesis[14]. Studies using knockout mice deficient in various cytokines showed that fibrogenesis, especially in the model of schistosomiasis-induced liver fibrosis, is strongly associated with a T helper 2 (Th2) CD4$^+$ cell response[15]. Th2 cells secrete IL-4, IL-5, IL-6, IL-10 and IL-13, and are responsible for humoral immunity. Although an equally potent inflammatory response develops when Th1 cells dominate, the development of tissue fibrosis is almost completely attenuated. Th1 cells are associated with cellular immunity and secrete IL-2, IL-12, TNF-α and interferon (IFN)-γ. Although many studies of fibrosis in mice deficient for Th2 or Th1 cytokines showed the importance of the Th1/Th2 homeostasis in liver fibrosis, there are many exceptions. While typical Th2 cytokines such as IL-4 and IL-13 show strong profibrogenic effects, IL-6 and IL-10 do not have this effect. IL-4 is increased in the peripheral blood mononuclear cells of patients with periportal liver fibrosis. Mice lacking IL-4 or IL-13 develop less liver fibrosis than wild-type mice in schistosomiasis-infected mice. IL-6, in contrast, has antifibrotic properties; it participates in tissue remodelling due to induction of matrix metalloproteinase (MMP)-13 gene transcription. Therefore, $IL6^{-/-}$ mice show a lower collagenolytic activity and develop more severe fibrosis[16,17]. IL-10 also induces antifibrogenic effects in fibrosing liver; it mediates a strong immunosuppressive effect and potentiates the effect of antifibrotic cytokines. Consistent with this, $IL-10^{-/-}$ mice exhibit increased liver fibrosis in response to injury[18]. IFN-γ is a potent antifibrogenic cytokine, as demonstrated in many different studies (reviewed in refs 19 and 20). In schistosomiasis-infected mice, treatment with IFN-γ or IL-12 showed no effect on inflammation, but collagen deposition associated with chronic granuloma formation was substantially reduced. Consistently IFN-$\gamma^{-/-}$ mice have accelerated development of liver fibrosis in response to injury[21].

MICROCIRCULATORY EFFECTS IN THE DEVELOPMENT OF LIVER FIBROSIS

Cytokines with vasoactive properties regulate liver fibrosis. Vasodilators such as nitric oxide or relaxin exert antifibrotic effects while vasoconstrictors (e.g. norepinephrine, angiotensin II) have opposite effects[22,23]. Nitric oxide synthetase isoforms, constitutively produced in the endothelium (eNOS) or induced (iNOS) are involved in the regulation of vascular resistance and portal hypertension, a leading cause of fibrogenesis. Genetic ablation of iNOS in mice, thereby abolishing its vasodilatory effect, leads to more severe liver fibrosis. In contrast, endothelin-1, a potent vasoconstrictor, stimulates fibrogenesis through its type A receptor. Therefore endothelin-1-deficient mice develop less fibrosis[24]. Among vasoactive cytokines angiotensin II plays a major role in the development of liver fibrosis. Angiotensinogen$^{-/-}$ mice develop less fibrosis in response to liver injury. Angiotensin II is the effector peptide of the renin–angiotensin sytem and a major vasoactive cytokine regulating arterial pressure homeostasis. Angiotensinogen is formed in the liver and cleaved by renin to form angiotensin I. In turn, angiotensin I is converted to angiotensin II by the angiotensin-converting enzyme (ACE). Angiotensin II binds to AT1 or AT2 plasma membrane receptors to mediate its biological activity. Mostly the AT1 receptor mediates the fibrotic potential of angiotensin II whereas this effect is generally opposed by AT2[25]. Recent studies from our laboratory have demonstrated that the renin–angiotensin-dependent pathway is also expressed locally in the injured liver. Activated HSC synthesize angiotensin II *de novo*, contributing to the profibrotic microenviroment in the injured liver by paracrine and autocrine stimulation[26,27]; therefore, angiotensin II also stimulates hepatic inflammation and stimulates multiple fibrogenic actions in activated HSC including cell proliferation, migration, secretion of proinflammatory cytokines and collagen synthesis.

OXIDATIVE STRESS, ROS AND NICOTINAMIDE ADENINE DINUCLEOTIDE PHOSPHATASE (NADPH) OXIDASES

ROS play an important role in liver fibrosis, being increased in situations of oxidative stress[28]. The ROS family includes superoxide, hydrogen peroxide, hydroxyl radicals and a variety of reaction products. Damaged hepatocytes, activated Kupffer cells and neutrophils contribute to intrahepatic ROS production. Derived from hepatocytes cytochrome 450 E1 ROS stimulate HSC in a paracrine manner through redox-sensitive intracellular pathways. This leads to the activation of HSC and subsequently to the increased deposition of collagen and the progression of fibrosis[29,30].

Furthermore biological effects of angiotensin II are mediated by ROS generated in fibrogenic cells by a non-phagocytic form of NADPH oxidases[31]. This is also the major source of ROS in HSC and Kupffer cells. In contrast to the phagocytic type, NADPH oxidases present in fibrogenic cells are constitutively active. They produce low levels of ROS under basal conditions and generate higher levels of oxidants in response to cytokines stimulating redox-sensitive intracellular pathways[32]. The activation of endogenous ROS formation is controlled by angiotensin II through second-messenger pathways. At least three signalling cascades need to be activated to result in the formation of NADPH oxidase. The cytosolic phagocytic oxidases p47phox and p67phox become phosphorylated by proteinkinase C and bind to membrane-bound heterodimeric flavocytochrome B consisting of gp91phox and p22phox. Together with the small GTPase Rac (Rac-1 or Rac-2), they form a complex and induce the membrane translocation of all cytosolic factors. Flavocytochrome B undergoes a conformational change induced by this event, thereby permitting the completion of the electron transfer from flavin adenine dinucleotide (FAD) to nicotinamide adenine dinucleotide (NADH) and ultimately to superoxide anion[26,33]. This directly induces the up-regulation of collagen-αI(I) gene expression[34]. Mice deficient for the angiotensin II receptor (AT1) or p47phox, one of the important subunits of NADPH oxidase, show significantly less fibrosis when subjected to prolonged alcohol intake or bile duct ligation. Antioxidants also have a protective effect on ROS-mediated liver fibrosis as well as ROS-scavenging enzymes such as superoxide dismutase (SOD1, SOD2, SOD3)[30]. As predicted from the genetic studies, drugs such as ACE inhibitors or AT1 receptor blockers have an antifibrotic effect[24].

ADIPOKINES

Adipokines, such as leptin, adiponektin and resistin, are cytokines originated from the adipose tissue. They are actively involved in lipid metabolism and contribute to liver fibrosis by activating HSC. Leptin is required for HSC activation and liver fibrogenesis[35,36]. Leptin- or leptin-receptor-deficient mice develop less severe liver fibrosis than wild-type mice. Resistin is able to activate HSC and induce the expression of proinflammatory chemokines such as MCP-1 and IL-8 through the activation of NF-κB-dependent pathway[37]. In contrast adiponektin inhibits liver fibrogenesis *in vivo* and *in vitro*[38].

INTRACELLULAR SIGNALLING PATHWAYS

HSC are the major population of collagen-producing cells in fibrotic liver. Activation of HSC is critical for pathogenesis of liver fibrosis. Many studies have investigated the intracellular signalling pathways that are involved in HSC activation[24]. TGF-β_1 is the most potent profibrogenic cytokine and strictly required for activation of HSC into collagen-expressing myofibroblasts. It mediates the crosstalk between parenchymal, inflammatory and collagen-expressing cells, it triggers apoptosis of hepatocytes and induces the activation and recruitment of inflammatory cells to the damaged liver tissue, as well as the differentiation of liver resident cells (fibroblasts, HSC, epithelial cells) into collagen-producing myofibroblasts. It is synthesized as a non-active proform, which forms a complex with two latent associated proteins LAP and LTBP, and is cleaved by the endopeptidase furin to produce a functionally active form[39]. Out of the three TGF-β isoforms (β_1, β_2, β_3) that have been identified up to now, TGF-β_1 is the only one linked to liver fibrosis. In spite of signalling through distinctive pathways in different cell types such as the Smad1/5/8, Smad2/3, MAP kinase and PI3 kinase pathway, it shows three major molecular effects on liver fibrosis: it activates HSC, stimulates ECM synthesis and suppresses ECM degradation[40].

However, mitogen-activated protein kinases (MAPK) have been shown to also play an important role in the activation of HSC. Platelet-derived growth factor (PDGF) is a potent mitogenic activator of stellate cells and leads to Ras activation followed by the sequential activation of Raf, mitogen-induced extracellular kinase (MEK), and extracellular signal regulated kinase (ERK)[41,42]. C-Jun nuclear kinase (JNK) regulates apoptosis of hepatocytes as well as the secretion of inflammatory cytokines by cultured HSC. It also leads to proliferation of HSC[43,44]. In contrast, p38, another MAPK member, has an inhibitory effect on HSC proliferation[45]. Further on PDGF activates and requires focal adhesion kinase (FAK) and phosphatidylinositol 3-kinase (PI3K) for HSC proliferation. This pathway mediates agonist-induced fibrogenic actions in HSC[42].

CELL DEATH AND LIVER FIBROSIS

Next to the activation of inflammatory processes by hepatocellular stress, and the recruitment of non-parenchymal cells to the injured liver tissue, cell death and apoptosis play an important role in starting and modulating hepatic fibrogenic processes. Upon liver injury an increased rate of intrahepatic apoptosis is likely to be the first cellular response to a broad spectrum of harmful events[46,47]. Hepatocytes are susceptible to toxic agents such as alcohol, bile acids or viral infections, and activate apoptosis pathways in response to irreversible injury. There are two different pathways by which apoptosis in hepatocytes can be triggered: the extrinsic death receptor-mediated pathway, or the intrinsic intracellular organelle-based pathway[48]. In the liver the death receptor-triggered pathway is the more common mechanism of hepatocyte apoptosis[49]; it requires activation of death receptors (DR) such as Fas/CD95, tumour necrosis factor receptor-1 (TNFR-1/CD120a), or tumour necrosis factor-associated apoptosis-inducing ligand receptors-1 and -2 (TRAIL-R1/DR4 and TRAIL-R2/DR5)[49]. These receptors are often up-regulated in fibrotic livers. Besides inducing programmed cell death these receptors also activate signalling pathways which stimulate the synthesis of proinflammatory mediators such as chemokine expression, infiltration of neutrophils and inflammation[50]. Moreover, crosslinked by TNF-α, TNFR-1/CD120a affects downstream activation of NF-κB, which in turn induces the expression of many proinflammatory cytokines[51]. Thus, damaged hepatocytes undergoing apoptosis also release ROS and secrete profibrogenic factors such as CXC chemokines (CXCL1, CXCL2). This, in turn, leads to the activation of HSC and other collagen-producing cells, and recruits inflammatory cells to the site of injury. Activated HSC then secrete TGF-β_1, CXCL1 and CXCL2, and further facilitate the hepatotoxic effect, accelerate hepatocyte damage and increase collagen production.

HEPATIC STELLATE CELLS

In the normal liver HSC reside in the space of Disse and store more than 80% of the total liver vitamin A. They share many characteristics of adipocytes and express PPARγ, SREB -1c and leptin. They also express several neural markers such as GFAP, synamin and synantrophysin, and secrete growth factors such as hepatocyte growth factor (HGF), stem cell factor (SCF), fibroblast growth factor 10 (FGF10) and brain-derived nerve growth factor (BDNF). This suggests their close interaction with liver progenitor cells which express many of the receptors for these growth factors. In the injured liver HSC undergo a phenotypic change from non-proliferating, retinoid-storage cells to proliferating activated myofibroblasts which are the major source of ECM production. This process is considered to be the key event in the pathogenesis of liver fibrosis and is induced by profibrogenic cytokines released from damaged hepatocytes, Kupffer cells and inflammatory cells, recruited to the injured liver tissue[52]. Activated HSC obtain myofibroblastic phenotype (transdifferentiation is a different process, HSC activate into myofibroblasts), induce expression of myogenic markers (collagen type I, α-SMA, c-myb, myocyte enhancer factor-2, desmin) and produce almost all of the ECM components present in fibrotic connective tissue. In addition, activated HSC secrete many different cytokines and chemokines. Among these inflammatory cytokines and chemokines are TGF-β_1, the most potent profibrotic cytokine, MCP-1, RANTES, IL-10 and IL-8. They up-regulate adhesion molecules such as integrins, VCAM-1, and ICAM-1, and thereby cause lymphocyte recruitment and activation[53]. Cultured myofibroblasts express HLA-II, CD40 and CD80 surface antigens and induce an allogenic response in T cells. This suggests that activated HSC are involved in antigen presentation and this is supported by the fact that activated HSC also express CD1b and CD1c, antigens involved in presentation of lipids and glycolipids to cells of the immune system and are capable of phagocytosis themselves[54].

TISSUE DEGENERATION

Liver fibrosis is a dynamic process and involves phases of progression and regression. In addition to increased matrix synthesis this pathological process involves major changes in the regulation of matrix degradation. In fibrotic liver the fibrillar matrix is composed predominantly of the interstitial collagens type I and III. These triple helical molecules are relatively resistant to protease activity but are cleaved by the interstitial collagenases matrix metalloprotease (MMP)-13 (in rats) and MMP-8[55]. The inhibition of this matrix degeneration is a key feature of the progression of liver fibrosis. These MMP are subject to TGF-β_1-induced inhibition; furthermore, expression of tissue inhibitor of matrix metalloprotease-1 (TIMP-1), a natural inhibitor of MMP, is also up-regulated during this process[56]. Studies of inducible TGF-β_1 transgenic mice demonstrated that elevated levels of TGF-β_1 have a strong regulatory effect on inhibition of MMP and up-regulation of TIMP-1; therefore, a modulated decrease in TGF-β_1 level is associated with improvement of liver fibrosis[57].

REVERSAL OF LIVER FIBROSIS

Until recently liver fibrosis was considered as an irreversible process[58,59]; however, reversal of cirrhosis has now been described in many patients with diverse liver diseases[60,61]. As previously discussed, HSC play a major role in progression of liver fibrogenesis, and they provide the major obstacle for regression of fibrosis (Figure 3). They are the major source not only for collagen production, but also for the secretion of profibrogenic and proinflammatory cytokines. They also produce TIMP, therefore disturbing the balance of ECM production and degradation[62,63]. Regression of liver fibrosis could be achieved by shifting the balance towards increased degradation of collagen and ECM. To achieve this, reduced levels of profibrogenic and proinflammatory cytokines are required. In this regard elimination of HSC cells is an important target in reversal of hepatic fibrosis. This can be achieved by NKT-dependent apoptosis of HSC (Figure 3).

HSC, other liver myofibroblasts and inflammatory cells contributing to liver fibrosis, including macrophages and Kupffer cells, express many matrix-degrading MMP (however, HSC are also the major source of TIMP)[64]. MMP are involved in the degradation of collagen and other ECM components. Unfortunately, in the fibrotic liver their activity is suppressed by powerful inhibitors such as TIMP-1 and TIMP-2[65]. In the resolution of liver fibrosis the expression of TIMP-1 and TIMP-2 decreases significantly while matrix-

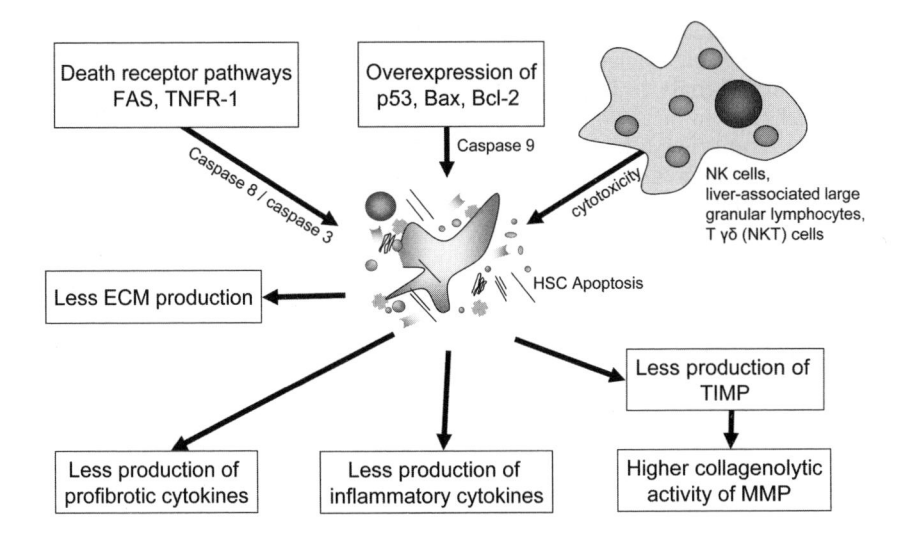

Figure 3 Apoptosis of hepatic stellate cells is a key feature of fibrosis resolution. Apoptosis can be initiated through death receptor pathways involving FAS and TNFR-1 or by overexpression of proapoptotic proteins such as p53, Bax and Bcl-2. NK cells, liver-associated large granular lymphocytes or T γδ (NKT) cells can also kill HSC in spite of expressing MHC I complex. HSC apoptosis leads to decreased ECM production, decreased production of profibrotic and inflammatory cytokines and higher collagenolytic activity of MMP because of decreased TIMP production

degrading MMP continue to be expressed. This leads to an increased collagenase activity and consequent matrix degradation within the liver[66].

The apoptosis of HSC plays a pivotal role in the resolution of liver fibrosis[67]. During ongoing liver injury, activated HSC are protected against apoptosis, probably through signals from soluble factors and changes in the surrounding matrix. When the injurious stimulus is withdrawn, and remodelling of matrix is required, the loss of these survival factors causes the activated HSC to undergo apoptosis, which facilitates the remodelling process by removing a major cellular source of collagen, profibrotic and inflammatory cytokines and TIMP[66]. HSC apoptosis can be induced by death receptor-mediated pathways. HSC increase expression of Fas or TNFR-1 receptor and their ligands and undergo a caspase 8/caspase 3-dependent apoptosis. Alternatively, overexpression of proapoptotic proteins such as p53, Bax and Bcl-2 leads to caspase-9-mediated programmed cell death[68]. In addition, hepatic natural killer (NK) cells serve as a key regulator in HSC apoptosis. NK cells induce apoptosis in a wide range of cells; they target tumour cells which have lost class I expression and up-regulate Rae1, therefore removing NK-inhibitory signals and expressing NK-activating signals[69]. But stimulation of NK cells through NKG2D enables these cells to induce apoptosis even in the presence of MHC class I on target cells. Therefore, they are able to kill activated HSC, known to express MCH I[70]. The required step to initiate cytotoxicity against HSC seems to be the up-regulation of Rae1 by HSC, suggesting that HSC trigger their own destruction in response to low levels of stimulatory signals[71]. In contrast to this TGF-β_1, which is expressed by activated HSC in large amounts, is a potent suppressor of NK cell production of IFN-γ and other NK cell functions[72]. Therefore cells overexpressing Rae1 might also have switched off TGF-β_1 production, thereby removing a potent NK cell-inhibitory signal[71].

The elimination of activated HSC, either through death receptor-mediated pathways or by cytotoxicity provided by NK cells (but also by a liver-associated population of large granular lymphocytes and liver-specific cells T $\gamma\delta$ (NKT) cells), is the key event in regression of liver fibrosis. It not only shifts the balance of ECM degrading and ECM producing towards collagenolytic processes by removing the main source of TIMP and thereby increasing the MMP activity; it also takes away the major source of collagen and the major source of profibrotic and inflammatory cytokines. Therefore the progression of liver fibrosis ceases and processes of fibrosis resolution are facilitated. This concept might also be a challenging therapeutic principle, allowing amelioration of liver fibrosis not only by avoiding hepatotoxic agents (e.g. alcohol, hepatitis C and hepatitis B virus) but actively inducing the resolution of fibrosis by targeting HSC directly.

References

1. Friedman SL. Liver fibrosis – from bench to bedside. J Hepatol. 2003;38(Suppl. 1):S38–53.
2. Arthur MJ. Fibrogenesis II. Metalloproteinases and their inhibitors in liver fibrosis. Am J Physiol Gastrointest Liver Physiol. 2000;279:G245–9.
3. Friedman SL, Roll FJ, Boyles J, Bissell DM. Hepatic lipocytes: the principal collagen-producing cells of normal rat liver. Proc Natl Acad Sci USA. 1985;82:8681–5.
4. Ramadori G, Saile B. Portal tract fibrogenesis in the liver. Lab Invest. 2004;84:153–9.
5. Russo FP, Alison MR, Bigger BW et al. The bone marrow functionally contributes to liver fibrosis. Gastroenterology. 2006;130:1807–21.
6. Ikegami T, Zhang Y, Matsuzaki Y. Liver fibrosis: possible involvement of EMT. Cells Tissues Organs. 2007;185:213–21.
7. Weiler-Normann C, Herkel J, Lohse AW. Mouse models of liver fibrosis. Z Gastroenterol. 2007;45:43–50.
8. Goetz M, Lehr HA, Neurath MF, Galle PR, Orth T. Long-term evaluation of a rat model of chronic cholangitis resembling human primary sclerosing cholangitis. Scand J Immunol. 2003;58:533–40.
9. Zimmerman HJ, Lewis JH. Chemical- and toxin-induced hepatotoxicity. Gastroenterol Clin N Am. 1995;24:1027–45.
10. de la M Hall P, Lieber CS, DeCarli LM et al. Models of alcoholic liver disease in rodents: a critical evaluation. Alcohol Clin Exp Res. 2001;25(5 Suppl. ISBRA):254S–61S.
11. Oz HS, Chen TS, Neuman M. Methionine deficiency and hepatic injury in a dietary steatohepatitis model. Dig Dis Sci. 2007 [Epub ahead of print].
12. Wynn TA, Thompson RW, Cheever AW, Mentink-Kane MM. Immunopathogenesis of schistosomiasis. Immunol Rev. 2004;201:156–67.
13. Imamura M, Ogawa T, Sasaguri Y, Chayama K, Ueno H. Suppression of macrophage infiltration inhibits activation of hepatic stellate cells and liver fibrogenesis in rats. Gastroenterology. 2005;128:138–46.
14. Wynn TA. Fibrotic disease and the T(H)1/T(H)2 paradigm. Nat Rev Immunol. 2004;4:583–94.
15. Wynn TA, Cheever AW, Jankovic D et al. An IL-12-based vaccination method for preventing fibrosis induced by schistosome infection. Nature. 1995;376:594–6.

16. Streetz KL, Tacke F, Leifeld L et al. Interleukin 6/gp130-dependent pathways are protective during chronic liver diseases. Hepatology. 2003;38:218–9.
17. Solis Herruzo JA, de la Torre P, Diaz Sanjuan T, Garcia Ruiz I, Munoz Yague T. IL-6 and extracellular matrix remodeling. Rev Esp Enferm Dig. 2005;97:575–95.
18. Zhang LJ, Wang XZ. Interleukin-10 and chronic liver disease. World J Gastroenterol. 2006;12:1681–5.
19. Weng H, Mertens PR, Gressner AM, Dooley S. IFN-gamma abrogates profibrogenic TGF-beta signaling in liver by targeting expression of inhibitory and receptor Smads. J Hepatol. 2007;46:295–303.
20. Watson MW, Jaksic A, Price P et al. Interferon-gamma response by peripheral blood mononuclear cells to hepatitis C virus core antigen is reduced in patients with liver fibrosis. J Infect Dis. 2003;188:1533–6. Erratum in: J Infect Dis. 2005;191:145.
21. Czaja MJ, Weiner FR, Takahashi S et al. Gamma-interferon treatment inhibits collagen deposition in murine schistosomiasis. Hepatology. 1989;10:795–800.
22. Williams EJ, Benyon RC, Trim N et al. Relaxin inhibits effective collagen deposition by cultured hepatic stellate cells and decreases rat liver fibrosis *in vivo*. Gut. 2001;49:577–83.
23. Oben JA, Roskams T, Yang S et al. Hepatic fibrogenesis requires sympathetic neurotransmitters. Gut. 2004;53:438–45.
24. Bataller R, Brenner DA. Liver fibrosis. J Clin Invest. 2005;115:209–18.
25. Xiao HD, Fuchs S, Frenzel K, Teng L, Bernstein KE. Circulating versus local angiotensin II in blood pressure control: lessons from tissue-specific expression of angiotensin-converting enzyme (ACE). Crit Rev Eukaryot Gene Expr. 2004;14:137–45.
26. De Minicis S, Brenner DA. NOX in liver fibrosis. Arch Biochem Biophys. 2007;462:266–72.
27. Bataller R, Schwabe RF, Choi YH et al. NADPH oxidase signal transduces angiotensin II in hepatic stellate cells and is critical in hepatic fibrosis. J Clin Invest. 2003;112:1383–94.
28. Siegmund SV, Brenner DA. Molecular pathogenesis of alcohol-induced hepatic fibrosis. Alcohol Clin Exp Res. 2005;29:102S–9S.
29. Adachi T, Togashi H, Suzuki A et al. NAD(P)H oxidase plays a crucial role in PDGF-induced proliferation of hepatic stellate cells. Hepatology. 2005;41:1272–81.
30. Svegliati-Baroni G, Saccomanno S, van Goor H, Jansen P, Benedetti A, Moshage H. Involvement of reactive oxygen species and nitric oxide radicals in activation and proliferation of rat hepatic stellate cells. Liver. 2001;21:1–12.
31. Paravicini TM, Touyz RM. Redox signaling in hypertension. Cardiovasc Res. 2006;71:247–58.
32. Brandes RP, Kreuzer J. Vascular NADPH oxidases: molecular mechanisms of activation. Cardiovasc Res. 2005;65:16–27.
33. Babior BM. NADPH oxidase: an update. Blood. 1999;93:1464–76.
34. Bataller R, Schwabe RF, Choi YH et al. NADPH oxidase signal transduces angiotensin II in hepatic stellate cells and is critical in hepatic fibrosis. J Clin Invest. 2003;112:1383–94.
35. Marra F. Leptin and liver fibrosis: a matter of fat. Gastroenterology. 2002;122:1529–32.
36. Ikejima K, Takei Y, Honda H et al. Leptin receptor-mediated signaling regulates hepatic fibrogenesis and remodeling of extracellular matrix in the rat. Gastroenterology. 2002;122:1399–410.
37. Bertolani C, Sancho-Bru P, Failli P et al. Resistin as an intrahepatic cytokine: overexpression during chronic injury and induction of proinflammatory actions in hepatic stellate cells. Am J Pathol. 2006;169:2042–53.
38. Kamada Y, Tamura S, Kiso S et al. Enhanced carbon tetrachloride-induced liver fibrosis in mice lacking adiponectin. Gastroenterology. 2003;125:1796–1807.
39. Gressner AM, Weiskirchen R. Modern pathogenetic concepts of liver fibrosis suggest stellate cells and TGF-beta as major players and therapeutic targets. J Cell Mol Med. 2006;10:76–99.
40. Sanderson N, Factor V, Nagy P et al. Hepatic expression of mature transforming growth factor β 1 in transgenic mice results in multiple tissue lesions. Proc Natl Acad Sci USA. 1995;92:2572–6.
41. Pinzani P, Marra FJ, Carloini V. Signal transduction in hepatic stellate cells. Liver. 1998;18:2–23.

42. Marra F, Arrighi MC, Fazi M et al. Extracellular signal-regulated kinase activation differentially regulates platelet-derived growth factor's actions in hepatic stellate cells, and is induced by *in vivo* liver injury in the rat. Hepatology. 1999;30:951–8.
43. Schwabe RF, Uchinami H, Qian T et al. Differential requirement for c-Jun NH2-terminal kinase in TNFalpha- and Fas-mediated apoptosis in hepatocytes. FASEB J. 2004;18:720–2.
44. Schwabe RF, Schnabl B, Kweon YO, Brenner DA. CD40 activates NF-kappa B and c-Jun N-terminal kinase and enhances chemokine secretion on activated human hepatic stellate cells. J Immunol. 2001;166:6812–19.
45. Schnabl B, Bradham CA, Bennett BL, Manning AM, Stefanovic B, Brenner DA. TAK1/ JNK and p38 have opposite effects on rat hepatic stellate cells. Hepatology. 2001;34:953–63.
46. Canbay A, Kip SN, Kahraman A, Gieseler RK, Nayci A, Gerken G. Apoptosis and fibrosis in non-alcoholic fatty liver disease. Turk J Gastroenterol. 2005;16:1–6.
47. Yoon JH, Gores GJ. Death receptor-mediated apoptosis and the liver. J Hepatol. 2002;37:400–10.
48. Green DR, Reed JC. Mitochondria and apoptosis. Science. 1998;281:1309–12.
49. Faubion WA, Gores GJ. Death receptors in liver biology and pathobiology. Hepatology. 1999;29:1–4.
50. Faouzi S, Burckhardt BE, Hanson JC et al. Anti-Fas induces hepatic chemokines and promotes inflammation by an NF-kappa B-independent, caspase-3-dependent pathway. J Biol Chem. 2001;276:49077–82.
51. Locksley RM, Killeen N, Lenardo MJ. The TNF and TNF receptor superfamilies: integrating mammalian biology. Cell. 2001;104:487–501.
52. Kisseleva T, Brenner DA. Role of hepatic stellate cells in fibrogenesis and the reversal of fibrosis. J Gastroenterol Hepatol. 2007;22(Suppl. 1):S73–8.
53. Knittel T, Dinter C, Kobold D et al. Expression and regulation of cell adhesion molecules by hepatic stellate cells (HSC) of rat liver: involvement of HSC in recruitment of inflammatory cells during hepatic tissue repair. Am J Pathol. 1999;154:153–67.
54. Vinas O, Bataller R, Sancho-Bru P et al. Human hepatic stellate cells show features of antigen-presenting cells and stimulate lymphocyte proliferation. Hepatology. 2003;38:919–29.
55. Arthur MJ. Fibrogenesis II. Metalloproteinases and their inhibitors in liver fibrosis. Am J Physiol Gastrointest Liver Physiol. 2000;279:G245–9.
56. Iredale JP, Benyon RC, Arthur MJP et al. Tissue inhibitor of metalloproteinase-1 messenger RNA expression is enhanced relative to interstitial collagenase messenger RNA in experimental liver injury and fibrosis. Hepatology. 1996;24:176–84.
57. Ueberham E, Low R, Ueberham U, Schonig K, Bujard H, Gebhardt R. Conditional tetracycline-regulated expression of TGF-beta1 in liver of transgenic mice leads to reversible intermediary fibrosis. Hepatology. 2003;37:1067–78.
58. Desmet V, Roskams T. Cirrhosis reversal: a duel between dogma and myth. J Hepatol. 2004;40:860–7.
59. Bonis PAL, Friedman SL, Kaplan MM. Is liver fibrosis reversible? N Engl J Med. 2001;344:452–4.
60. Hammel P, Couvelard A, O'Toole D et al. Regression of liver fibrosis after biliary drainage in patients with chronic pancreatitis and stenosis of the common bile duct. N Engl J Med. 2001;344:418–23.
61. Poynard T, McHutchison J, Manns M et al. Impact of pegylated interferon alfa-2b and ribavirin on liver fibrosis in patients with chronic hepatitis C. Gastroenterology. 2002;122:1303–13.
62. Tsukada S, Parsons CJ, Rippe RA. Mechanisms of liver fibrosis. Clin Chim Acta. 2006;364:33–60.
63. Friedman SL. Mechanisms of disease: mechanisms of hepatic fibrosis and therapeutic implications. Nat Clin Pract Gastroenterol Hepatol. 2004;2:98–105.
64. Benyon RC, Arthur MJP. Extracellular matrix degradation and the role of hepatic stellate cells. Semin Liver Dis. 2001;21:373–84.
65. Benyon RC, Iredale JP, Goddard S, Winwood PJ, Arthur MJP. Expression of tissue inhibitor of metalloproteinases-1 and -2 is increased in fibrotic human liver. Gastroenterology. 1996;110:821–31.

66. Henderson NC, Iredale JP. Liver fibrosis: cellular mechanisms of progression and resolution. Clin Sci (Lond). 2007;112:265–80.
67. Murphy FR, Issa R, Zhou X et al. Inhibition of apoptosis of activated hepatic stellate cells by tissue inhibitor of metalloproteinase-1 is mediated via effects on matrix metalloproteinase inhibition: implications for reversibility of liver fibrosis. J Biol Chem. 2002;277:11069–76.
68. Iredale JP. Hepatic stellate cell behavior during resolution of liver injury. Semin Liver Dis. 2001;21:427–36.
69. Moretta A. Natural killer cells and dendritic cells: rendezvous in abused tissues. Nat Rev Immunol. 2002;2:957–64.
70. Laouar Y, Sutterwala FS, Gorelik L, Flavell RA. Transforming growth factor-beta controls T helper type 1 cell development through regulation of natural killer cell interferon-gamma. Nat Immunol. 2005;6:600–7.
71. Mehal WZ. Activation-induced cell death of hepatic stellate cells by the innate immune system. Gastroenterology. 2006;130:600–3.
72. Shi Z, Wakil AE, Rockey DC. Strain-specific differences in mouse hepatic wound healing are mediated by divergent T helper cytokine responses. Proc Natl Acad Sci USA. 1997;94:10663–8.

13
Hepatic fibrogenesis and carcinogenesis: Krüppel-like factors and beyond

S. L. FRIEDMAN

INTRODUCTION

The understanding of hepatic fibrosis, or the liver's scarring response has emerged as a major focus of current research in hepatology. In particular, hepatic stellate cell activation is a central event in fibrogenesis, and has contributed to a detailed understanding of fibrosis pathogenesis. What is less clear, however, is why the fibrotic milieu accelerates emergence of hepatocellular carcinoma.

PATHOGENESIS OF HEPATIC FIBROSIS

Hepatic stellate cells (HSC) are the primary source of extracellular matrix in normal and fibrotic liver. They undergo an 'activation' or transdifferentiation in progressive stages yielding a cell type that is highly proliferative, fibrogenic and contractile[1]. Activation of HSC is the central event of fibrogenesis. Exciting progress has been made in understanding the molecular basis of this process. Major advances include: (a) elucidation of effects of key cytokines on and their signalling pathways in HSC; (b) understanding of transcriptional regulation of HSC activation; (c) characterization of matrix proteases and their inhibitors; (d) demonstration of apoptosis as an important event in resolution of hepatic fibrosis and identification of its mediators; (e) elucidation of the complex and dynamic interaction between HSC and matrix; (f) understanding of the role of other cellular elements in hepatic fibrosis and their interaction with HSC. In addition, clinical studies have begun to identify host genetic polymorphisms that may soon predict risk of fibrosis progression.

Recent studies have underscored the heterogeneity of mesenchymal populations in liver ranging from classic vitamin A-storing stellate cells to portal fibroblasts[2], with the variable expression of neural[3], angiogenic[4], contractile[5] and even bone-marrow-derived[6] markers. Moreover, experimental genetic 'marking' of stellate cells, by expressing fluorescent proteins downstream of either fibrogenic or contractile gene promoters, illustrates the plasticity of fibrogenic cell populations *in vivo*[7].

CELLULAR AND MOLECULAR FEATURES OF STELLATE CELL ACTIVATION

The fundamental features of stellate cell activation appear to be similar regardless of the initial cause of injury although, increasingly, disease-specific mechanisms of stellate cell activation have also begun to emerge, especially for HCV infection[8,9] and non-alcoholic steatohepatitis[10,11]. Activation occurs in two phases, initiation and perpetuation, followed by resolution if liver injury is abrogated. Initiation is mediated primarily by paracrine stimuli (oxidative stress, apoptotic fragments and cytokines) from injured neighbouring liver cells and infiltrating inflammatory cells. Perpetuation connotes those responses to cytokines that collectively enhance scar formation (see below). Resolution refers to the fate of activated stellate cells when the primary insult is withdrawn or attenuated (reviewed in refs 12 and 13).

The perpetuation of stellate cell activation can be further subdivided into at least seven distinct events, which can occur simultaneously. Specific pathways and mediators contributing to these responses include:

1. Proliferation, due to several mitogenic cytokines, including platelet-derived growth factor (PDGF)[14], fibroblast growth factor (FGF), thrombin[15] and vascular endothelial growth factor (VEGF)[17];

2. Chemotaxis and migration is an equally important mechanism of stellate cell accumulation, which has been attributed to cytokines (e.g. PDGF, transforming growth factor beta 1 (TGF-β_1), endothelin-1 (ET-1))[16,17] and altered cell–matrix interactions;

3. Fibrogenesis, which is largely driven by the cytokine TGF-β_1, whose activity is amplified by increased production[18], increased activation of the latent form[19] and enhanced receptor expression[20];

4. Release of proinflammatory, profibrogenic and pro-mitogenic cytokines (in particular monocyte chemotactic peptide (MCP-1), which increase the accumulation of inflammatory cells and stimulate extracellular matrix (ECM) production via autocrine pathways, especially through the actions of TGF-β_1 and PDGF[21];

5. Contractility, which confers upon the cells the potential to constrict sinusoids and reduce blood flow. Actions of endothelin-1 are key components of this response, which probably contributes to increased portal pressure in patients with chronic liver disease[5,22];

6. Degradation of the liver's normal matrix, thereby disrupting the delicate scaffolding required to preserve liver function (see ref. 23 for review);

7. Loss of vitamin A droplets, whose functional role is not clear, but may involve altered retinoid receptor signalling[24-29].

KRÜPPEL-LIKE FACTORS (KLF) – OVERVIEW

The family of Krüppel-like zinc finger transcription factors currently includes at least 15 members that regulate remarkably diverse processes including cell growth, signal transduction and differentiation[30-34]. KLF genes are highly conserved evolutionarily, with homologues expressed in zebrafish[35] and *Xenopus*[36]. All KLF members possess a tightly-conserved C-terminal 81 amino acid zinc finger DNA-binding domain that can interact with 'GC-box' or 'CACC-box' DNA motifs in responsive promoters, with each KLF having a distinct N-terminal activation domain[32].

While the DNA binding domains of KLF are identical, their divergent activation domains account for a remarkably broad range of biological activities. Indeed, few generalizations can be made about the family apart from their structural similarity. Some are transcriptional activators; others are repressors; while still others, for example KLF6, are bifunctional in *trans*-repressing some genes while *trans*-activating others[30]. The proteins may be phosphorylated, acetylated[37,38], or ubiquitinylated[39].

KLF play key developmental roles based on studies in both lower species[35] and rodents, and our finding of lethality of KLF6$^{-/-}$ mice conforms to this paradigm (see ref. 40). Knockout mouse models have revealed roles of KLF in T-cell activation (KLF2)[41], blood vessel stability (KLF2)[42], erythropoiesis[43-45], olfactory differentiation[46] and epithelial barrier integrity (KLF4)[47,48]. These developmental activities are ascribed to those KLF that are tissue-restricted as well as those that are ubiquitously expressed. For example, KLF4 and KLF6 are both widely expressed, yet their developmental expression is restricted[49-52]. While KLF4$^{-/-}$ mice are viable, they display increased gastric epithelial growth with premalignant lesions with loss of differentiation[53], associated with loss of goblet cells in the colon[54]. KLF4 has also been described as one of four essential factors determining pluripotency in embryonic stem cells[55,56]. Importantly, even heterozygous KLF gene-deleted mice may have a phenotype, as in KLF5$^{+/-}$ mice, which have defective vascular remodelling[57].

KLF6 – GENERAL FEATURES AND ROLE IN LIVER BIOLOGY

Within this broader context much has been learned about the biology of KLF6 since our cloning of this molecule as an immediate–early gene induced in response to injury in hepatic stellate cells, and in hepatocytes following partial hepatectomy[58-60]. KLF6, like the KLF family in general, can assume a remarkable range of functions that may be temporally, spatially, cell context or developmentally restricted. KLF6 is a 283 amino acid protein with a 202 residue N-terminal activation domain and a classic Krüppel-like 81 amino acid C-terminal DNA binding domain. The activation domain is proline- and serine-rich with multiple potential phosphorylation sites, and a PEST sequence defining possible proteasomal targeting[58]. Initially described as a *trans*-activator of collagen I[58], HIV[60] and a pregnancy-specific glycoprotein[59] its list of transcriptional targets now includes p21[61], TGF-β_1 and its receptors[62], a collagen chaperone protein HSP-47[63], nitric oxide synthase[64], urokinase type plasminogen activator[65], leukotriene C synthase[66], keratin genes[67,68], acid ceramidase[69], multi-drug resistance genes[70] and cyclin D1 (unpublished data). Of equal importance, KLF6 is induced during adipogenesis[71], and regulates adipocyte differentiation. During injury responses, KLF6 is induced as an immediate–early gene in several contexts including stellate cell activation following liver injury[58], endothelial cell wounding[72], or hepatic regeneration. We have uncovered the anti-proliferative activity of KLF6 based on its ability to significantly suppress hepatocellular growth when expressed in hepatocytes of transgenic mice through p53-independent *trans*-activation of the cdk/cyclin inhibitor, p21[73].

Our recent investigations of fibrosis have focused on the role of Krüppel-like factor 6 (KLF6), in stellate cell activation. For several years we were puzzled by the paradoxical findings that KLF6 is growth-suppressive and a *bona-fide* tumour-suppressor gene, yet it was induced during a growth burst in this cell type. The paradox has been resolved with the finding that KLF6 is alternatively spliced, and studies to date indicate that early stellate cell activation is marked by induction of splice forms of KLF6, which have dominant negative, growth-promoting activities. Splicing is also enhanced by oxidant stress and occurs *in vivo* and in culture. These findings point to a novel mechanism of transcriptional/post-transcriptional gene regulation in hepatic stellate cells, and add to the complexity underlying regulation of this fascinating cell type's behaviour.

At the same time we have explored the role of KLF6 in hepatic carcinogenesis, since the molecule is ubiquitously expressed, is up-regulated during liver injury, and has been established as a tumour-suppressor gene in a number of cancers, including HCC. Initial studies analysing 41 HCC of different aetiologies confirmed a high degree of KLF6 LOH but very few inactivating mutations[74,75]. We next compared mRNA expression of full-length KLF6 and KLF6 splice form mRNA between either dysplasia or HCC and surrounding tissue in HCV-infected patients, as well as in a cohort of HBV patients. Expression of KLF6 mRNA was decreased in 73% of HBV-associated HCC compared to matched surrounding tissue (ST), with reductions of ~80% in one-third of the patients. KLF6 mRNA expression was also reduced in dysplastic nodules from patients with HCV compared to cirrhotic livers with an additional, marked decrease in the very advanced, metastatic stage. An increased ratio of KLF6SV1/wt KLF6 was present in a subset of the HBV-related HCC compared to matched ST, but this was not associated with any specific histological subgroups in the HCV subset. Reconstituting KLF6 in HepG2 cells by retroviral infection decreased proliferation and related markers including cyclin D1, and β-catenin, increased cellular differentiation based on induction of albumin, E-cadherin, and decreased α-fetoprotein. These data indicated that reduced KLF6 expression is common in both HBV- and HCV-related HCC and occurs at critical stages during cancer progression. Effects of KLF6 were attributable at least in part to regulation of genes controlling hepatocyte growth and differentiation.

These findings underscore the dual role of a transcription factor (KLF6) in directing the response to liver injury and contributing to hepatocarcinogenesis by divergent regulation in different liver cell types. Moreover, the findings establish a paradigm wherein alternative splicing may contribute to the response to injury as well as the progression of carcinoma. Other transcription factors may follow similar pathways of dysregulation in cancer, in particular other Krüppel-like factors, (e.g. KLF4).

HOW DOES HEPATIC FIBROGENESIS PROMOTE HCC?

It remains unclear whether these findings contribute to our understanding of how fibrosis accelerates carcinogenesis in liver. Traditional explanations have included: (1) enhanced survival signals released by fibrotic matrix that prevent death of hepatocytes after DNA damage; (2) reduced NK cell number and activity, leading to diminished tumour surveillance as fibrosis progresses; (3) decreased telomere length during carcinogenesis.

Further advances in the understanding of the molecular biology of hepatic fibrosis are critical not only to the development of effective, targeted antifibrotic therapies, but also to our understanding of hepatocarcinogenesis. Effective antifibrotic therapies may ultimately reduce the incidence of HCC but clinical trials are needed to establish this possibility. Continued insights into signalling and gene regulation may ultimately yield new therapies that are both antifibrotic and antineoplastic.

References

1. Friedman SL. Molecular regulation of hepatic fibrosis, an integrated cellular response to tissue injury. J Biol Chem. 2000;275:2247–50.
2. Kinnman N, Francoz C, Barbu V et al. The myofibroblastic conversion of peribiliary fibrogenic cells distinct from hepatic stellate cells is stimulated by platelet-derived growth factor during liver fibrogenesis. Lab Invest. 2003 Feb;83:163–73.
3. Cassiman D, Libbrecht L, Desmet V, Denef C, Roskams T. Hepatic stellate cell/myofibroblast subpopulations in fibrotic human and rat livers. J Hepatol. 2002;36:200–9.
4. Corpechot C, Barbu V, Wendum D et al. Hypoxia-induced VEGF and collagen I expressions are associated with angiogenesis and fibrogenesis in experimental cirrhosis. Hepatology. 2002 May;35:1010–21.
5. Rockey DC. Vascular mediators in the injured liver. Hepatology. 2003;37:4–12.
6. Forbes SJ, Russo FP, Rey V et al. A significant proportion of myofibroblasts are of bone marrow origin in human liver fibrosis. Gastroenterology. 2004;126:955–63.
7. Magness ST, Bataller R, Yang L, Brenner DA. A dual reporter gene transgenic mouse demonstrates heterogeneity in hepatic fibrogenic cell populations. Hepatology. 2004;40:1151–9.
8. Schulze-Krebs A, Preimel D, Popov Y et al. Hepatitis C virus-replicating hepatocytes induce fibrogenic activation of hepatic stellate cells. Gastroenterology. 2005;129:246–58.
9. Bataller R, Paik YH, Lindquist JN, Lemasters JJ, Brenner DA. Hepatitis C virus core and nonstructural proteins induce fibrogenic effects in hepatic stellate cells. Gastroenterology. 2004;126:529–40.

10. Schaffler A, Scholmerich J, Buchler C. Mechanisms of disease: adipocytokines and visceral adipose tissue – emerging role in nonalcoholic fatty liver disease. Nat Clin Pract Gastroenterol Hepatol. 2005;2:273–80.
11. Kaser S, Moschen A, Cayon A et al. Adiponectin and its receptors in non-alcoholic steatohepatitis. Gut. 2005;54:117–21.
12. Friedman SL. Mechanisms of hepatic fibrosis and therapeutic implications. Nature Clin Pract Gastroenterol Hepatol. 2004;1:98–105.
13. Iredale JP. Hepatic stellate cell behavior during resolution of liver injury. Semin Liver Dis. 2001;21:427–36.
14. Pinzani M. PDGF and signal transduction in hepatic stellate cells. Front Biosci. 2002;7: d1720–6.
15. Marra F, Grandaliano G, Valente AJ, Abboud HE. Thrombin stimulates proliferation of liver fat-storing cells and expression of monocyte chemotactic protein-1: potential role in liver injury. Hepatology. 1995;22:780–7.
16. Ikeda K, Wakahara T, Wang YQ, Kadoya H, Kawada N, Kaneda K. *In vitro* migratory potential of rat quiescent hepatic stellate cells and its augmentation by cell activation. Hepatology. 1999;29:1760–7.
17. Tangkijvanich P, Tam SP, Yee HF Jr. Wound-induced migration of rat hepatic stellate cells is modulated by endothelin-1 through rho-kinase-mediated alterations in the acto-myosin cytoskeleton. Hepatology. 2001;33:74–80.
18. Bissell DM, Roulot D, George J. Transforming growth factor beta and the liver. Hepatology. 2001;34:859–67.
19. Dooley S, Delvoux B, Lahme B, Mangasser-Stephan K, Gressner AM. Modulation of transforming growth factor beta response and signaling during transdifferentiation of rat hepatic stellate cells to myofibroblasts. Hepatology. 2000;31:1094–106.
20. Friedman SL, Yamasaki G, Wong L. Modulation of transforming growth factor beta receptors of rat lipocytes during the hepatic wound healing response. Enhanced binding and reduced gene expression accompany cellular activation in culture and *in vivo*. J Biol Chem. 1994;269:10551–8.
21. Pinzani M, Marra F. Cytokine receptors and signaling in hepatic stellate cells. Semin Liver Dis. 2001;21:397–416.
22. Ikura Y, Ohsawa M, Naruko T et al. Expression of the hepatic endothelin system in human cirrhotic livers. J Pathol. 2004;204:304–10.
23. Iredale JP. Cirrhosis: new research provides a basis for rational and targeted treatments. Br Med J. 2003;327:143–7.
24. Okuno M, Kojima S, Akita K et al. Retinoids in liver fibrosis and cancer. Front Biosci. 2002;7:d204–18.
25. Okuno M, Moriwaki H, Imai S et al. Retinoids exacerbate rat liver fibrosis by inducing the activation of latent TGF-beta in liver stellate cells. Hepatology. 1997;26:913–21.
26. Li H, Zhang J, Huang G et al. Effect of retinoid kappa receptor alpha (RXRalpha) transfection on the proliferation and phenotype of rat hepatic stellate cells *in vitro*. Chin Med J (Engl). 2002;115:928–32.
27. Wang L, Tankersley LR, Tang M, Potter JJ, Mezey E. Regulation of the murine alpha(2)(I) collagen promoter by retinoic acid and retinoid X receptors. Arch Biochem Biophys. 2002;401:262–70.
28. Natarajan SK, Thomas S, Ramachandran A, Pulimood AB, Balasubramanian KA. Retinoid metabolism during development of liver cirrhosis. Arch Biochem Biophys. 2005;443:93–100.
29. Hellemans K, Verbuyst P, Quartier E et al. Differential modulation of rat hepatic stellate phenotype by natural and synthetic retinoids. Hepatology. 2004;39:97–108.
30. Bieker JJ. Kruppel-like factors: three fingers in many pies. J Biol Chem. 2001;276:34355–8.
31. Black BE, Levesque L, Holaska JM, Wood TC, Paschal BM. Identification of an NTF2-related factor that binds Ran-GTP and regulates nuclear protein export. Mol Cell Biol. 1999;19:8616–24.
32. Philipsen S, Suske G. A tale of three fingers: the family of mammalian Sp/XKLF transcription factors. Nucleic Acids Res. 1999;27:2991–3000.
33. Kaczynski J, Cook T, Urrutia R. Sp1- and Kruppel-like transcription factors. Genome Biol. 2003;4:206.

34. Dang DT, Pevsner J, Yang VW. The biology of the mammalian Kruppel-like family of transcription factors. Int J Biochem Cell Biol. 2000;32:1103–21.
35. Oates AC, Pratt SJ, Vail B et al. The zebrafish klf gene family. Blood. 2001;98:1792–801.
36. Huber TL, Perkins AC, Deconinck AE, Chan FY, Mead PE, Zon LI. Neptune, a Krüppel-like transcription factor that participates in primitive erythropoiesis in *Xenopus*. Curr Biol. 2001;11:1456–61.
37. Zhang W, Kadam S, Emerson BM, Bieker JJ. Site-specific acetylation by p300 or CREB binding protein regulates erythroid Kruppel-like factor transcriptional activity via its interaction with the SWI–SNF complex. Mol Cell Biol. 2001;21:2413–22.
38. Li D, Yea S, Dolios G et al. Regulation of Kruppel-like factor 6 tumor suppressor activity by acetylation. Cancer Res. 2005;65:9216–25.
39. Banck MS, Beaven SW, Narla G, Walsh MJ, Friedman SL, Beutler AS. KLF6 degradation after apoptotic DNA damage. FEBS Lett. 2006;580:6981–6.
40. Matsumoto N, Kubo A, Liu H et al. Developmental regulation of yolk sac hematopoiesis by Kruppel-like factor 6. Blood. 2006;107:1357–65.
41. Kuo CT, Veselits ML, Leiden JM. LKLF: a transcriptional regulator of single-positive T cell quiescence and survival. Science. 1997;277:1986–90.
42. Kuo CT, Veselits ML, Barton KP, Lu MM, Clendenin C, Leiden JM. The LKLF transcription factor is required for normal tunica media formation and blood vessel stabilization during murine embryogenesis. Genes Dev. 1997;11:2996–3006.
43. Perkins AC, Sharpe AH, Orkin SH. Lethal beta-thalassaemia in mice lacking the erythroid CACCC-transcription factor EKLF. Nature. 1995;375:318–22.
44. Nuez B, Michalovich D, Bygrave A, Ploemacher R, Grosveld F. Defective haematopoiesis in fetal liver resulting from inactivation of the EKLF gene. Nature. 1995;375:316–18.
45. Emery DW, Gavriilidis G, Asano H, Stamatoyannopoulos G. The transcription factor KLF11 can induce gamma-globin gene expression in the setting of *in vivo* adult erythropoiesis. J Cell Biochem. 2007;100:1045–55.
46. Kajimura D, Dragomir C, Ramirez F, Laub F. Identification of genes regulated by transcription factor KLF7 in differentiating olfactory sensory neurons. Gene. 2007;388:34–42.
47. Swamynathan SK, Katz JP, Kaestner KH, Ashery-Padan R, Crawford MA, Piatigorsky J. Conditional deletion of the mouse Klf4 gene results in corneal epithelial fragility, stromal edema, and loss of conjunctival goblet cells. Mol Cell Biol. 2007;27:182–94.
48. Segre JA, Bauer C, Fuchs E. Klf4 is a transcription factor required for establishing the barrier function of the skin. Nat Genet. 1999;22:356–60.
49. Laub F, Aldabe R, Ramirez F, Friedman S. Embryonic expression of Kruppel-like factor 6 in neural and non-neural tissues. Mech Dev. 2001;106:167–70.
50. Fischer EA, Verpont MC, Garrett-Sinha LA, Ronco PM, Rossert JA. Klf6 is a zinc finger protein expressed in a cell-specific manner during kidney development. J Am Soc Nephrol. 2001;12:726–35.
51. Blanchon L, Bocco JL, Gallot D et al. Co-localization of KLF6 and KLF4 with pregnancy-specific glycoproteins during human placenta development. Mech Dev. 2001;105:185–9.
52. Ton-That H, Kaestner KH, Shields JM, Mahatanankoon CS, Yang VW. Expression of the gut-enriched Kruppel-like factor gene during development and intestinal tumorigenesis. FEBS Lett. 1997;419:239–43.
53. Katz JP, Perreault N, Goldstein BG et al. Loss of Klf4 in mice causes altered proliferation and differentiation and precancerous changes in the adult stomach. Gastroenterology. 2005;128:935–45.
54. Katz JP, Perreault N, Goldstein BG et al. The zinc-finger transcription factor Klf4 is required for terminal differentiation of goblet cells in the colon. Development. 2002;129:2619–28.
55. Yamanaka S. Strategies and new developments in the generation of patient-specific pluripotent stem cells. Cell Stem Cell. 2007;1:39–49.
56. Takahashi K, Yamanaka S. Induction of pluripotent stem cells from mouse embryonic and adult fibroblast cultures by defined factors. Cell. 2006;126:663–76.
57. Shindo T, Manabe I, Fukushima Y et al. Kruppel-like zinc-finger transcription factor KLF5/BTEB2 is a target for angiotensin II signaling and an essential regulator of cardiovascular remodeling. Nat Med. 2002;8:856–63.

58. Ratziu V, Lalazar A, Wong L et al. Zf9, a Kruppel-like transcription factor up-regulated *in vivo* during early hepatic fibrosis. Proc Natl Acad Sci USA. 1998;95:9500–5.
59. Koritschoner NP, Bocco JL, Panzetta-Dutari GM, Dumur CI, Flury A, Patrito LC. A novel human zinc finger protein that interacts with the core promoter element of a TATA box-less gene. J Biol Chem. 1997;272:9573–80.
60. Suzuki T, Yamamoto T, Kurabayashi M, Nagai R, Yazaki Y, Horikoshi M. Isolation and initial characterization of GBF, a novel DNA-binding zinc finger protein that binds to the GC-rich binding sites of the HIV-1 promoter. J Biochem (Tokyo). 1998;124:389–95.
61. Narla G, Heath KE, Reeves HL et al. KLF6, a candidate tumor suppressor gene mutated in prostate cancer. Science. 2001;294:2563–6.
62. Kim Y, Ratziu V, Choi SG et al. Transcriptional activation of transforming growth factor beta1 and its receptors by the Kruppel-like factor Zf9/core promoter-binding protein and Sp1. Potential mechanisms for autocrine fibrogenesis in response to injury. J Biol Chem. 1998;273:33750–8.
63. Yasuda K, Hirayoshi K, Hirata H, Kubota H, Hosokawa N, Nagata K. The Kruppel-like factor Zf9 and proteins in the Sp1 family regulate the expression of HSP47, a collagen-specific molecular chaperone. J Biol Chem. 2002;277:44613–22.
64. Warke VG, Nambiar MP, Krishnan S et al. Transcriptional activation of the human inducible nitric-oxide synthase promoter by Kruppel-like factor 6. J Biol Chem. 2003;278:14812–19.
65. Kojima S, Hayashi S, Shimokado K et al. Transcriptional activation of urokinase by the Kruppel-like factor Zf9/COPEB activates latent TGF-beta1 in vascular endothelial cells. Blood. 2000;95:1309–16.
66. Zhao JL, Austen KF, Lam BK. Cell-specific transcription of leukotriene C(4) synthase involves a Kruppel-like transcription factor and Sp1. J Biol Chem. 2000;275:8903–10.
67. Okano J, Opitz OG, Nakagawa H, Jenkins TD, Friedman SL, Rustgi AK. The Kruppel-like transcriptional factors Zf9 and GKLF coactivate the human keratin 4 promoter and physically interact. FEBS Lett. 2000;473:95–100.
68. Chiambaretta F, Blanchon L, Rabier B et al. Regulation of corneal keratin-12 gene expression by the human Kruppel-like transcription factor 6. Invest Ophthalmol Vis Sci. 2002;43:3422–9.
69. Park JH, Eliyahu E, Narla G, DiFeo A, Martignetti JA, Schuchman EH. KLF6 is one transcription factor involved in regulating acid ceramidase gene expression. Biochim Biophys Acta. 2005;1732:82–7.
70. Ho EA, Piquette-Miller M. KLF6 and HSF4 transcriptionally regulate multidrug resistance transporters during inflammation. Biochem Biophys Res Commun. 2007;353:679–85.
71. Inuzuka H, Wakao H, Masuho Y, Muramatsu MA, Tojo H, Nanbu-Wakao R. cDNA cloning and expression analysis of mouse zf9, a Kruppel-like transcription factor gene that is induced by adipogenic hormonal stimulation in 3T3-L1 cells. Biochim Biophys Acta. 1999;1447:199–207.
72. Botella LM, Sanchez-Elsner T, Sanz-Rodriguez F et al. Transcriptional activation of endoglin and transforming growth factor-beta signaling components by cooperative interaction between Sp1 and KLF6: their potential role in the response to vascular injury. Blood. 2002;100:4001–10.
73. Narla G, Kremer-Tal S, Matsumoto N et al. *In vivo* regulation of p21 by the Kruppel-like factor 6 tumor-suppressor gene in mouse liver and human hepatocellular carcinoma. Oncogene. 2007;26:4428–34.
74. Kremer-Tal S, Reeves HL, Narla G et al. Frequent inactivation of the tumor suppressor Kruppel-like factor 6 (KLF6) in hepatocellular carcinoma. Hepatology. 2004;40:1047–52.
75. Kremer-Tal S, Narla G, Chen Y et al. Downregulation of KLF6 is an early event in hepatocarcinogenesis, and stimulates proliferation while reducing differentiation. J Hepatol. 2007;46:645–54.

Section IV
Clinical management of progressive liver fibrosis

Chair: G RAMADORI and C TRAUTWEIN

14
Biomarkers of liver fibrosis

D. THABUT and M. SIMON-RUDLER

INTRODUCTION

The consensus conference statements recommended liver biopsy in the management of almost all patients with chronic liver diseases related to hepatitis C, hepatitis B, alcoholic and non-alcoholic fatty liver disease, but also underlined the necessity of developing reliable non-invasive tests[1]. However, liver biopsy has several well-known limitations, i.e. sampling error and intra- and inter-observer variability[2-8] and risks, i.e. morbidity ranging from 0.3% to 0.6%, and mortality (0.05%)[9]. Moreover, it is costly. Hence, in the past five years there has been an increasing desire for non-invasive tests to assess the stage of liver fibrosis. Ideally, non-invasive methods should be repeatable, with no sampling error or observer variability, and be less expensive than liver biopsy. There are two categories of non-invasive test: serum markers and methodologies related to liver imaging technique (the most innovative being the measurement of transient elastography). The aim of this chapter is to describe the different serum markers of liver fibrosis and their performance, and the chapter will focus on hepatitis C virus (HCV) patients, because the tests were generally constructed on that population.

Serum markers can be direct or indirect. Direct markers measure components of extracellular matrix in serum (e.g. hyaluronic acid, collagen IV, etc.) as well as cytokines involved in the fibrogenetic and fibrolysis process. Indirect markers include markers of liver function and liver inflammation and comprise routinely available tests. Since the first publication in 1991 of the PGA index[10], more than 400 original articles have been published describing non-invasive markers of liver fibrosis, and 16 tests were validated at least twice in HCV patients[11-26] (Table 1). Before comparing tests, the validation of each test must be considered. First there is an exploratory phase, which is the construction of the test. Of major importance is then the validation step, which can be internal or external. Before its current use in clinical practice an external independent and prospective validation is mandatory. Also necessary is determination of pre-analytical and analytical recommendations, precautions of use and security algorithms for false-negative and false-positive. Then the test can be patented and commercialized. To date five tests are on the market: FibroTest–FibroSure, ELF index, Fibrometer, FibroSpect II

Table 1 Serum markers of hepatic fibrosis with at least two validations in HCV patients

Test	Year of first publication	Key leader	Components	Liver disease
AP[22]	1997	Poynard	Age, Plt	HCV
Bonacini[12]	1997	Lindsay	Plt, AST, ALT	HCV
Pohl[21]	2001	Pohl	Plt, AST	HCV
Forns[14]	2002	Forns	Plt, cholesterol, age	HCV
APRI[24]	2003	Lok	Plt, AST	HCV
MP3[19]	2004	Leroy	PIIINP, MMP1	HCV
Hui[15]	2005	Hui	BMI, Plt, albumin, Bili	HBV
SHASTA[17]	2005	Kelleher	HA, AST, albumin	HCV/HIV
AST/ALT[20]	2005	Park	AST, ALT	HCV
FIB-4[23]	2006	Sterling	Plt, AST, ALT, age	HCV/HIV
Fibroindex[18]	2007	Koda	Plt, AST, gamma-globulins	HCV
FibroTest/Fibrosure[16]	2001	Poynard	A2M, haptoglobin, ApoA1, Bili, GGT, age, gender	HCV
FibroSpectII[26]	2004	Oh	A2M, HA, TIMP1	HCV
ELF[25]	2004	Rosenberg	HA, PIIINP, TIMP	HCV
FibroMeter[13]	2005	Cales	Plt, AST, A2M, HA, PT, mixed age, gender	Mixed
HepaScore[11]	2005	Adams	A2M, HA, GGT, age, gender	HCV

and HepaScore[11,13,16,25,26]. For these tests we will try to answer the following questions: how are they validated; what is their diagnostic performance, i.e. is there a 'better test'; is there a way to optimize their performance, and can we expect more from non-invasive tests?

HOW ARE THE PATENTED SERUM MARKERS OF FIBROSIS VALIDATED?

Table 2 shows the number of validation studies published of each test and the number of independent validations and patients included in October 2007. Until now the FibroTest is the most validated test, with 12 independent validation studies[13,27–37].

What is the diagnostic performance of the patented serum markers of fibrosis, and is there a 'better test'?

Usually the performance of a test is studied with the area under the receiving operating curve (AUROC), which reflects the specificity and sensitivity of the test. However, this index has several pitfalls, one being that the liver biopsy, which is considered as the gold standard, is a poor reference standard. Another problem is the bivarial categorization of liver biopsy into two groups, that can be F0F1 vs F2F3F4 if the test aims to detect significant fibrosis, F0F1F2 vs F3F4 to detect severe fibrosis and F0F1F2F3 vs F4 to detect cirrhosis. When looking at the areas of fibrosis[2], grouping different stages may not be relevant; moreover, the AUROC will depend on the prevalence of each fibrosis stage in the studied population. For example, the AUROC for the detection of significant fibrosis will be higher if the population sampled is mainly composed of F0 and F4 patients, rather than of F1 and F2 patients[38]. Therefore, comparison of different tests must be performed on the same population, and comparison of AUROC provided by different studies makes no sense.

A recent overview found no significant difference between the AUROCs for advanced fibrosis among the patented biomarkers. Because of the limited number of patients included in the direct comparisons a clinically significant difference cannot be excluded, particularly between Hepascore with a possible

Table 2 Validation of the five patented biomarkers

Test	No. of studies published	No. of independent studies published	No. of patients
FibroTest	33	12	2256
FibroSpect	3	3	321
FibroMeter	3	2	536
ELF	3	1	120
HepaScore	3	2	536

smaller AUROC (0.04 difference) vs FibroTest and Fibrometer[39]. To date two independent studies have compared three of the five patented tests[31,33], i.e. FibroTest, Fibrometer and Hepascore. There was no difference between any test, when considering the AUROC for the detection of significant fibrosis, severe fibrosis or cirrhosis.

Another way to compare the tests could be to compare their accuracy, or its opposite, the proportion of misclassified patients, for each stage of fibrosis. Then a profile performance test can be established. This was done by Halfon et al. for FibroTest and Fibrometer. In that study, when the accuracy is similar between the two tests (71% and 72% all stages together, p = n.s.), the FibroTest appears to be the better performer in classifying correctly F1 patients, whereas Fibrometer classifies better F2 and F3 patients[31]. These results have to be confirmed by other studies.

The study of discordant cases is of major importance when interpreting the results of a test. Until now the FibroTest is the test where discordances were the best studied. Overall, 18–24% discordances are reported[40]. The classical causes of false-positives (haemolysis, Gilbert syndrome and sepsis) and false-negatives (inflammation) of the FibroTest are now well described. In an independent study discordances were imputable to the FibroTest in 29% of cases (5% of the entire population), 21% to liver biopsy, and the remaining discordant cases were undetermined. Not surprisingly, the main factor of discordance was being at an intermediate stage of fibrosis[32]. However, one must consider the performance of liver biopsy between two intermediate stages, which is rather poor[2]. Indeed, the entire liver is certainly the gold standard, but a liver biopsy of 15 mm (the median biopsy length in tertiary centres) has an AUROC of 0.82 between F1 and F2, being around 20% of false-positives or false-negatives[2]. Therefore, a test with an AUROC of 0.66 (usually described as a 'weak' value when using a true gold standard) between F1 and F2 has a relative AUROC vs the best AUROC possible of $0.66/0.82 = 0.80$, which is in the end acceptable for a non-invasive test. The size of liver biopsy has been reported inconstantly to be a factor of discordance[40].

The number of liver biopsies avoided could also represent a target for comparing tests. However, one must be aware of the fact that the number of biopsies avoided depends on the specificity and sensitivity asked for a test. For example, in the first publication of the FibroTest by Imbert-Bismuth et al., demanding a specificity of 95% and a sensitivity of 100% for the diagnosis of significant liver fibrosis, only 46% of biopsies could be avoided[16]. Similarly, Parkes et al. arbitrarily defined an 'inaccurate' zone of a marker when it 'cannot reliably attribute results for tests as tests perform with lower sensitivities/ specificities at thresholds, where positive predictive value <90%, negative predictive value >95%'[41]. Choosing these thresholds could be acceptable if a true gold standard existed. However, if this definition was applied to 15 mm liver biopsies the biopsy would be inaccurate in 40% of cases for a diagnosis between F1 and F2.

In summary, tests are difficult to compare, and independent validations did not identify a better test. Tests may have different profiles, and the overall proportion of discordances ranges 20%.

IS THERE A WAY TO OPTIMIZE THE PERFORMANCES OF THE TESTS?

The combination of different serum markers together with transient elastometry is certainly a good way to go. Sebastiani et al. proposed stepwise algorithms in patients with compensated chronic hepatitis C, by performing sequentially APRI, FibroTest and in the remaining patients liver biopsy. With this approach, liver biopsy could be avoided in 71% of cases with an accuracy of 93%[36]. Castera et al. proposed the combination of FibroTest and transient elastometry, and this significantly improved the performance of each non-invasive test alone, with an accuracy of 84% when combining the tests[28]. This is probably the most promising approach.

CAN WE EXPECT MORE FROM NON-INVASIVE TESTS?

Due to the low performance of liver biopsy, the correct way to evaluate a test could be to consider its prognostic value. The FibroTest has been shown to have an excellent prognostic value, predicting survival without HCV complications in a series of 537 patients[42]. Similarly, the ELF score could predict liver-related morbidity and mortality with a better sensitivity than liver biopsy[25].

Non-expert physicians and patients are waiting for an almost perfect test, which is a biomarker with less than 10% of false-positive or false-negative results and more than 99% applicability. This is not possible, even with liver biopsy[43]. A 25 mm non-fragmented biopsy is obtained in less than 50% of all large series[40] and the rate of false-positive/negative of such a 25 mm non-fragmented biopsy is still around 20%, for the diagnosis of advanced fibrosis, in comparison with the true gold standard which is the whole liver[2]. Among the discordances observed between biopsy and biomarker estimates of fibrosis, the cause of failure is frequently biopsy failure[40,42]. Therefore, we believe that it is an illusion to wait for an almost perfect biomarker with an AUROC greater than 90% for the diagnosis of advanced fibrosis. Hence, in France, practices are evolving rapidly and a nationwide survey recently found that, among 546 hepatologists, 81% used a non-invasive biomarker (FibroTest–ActiTest) and 32% used elastography (Fibroscan), with a dramatic decrease in the use of liver biopsy for more than 50% of patients with chronic hepatitis C, and with a subsequent increase in the number of patients treated[44]. A recent overview by French health authorities officially approved non-invasive biomarkers Fibro-Test and transient elastometry-Fibroscan as first-line estimates of fibrosis in patients with chronic hepatitis C, recommended reimbursement by social security and approved liver biopsy only as second-line estimate in case of discordance or non-interpretability of non-invasive markers[45].

In conclusion, during the past 5 years there has been a major improvement in the non-invasive diagnosis of liver fibrosis, especially for chronic hepatitis C patients. Independent validations, assessment of pre-analytical and analytical recommendations and study of discordances are of major importance before considering use of a test in clinical practice. All the patented tests seem to be comparable, and have rather good performances. Because of the low performance of liver biopsy, the existence of a perfect test is unlikely. Liver biopsy should no longer be considered mandatory as a first-line estimate of fibrosis in HCV patients.

References

1. Bravo AA, Sheth SG, Chopra S. Liver biopsy. N Engl J Med. 2001;344:495–500.
2. Bedossa P, Dargere D, Paradis V. Sampling variability of liver fibrosis in chronic hepatitis C. Hepatology. 2003;38:1449–57.
3. Bedossa P, Poynard T, Naveau S, Martin ED, Agostini H, Chaput JC. Observer variation in assessment of liver biopsies of alcoholic patients. Alcohol Clin Exp Res. 1988;12:173–8.
4. Colloredo G, Guido M, Sonzogni A, Leandro G. Impact of liver biopsy size on histological evaluation of chronic viral hepatitis: the smaller the sample, the milder the disease. J Hepatol. 2003;39:239–44.
5. Labayle D, Chaput JC, Albuisson F, Buffet C, Martin E, Etienne JP. [Comparison of the histological lesions in tissue specimens taken from the right and left lobe of the liver in alcoholic liver disease (author's transl)]. Gastroenterol Clin Biol. 1979;3:235–40.
6. McHutchison J, Poynard T, Afdhal N. Fibrosis as an end point for clinical trials in liver disease: a report of the international fibrosis group. Clin Gastroenterol Hepatol. 2006;4:1214–20.
7. Ratziu V, Charlotte F, Heurtier A et al. Sampling variability of liver biopsy in nonalcoholic fatty liver disease. Gastroenterology. 2005;128:1898–906.
8. Regev A, Berho M, Jeffers LJ et al. Sampling error and intraobserver variation in liver biopsy in patients with chronic HCV infection. Am J Gastroenterol. 2002;97:2614–18.
9. Poynard T, Ratziu V, Bedossa P. Appropriateness of liver biopsy. Can J Gastroenterol. 2000;14:543–8.
10. Poynard T, Aubert A, Bedossa P et al. A simple biological index for detection of alcoholic liver disease in drinkers. Gastroenterology. 1991;100:1397–402.
11. Adams LA, Bulsara M, Rossi E et al. Hepascore: an accurate validated predictor of liver fibrosis in chronic hepatitis C infection. Clin Chem. 2005;51:1867–73.
12. Bonacini M, Hadi G, Govindarajan S, Lindsay KL. Utility of a discriminant score for diagnosing advanced fibrosis or cirrhosis in patients with chronic hepatitis C virus infection. Am J Gastroenterol. 1997;92:1302–4.
13. Cales P, Oberti F, Michalak S et al. A novel panel of blood markers to assess the degree of liver fibrosis. Hepatology. 2005;42:1373–81.
14. Forns X, Ampurdanes S, Llovet JM et al. Identification of chronic hepatitis C patients without hepatic fibrosis by a simple predictive model. Hepatology. 2002;36:986–92.
15. Hui AY, Chan HL, Wong VW et al. Identification of chronic hepatitis B patients without significant liver fibrosis by a simple noninvasive predictive model. Am J Gastroenterol. 2005;100:616–23.
16. Imbert-Bismut F, Ratziu V, Pieroni L, Charlotte F, Benhamou Y, Poynard T. Biochemical markers of liver fibrosis in patients with hepatitis C virus infection: a prospective study. Lancet. 2001;357:1069–75.
17. Kelleher TB, Mehta SH, Bhaskar R et al. Prediction of hepatic fibrosis in HIV/HCV co-infected patients using serum fibrosis markers: the SHASTA index. J Hepatol. 2005;43:78–84.
18. Koda M, Matunaga Y, Kawakami M, Kishimoto Y, Suou T, Murawaki Y. FibroIndex, a practical index for predicting significant fibrosis in patients with chronic hepatitis C. Hepatology. 2007;45:297–306.
19. Leroy V, Monier F, Bottari S et al. Circulating matrix metalloproteinases 1, 2, 9 and their inhibitors TIMP-1 and TIMP-2 as serum markers of liver fibrosis in patients with chronic hepatitis C: comparison with PIIINP and hyaluronic acid. Am J Gastroenterol. 2004;99:271–9.
20. Park G, Jones DB, Katelaris P. Value of AST/ALT ratio as fibrotic predictor in chronic hepatitis C. Am J Gastroenterol. 2005;100:1623–4; author reply 4.

21. Pohl A, Behling C, Oliver D, Kilani M, Monson P, Hassanein T. Serum aminotransferase levels and platelet counts as predictors of degree of fibrosis in chronic hepatitis C virus infection. Am J Gastroenterol. 2001;96:3142–6.
22. Poynard T, Bedossa P. Age and platelet count: a simple index for predicting the presence of histological lesions in patients with antibodies to hepatitis C virus. METAVIR and CLINIVIR Cooperative Study Groups. J Viral Hepat. 1997;4:199–208.
23. Sterling RK, Lissen E, Clumeck N et al. Development of a simple noninvasive index to predict significant fibrosis in patients with HIV/HCV coinfection. Hepatology. 2006;43:1317–25.
24. Wai CT, Greenson JK, Fontana RJ et al. A simple noninvasive index can predict both significant fibrosis and cirrhosis in patients with chronic hepatitis C. Hepatology. 2003;38:518–26.
25. Rosenberg WM, Voelker M, Thiel R et al. Serum markers detect the presence of liver fibrosis: a cohort study. Gastroenterology. 2004;127:1704–13.
26. Zaman A, Rosen HR, Ingram K, Corless CL, Oh E, Smith K. Assessment of FIBROSpect II to detect hepatic fibrosis in chronic hepatitis C patients. Am J Med. 2007;120:280e9–14.
27. Bourliere M, Penaranda G, Renou C et al. Validation and comparison of indexes for fibrosis and cirrhosis prediction in chronic hepatitis C patients: proposal for a pragmatic approach classification without liver biopsies. J Viral Hepat. 2006;13:659–70.
28. Castera L, Vergniol J, Foucher J et al. Prospective comparison of transient elastography, Fibrotest, APRI, and liver biopsy for the assessment of fibrosis in chronic hepatitis C. Gastroenterology. 2005;128:343–50.
29. Colletta C, Smirne C, Fabris C et al. Value of two noninvasive methods to detect progression of fibrosis among HCV carriers with normal aminotransferases. Hepatology. 2005;42:838–45.
30. Grigorescu M, Rusu M, Neculoiu D et al. The FibroTest value in discriminating between insignificant and significant fibrosis in chronic hepatitis C patients. The Romanian experience. J Gastrointest Liver Dis. 2007;16:31–7.
31. Halfon P, Bacq Y, De Muret A et al. Comparison of test performance profile for blood tests of liver fibrosis in chronic hepatitis C. J Hepatol. 2007;46:395–402.
32. Halfon P, Bourliere M, Deydier R et al. Independent prospective multicenter validation of biochemical markers (fibrotest-actitest) for the prediction of liver fibrosis and activity in patients with chronic hepatitis C: the fibropaca study. Am J Gastroenterol. 2006;101:547–55.
33. Leroy V, Hilleret MN, Sturm N et al. Prospective comparison of six non-invasive scores for the diagnosis of liver fibrosis in chronic hepatitis C. J Hepatol. 2007;46:775–82.
34. Morali G, Maor Y, Klar R et al. Fibrotest-Actitest: the biochemical marker of liver fibrosis – the Israeli experience. Isr Med Assoc J. 2007;9:588–91.
35. Rossi E, Adams L, Prins A et al. Validation of the FibroTest biochemical markers score in assessing liver fibrosis in hepatitis C patients. Clin Chem. 2003;49:450–4.
36. Sebastiani G, Vario A, Guido M et al. Stepwise combination algorithms of non-invasive markers to diagnose significant fibrosis in chronic hepatitis C. J Hepatol. 2006;44:686–93.
37. Varaut A, Fontaine H, Serpaggi J et al. Diagnostic accuracy of the fibrotest in hemodialysis and renal transplant patients with chronic hepatitis C virus. Transplantation. 2005;80:1550–5.
38. Poynard T, Halfon P, Castera L et al. Standardization of ROC curve areas for diagnostic evaluation of liver fibrosis markers based on prevalences of fibrosis stages. Clin Chem. 2007;53:1615–22.
39. Poynard T, Morra R, Halfon P et al. Meta-analyses of Fibrotest diagnostic value in chronic liver disease. BMC Gastroenterol. 2007;7:40.
40. Poynard T, Munteanu M, Imbert-Bismut F et al. Prospective analysis of discordant results between biochemical markers and biopsy in patients with chronic hepatitis C. Clin Chem. 2004;50:1344–55.
41. Parkes J, Guha IN, Roderick P, Rosenberg W. Performance of serum marker panels for liver fibrosis in chronic hepatitis C. J Hepatol. 2006;44:462–74.
42. Ngo Y, Munteanu M, Messous D et al. A prospective analysis of the prognostic value of biomarkers (FibroTest) in patients with chronic hepatitis C. Clin Chem. 2006;52:1887–96.

43. Poynard T, Ratziu V, Benhamou Y, Thabut D, Moussalli J. Biomarkers as a first-line estimate of injury in chronic liver diseases: time for a moratorium on liver biopsy? Gastroenterology. 2005;128:1146–8; author reply 8.
44. Castera L, Denis J, Babany G, Roudot-Thoraval F. Evolving practices of non-invasive markers of liver fibrosis in patients with chronic hepatitis C in France: time for new guidelines? J Hepatol. 2007;46:528–9; author reply 9–30.
45. La Haute Autorité de Santé (HAS) in France – The HAS recommendations for the management of the chronic hepatitis C using non-invasive biomarkers. http://www.has-sante.fr/portail/display.jsp?id=c.476486 (Accessed August 2007).

15
Clinical evaluation of disease progression in chronic liver disease: towards an integrated system?

M. PINZANI and F. VIZZUTTI

INTRODUCTION

Progressive fibrosis and cirrhotic transformation of liver tissue are common pathological outcomes of most chronic liver diseases (CLD). Although the histopathological analysis of liver tissue still represents the reference standard for the evaluation of disease progression in CLD, a distinct change in clinical practice is currently occurring and the tendency to substitute liver biopsy with 'non-invasive methods' has grown to a level of complexity that needs clarification and guidance.

The aim of this chapter is to provide an overview on the proposed non-invasive diagnostic methodologies and their possible integration with standard invasive procedures for the evaluation of disease progression, i.e. liver biopsy and the measurement of portal pressure.

LACK OF A TRUE GOLD STANDARD

The introduction and evaluation of different non-invasive measures for assessing disease progression in CLD is based on the key limitation of using liver biopsy as a reference standard. Indeed, several limitations of liver biopsy, and particularly the fact that a single bioptic cylinder is representative of no more than 1/50 000 of the whole liver, make a fair comparison with a serum marker or liver stiffness measurement (LSM) rather difficult. This also considering that standard hystopathological analysis may have the same difficulty of non-invasive estimates in discriminating adjacent stages of fibrosis, i.e. F2 vs F1 or F3 vs F2[1,2]. To minimize these limitations it is absolutely important that histopathological staging is assessed with all the proposed recommendations concerning the size of the biopsy and the number of analysed portal tracts[1,3], and that the non-invasive methodology (blood test, LSM, etc.) is tested within a reasonable time from the liver biopsy, ideally within 24 h and certainly not within 3–6 months as often reported. In addition, there is need for amelioration and further development of the current histopathological scoring systems. For example, efforts should be directed at staging fibrosis beyond stage F4 since the current system makes no distinction between initial cirrhosis (i.e. thin bridging fibrous septa, with limited or no neo-angiogenesis, surrounding large parenchymal nodules) and advanced and end-stage cirrhosis where the tissue angio-architecture is largely altered[4].

Measurement of the hepatic venous pressure gradient (HVPG), currently employed for the evaluation of portal hypertension, has been suggested as a reliable endpoint to assess the therapeutic benefit of antiviral therapy in patients with advanced hepatic fibrosis due to chronic hepatitis C virus (HCV) infection[5–9]. In the absence of significant fibrotic evolution HVPG does not exceed 5 mmHg, whereas a gradient of more than 5 mmHg is always associated with significant fibrosis. Therefore, when considering the treatment of patients with advanced fibrosis with an HVPG in the range between 5 and 10 mmHg, measurement of HVPG could provide relevant indications about improvement, stabilization or worsening within the stage of compensated cirrhosis. In view of the fact that, within the range 5–10 mmHg, portal hypertension is a direct consequence of the fibrotic/cirrhotic transformation of liver tissue, measurement of HVPG could represent a reference standard superior to liver biopsy in advanced stages, although this is still controversial and needs to be further substantiated in prospective studies including a larger number of patients. Overall, it appears that the major limitation of HVPG measurement relies on logistics: it is expensive, requires a dedicated setting and very experienced operators and hence is available only in specialized centres.

BIOCHEMICAL MARKERS

A large scientific and commercial investment has been made in the past 10 years in order to develop serum markers able to predict the fibrotic stage of CLD. Among the proposed markers, some reflect alterations in hepatic function but do not directly reflect extracellular matrix (ECM) metabolism: 'indirect markers'. Others are directly linked to the modifications in ECM turnover occurring during fibrogenesis: 'direct markers'[10–27]. In most of the studies so far published, the AUC (area under the curve) for the ROC (receiver operating characteristic) curve is employed as a measure of test performance, with optimal values being as close to 1.0 as possible. Nevertheless, the reported median AUC in differentiating mild/no fibrosis and significant fibrosis in validation populations is around 0.77, which is far from high diagnostic accuracy. However, all tests show an improved performance when the endpoint is to differentiate cirrhosis/non-cirrhosis with median AUC in validation sets of approximately 0.87. In a recent modelling analysis including the majority of the proposed serum marker panels, Parkes and co-workers showed that, when positive and negative predictive values (PPV and NPV, respectively) thresholds of 90% and 95% were considered, liver biopsy could have been correctly avoided only in an average 35% of the study population, with 20% of patients misclassified and the remaining impossible to classify because of intermediate values[28].

Overall it is very important to note that, although direct, indirect and combined serum marker systems measure rather different biomarkers, they are all characterized by an AUC for the ROC clustering around 0.85. As already pointed out, it is likely that the explanation of this diagnostic equivalency lies in the inaccuracy of liver biopsy as reference standard either in absolute terms or relative to the lack of adequate standards in the so-far-performed validation studies[29]. A relevant interpretation problem concerns the different spectrum of fibrosis stages ('spectrum bias') that accounts for most of the heterogeneity between studies. For example, if a study is over-represented in extreme stages (i.e. F0 and F4) its specificity and sensitivity will be automatically higher than in a study including only adjacent stages. Therefore, sensitivity and/or standardization analysis should be performed according to these differences in stage prevalence defining advanced (i.e. ⩾F3) and non-advanced (i.e. ⩽F2) fibrosis.

A better definition of serum tests could derive from their evaluation in prospective studies employing a combination of different tests. Along these lines, Sebastiani and co-workers reported that a stepwise combination of different algorithms (APRI, FibroTest, Forns' index) in cohorts of patients with chronic HCV or HBV hepatitis may reduce the need for liver biopsy in 50–70% and 50–80% of cases, respectively[30,31]. Moreover, Leroy and co-workers prospectively compared six non-invasive scores for the diagnosis of liver fibrosis in chronic HCV hepatitis[32]. They found that the best combination (including MP3, FibroTest and APRI) could select one-third of patients with either absence of significant fibrosis or presence of advanced fibrosis with more than 90% certainty.

In summary, at the present stage of development we can conclude that the diagnostic accuracy of systems employing serum biomarkers has been proved useful for the detection (or exclusion) of significant fibrosis or cirrhosis mainly in patients with chronic HCV infection. However, it is rather clear that these tests may reduce but not eliminate the need for liver biopsy and that platelet count *per se* allows the exclusion of cirrhosis with a fairly similar degree of accuracy[33,34].

TRANSIENT ELASTOGRAPHY

In the past 5 years a non-invasive medical device based on transient elastography (Fibroscan®, Echosense, Paris, France) has received increasing interest. This system has been proposed for the measurement of liver stiffness, considered as a direct consequence of the fibrotic evolution of CLD[35]. As a result, several studies aimed at evaluating the clinical usefulness and diagnostic accuracy of LSM have been published in the past 2 years. These studies are listed in Table 1 with the proposed AUC, cut-off and predictive values. The results of the two pioneer studies performed in cohorts of patients with chronic hepatitis C suggested that this system could be useful in assessing the presence of significant fibrosis (i.e. ⩾F2) and in suggesting the presence of cirrhosis[36,44].

In a recent report Fraquelli and co-workers have provided important information for the establishment of practical guidelines in the use of LSM as

Table 1 Proposed liver stiffness measurement cut-off values for the prediction of different stages of fibrosis in chronic liver disease

Reference	Aetiology	LSM cut-off values (kPa) <F2	≥F2	≥F3	F4	PPV/NPV (%)*	AUC
Castera et al.[36]	HCV		7.1	9.5	12.5	95/48 87/81 77/95	0.83 ≥ F2 0.90 ≥ F3 0.95 = F4
Carrion et al.[37]	HCV post-OLT		8.5		12.5	79/92 50/100	0.90 ≥ F2 0.93 ≥ F3 0.98 = F4
Foucher et al.[38]	CLD		7.2	12.5	17.6	90/52 90/80 91/92	0.80 ≥ F2 0.90 ≥ F3 0.96 = F4
Gomez-Dominguez et al.[39]	CLD		4	11	16	88/50 78/76 80/98	0.74 ≥ F2 0.72 ≥ F3 0.94 = F4
Ganne-Carrie et al.[40]	CLD				14.6	74/96	0.95 = F4
de Ledinghen et al.[41]	HCV-HIV	4.5			14.5	NR 88/96	0.72 ≥ F2 0.91 ≥ F3 0.97 = F4
Kim et al.[42]	CLD		7.3	8.8	15	96/50 78/95 33/97	0.77 ≥ F2 0.92 ≥ F3 0.80 = F4

Table 1 (continued)

Reference	Aetiology	LSM cut-off values (kPa)				PPV/NPV (%)*	AUC
		<F2	≥F2	≥F3	F4		
Yoneda et al.[43]	NAFLD	5.6	6.6	8	17	93.5/59.1 90/83.3 63.6/95.6 83.3/100	0.88 ≥ F1 0.87 ≥ F2 0.91 ≥ F3 0.99 = F4
Ziol et al.[44]	HCV		8.8	9.6	14.6	88/56 71/93 78/97	0.79 ≥ F2 0.91 ≥ F3 0.97 = F4
Fraquelli et al.[45]	CLD		7.9	10.3	11.9	NR NR NR	0.86 ≥ F2 0.87 ≥ F3 0.90 = F4
Corpechot et al.[46]	PBC/PSC		7.3	9.8	17.3	91/79 84/95 78/99	0.92 ≥ F2 0.95 ≥ F3 0.96 = F4

LSM, liver stiffness measurement; CLD, chronic liver disease, i.e. HCV, HBV, ethanol, and NASH; PPV and NPV, positive and negative predictive values; AUC, area under the ROC curve; NR, not reported; NAFLD, non-alcoholic fatty liver disease.
*Importantly predictive values (PPV and NPV) vary based on the prevalence of the disease.

a diagnostic tool in CLD[45]. First, LSM is characterized by high intra- and inter-observer agreement (0.98), that probably makes this system the most reproducible among those currently available. Importantly, the inter-observer, and, most importantly, the intra-observer agreement are influenced by variables such as body mass index (BMI) (particularly when ≥28) and hepatic steatosis; therefore LSM should be used cautiously as a surrogate of liver biopsy for assessing liver fibrosis in the presence of these clinical features. This study also strongly suggests that factors other than fibrosis may impact on the results of LSM. Indeed, the extent of necroinflammatory activity influences LSM with a steady increase of LSM values in parallel with the degree of histological activity. This possibility is also strongly suggested by a recent report showing significant variations in liver stiffness occurring during ALT flares in patients with chronic viral hepatitis[47], and confirmed by recent results obtained by our group in patients with acute viral hepatitis[48]. Two considerations are inspired by the analysis of the data reported in Table 1. For degrees of fibrosis preceding the cirrhotic stage, and particularly in HCV-related CLD, reported LSM values are not very discrepant in the different series. However, values become very discrepant for the prediction of F4, probably caused by the difficulty of assessing the degree of fibrotic evolution beyond this stage. This last point raises the issue of the potential utility of LSM in the evaluation of disease progression in patients with histologically proven cirrhosis, i.e. a clinical stage similarly lacking adequate diagnostic implementation. Overall it is more and more evident that the use of LSM will allow a broader diagnostic flexibility and possibility of integration with other diagnostic methodologies for the clinical assessment of patients with advanced fibrosis and cirrhosis.

NON-INVASIVE STAGING IN PATIENTS WITH ADVANCED FIBROSIS/ CIRRHOSIS

Overall it is rather clear that serum markers, LSM as well as standard imaging techniques, perform quite well in advanced fibrosis and cirrhosis and, accordingly, these systems could be proposed for the clinical workout of advanced CLD. Indeed, there is need to differentiate advanced fibrosis (i.e. ≥F3–F4) and beyond, i.e. when the patient is in a clinical stage defined as 'compensated cirrhosis' and, subsequently, when clinically significant portal hypertension and relative complications develop. The current histological assessment of the fibrotic development of CLD tends to define METAVIR F4 as a sort of end-stage of the fibrogenic process, i.e. the cirrhotic transformation of liver tissue. However, the transition from this initial stage of cirrhosis to clinical decompensation may need several years or even decades. In this stage of CLD no effective diagnostic tools are available as an alternative or as an integration to the measurement of the HVPG.

Carrion and co-workers[37] reported that LSM reflects both the extent of fibrosis and the elevation of portal pressure in terms of HVPG in recurrent hepatitis C after liver transplantation. Recent results from our group have confirmed an excellent correlation between LSM and HPVG values <10

DISEASE PROGRESSION IN CLD

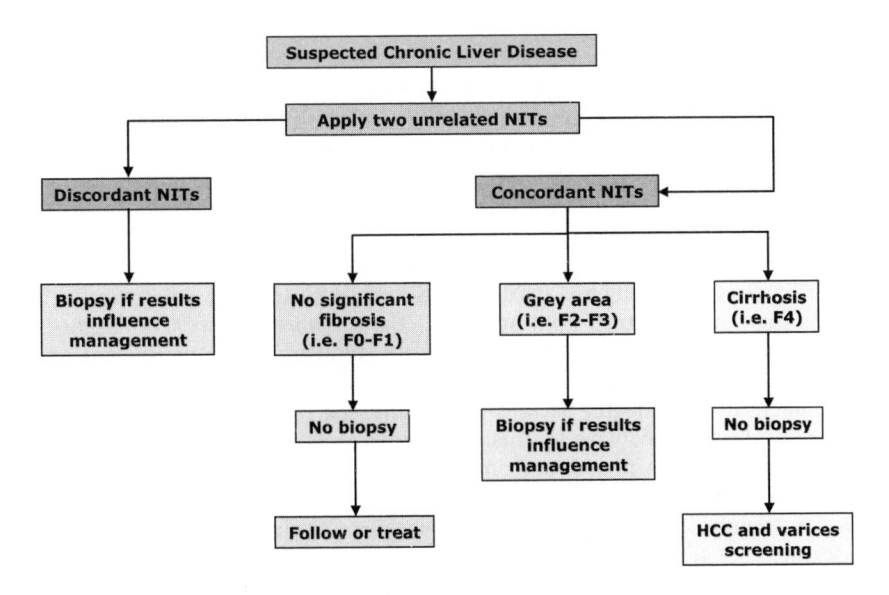

```
Suspected Chronic Liver Disease
            ↓
   Apply two unrelated NITs
      ↓              ↓
Discordant NITs   Concordant NITs
      ↓              ↓
Biopsy if results  ┌──────────┬──────────┬──────────┐
influence          No significant  Grey area   Cirrhosis
management         fibrosis        (i.e. F2-F3) (i.e. F4)
                   (i.e. F0-F1)
                        ↓              ↓              ↓
                   No biopsy    Biopsy if results  No biopsy
                                influence
                                management
                        ↓                             ↓
                   Follow or treat              HCC and varices
                                                screening
```

Figure 1 Proposed flowchart for the non-invasive assessment of fibrosis evolution in chronic HCV patients. NITs, non-invasive tests (including serum biomarkers and transient elastography); HCC, hepatocellular carcinoma; ALT, alanine aminotransferase

mmHg, whereas this correlation becomes poor for values $\geqslant 12$ mmHg[49]. Although this correlation needs to be further substantiated in a larger cohort of patients, it may have implications for the clinical assessment of patients at stages of evolution of CLD preceding the development of clinically significant portal hypertension. In this context transient elastography could be useful in differentiating stages of the progressive cirrhotic evolution of liver tissue once the histological stage of cirrhosis has been reached. In some studies this possibility has been extended to the prediction of the most common complication of cirrhosis. Foucher et al. have proposed the use of transient elastography for the detection of cirrhosis and prediction of related complications including the presence of oesophageal varices and variceal bleeding[50]. Other authors have suggested that LSM is able to predict the presence of large oesophageal varices and could be useful for selecting patients for endoscopic evaluation[51]. However, the poor correlation existing between LSM and HVPG values $\geqslant 12$ mmHg makes the possibility of predicting the presence and size of oesophageal varices with a sufficient degree of accuracy rather unlikely[49].

CONCLUSIONS

The present status of development of different non-invasive tools testifies the large effort for a better clinical definition of the fibrogenic progression of chronic hepatitis C as well as other liver fibrogenic disorders. Some major considerations arise from the experience so far accumulated. First, all non-invasive methodologies are characterized by a sufficient to excellent diagnostic accuracy for the detection (or exclusion) of advanced fibrosis and cirrhosis and none is able to allow a stepwise follow-up of the fibrogenic evolution of CLD according to the existing histopathological staging systems. In other words, due to the absence of a true gold standard, the definition of a 90% diagnostic accuracy remains a goal for the future. In addition, none of the currently available tests has a well-defined prognostic value such as the prediction of decompensation or death, Second, due to the 'spectrum bias' and the possible causes of discordance with the histopathological assessment, the applicability of the different proposed cut-off values in clinical practice is presently hazardous. Third, the combination of two unrelated non-invasive tests (i.e. one biochemical test with LSM) may provide a useful system for the initial assessment of fibrosis evolution in patients with CLD. Figure 1 illustrates a flow chart for chronic HCV hepatitis which is proposed in order to stimulate a constructive debate. The definition of intermediate stages of fibrosis (i.e. F2 and F3) as 'grey areas' highlights the current difficulty in the clinical use of the proposed non-invasive tests. Regardless, it is more and more evident that a rational and prudent use of the proposed methodologies will reduce the need for liver biopsy in a significant percentage of patients, and represents a diagnostic advantage.

Acknowledgements

The authors wish to thank Dr Umberto Arena and Professor Fabio Marra for their enthusiasm and efforts in this area of clinical research.

References

1. Regev A, Berho M, Jeffers LJ et al. Sampling error and intraobserver variation in liver biopsy in patients with chronic HCV infection. Am J Gastroenterol. 2002;97:2614–18.
2. Bedossa P, Dargère D, Paradis V. Sampling variability of liver fibrosis in chronic hepatitis C. Hepatology. 2003;38:1449–57.
3. Cadranel JF, Rufat P, Degos F. Practices of liver biopsy in France: results of a prospective nationwide survey. Hepatology. 2000;32:477–81.
4. Standish RA, Cholongitas E, Dhillon A, Burroughs AK, Dhillon AP. An appraisal of the histopathological assessment of liver fibrosis. Gut. 2006;55:569–78.
5. Samonakis DN, Cholongitas E, Thalheimer U et al. Hepatic venous pressure gradient to assess fibrosis and its progression after liver transplantation for HCV cirrhosis. Liver Transplant. 2007;13:1305–11.
6. Burroughs AK, Groszmann R, Bosch J et al. Assessment of therapeutic benefit of antiviral therapy in chronic hepatitis C: is hepatic venous pressure gradient a better end point? Gut. 2005;50:425–7.
7. Rincon D, Ripoll C, Lo Iacono Q et al. Antiviral therapy decreases hepatic venous pressure gradient in patients with chronic hepatitis C and advanced fibrosis. Am J Gastroenterol. 2006;101:2269–74.

8. Senzolo M, Burra P, Cholongitas E et al. The transjugular route: the key hole to the liver world. Dig Dis Sci. 2006;39:105–16.
9. Carrion JA, Navasa M, García-Retortillo M et al. Efficacy of antiviral therapy on hepatitis C recurrence after liver transplantation: a randomized controlled study. Gastroenterology. 2007;132:1746–56.
10. Forns X, Ampurdanès S, Llovet JM et al. Identification of chronic hepatitis C patients without hepatic fibrosis by a simple predictive model. Hepatology. 2002;36:986–92.
11. Wai CT, Greenson JK, Fontana RJ et al. A simple non-invasive index can predict both significant fibrosis and cirrhosis in patients with chronic hepatitis C. Hepatology. 2003;38:518–26.
12. Imbert-Bismut F, Ratziu V, Pieroni L, Charlotte F, Benhamou Y, Poynard T; MULTIVIRC Group. Biochemical markers of liver fibrosis in patients with hepatitis C virus infection: a prospective study. Lancet. 2001;357:1069–75.
13. Koda M, Matunaga Y, Kawakami M, Kishimoto Y, Suou T, Murawaki Y. FibroIndex, a practical index for predicting significant fibrosis in patients with chronic hepatitis C. Hepatology. 2007;45:297–306.
14. Testa R, Testa E, Giannini E et al. Non-invasive ratio indexes to evaluate fibrosis staging in chronic hepatitis C: role of platelet count/spleen diameter ratio index. J Intern Med. 2006;260:142–50.
15. Sud A, Hui JM, Farrell GC et al. Improved prediction of fibrosis in chronic hepatitis C using measures of insulin resistance in a probability index. Hepatology. 2004;39:1239–47.
16. Sterling RK, Lissen E, Clumeck N et al. Development of a simple non-invasive index to predict significant fibrosis in patients with chronic hepatitis C. Hepatology. 2006;43:1317–25.
17. Bonacini M, Hadi G, Govindarajan S, Lindsay KL. Utility of a discriminant score for diagnosing advanced fibrosis or cirrhosis in patients with chronic hepatitis C infection. Am J Gastroenterol. 1997;92:1302–14.
18. Pohl A, Behling C, Oliver D, Kilani M, Monson P, Hassanein T. Serum aminotransferase levels and platelet counts as predictors of degree of fibrosis in chronic hepatitis C virus infection. Am J Gastroenterol. 2001;96:3142–6.
19. Sheth SG, Flamm SL, Gordon FD, Chopra S. AST/ALT ratio predicts cirrhosis in patients with chronic hepatitis C virus infection. Am J Gastroenterol. 1998;93:44–8.
20. Park JH, Lin BP, Ngu MC, Jones DB, Katelaris PH. Aspartate aminotransferase, alanine aminotransferase ratio in chronic hepatitis C infection: Is it a useful predictor of cirrhosis? J Gastroenterol Hepatol. 2000;15:386–90.
21. Poynard T, Bedossa P. Age and platelet count: a simple index for predicting the presence of histological lesions in patients with antibodies to hepatitis C virus. METAVIR and CLINIVIR Cooperative Study Groups. J Viral Hepat. 1997;4:199–208.
22. Leroy V, Monier F, Bottari S et al. Circulating matrix metalloproteinases 1, 2, 9 and their inhibitors TIMP-1 and TIMP-2 as serum markers of liver fibrosis in patients with chronic hepatitis C: Comparison with PIIINP and hyaluronic acid. Am J Gastroenterol. 2004;99:271–9.
23. Rosenberg WM, Voelker M, Thiel R et al. Serum markers detect the presence of liver fibrosis: a cohort study. Gastroenterology. 2004;127:1704–13.
24. Kellher TB, Mehta SH, Bhaskar R et al. Prediction of hepatic fibrosis in HIV/HCV co-infected patients using serum fibrosis markers: the SHASTA index. J Hepatol. 2005;43:78–84.
25. Calès P, Oberti F, Michalak S et al. A novel panel of blood markers to assess the degree of liver fibrosis. Hepatology. 2005;42:1373–81.
26. Adams LA, Bulsara M, Rossi E et al. Hepascore: an accurate validated predictor of liver fibrosis in chronic hepatitis C infection. Clin Chem. 2005;51:1867–73.
27. Patel K, Gordon SC, Jacobson I et al. Evaluation of a panel of non-invasive serum markers to differentiate mild from moderate-to-advanced liver fibrosis in chronic hepatitis C patients. J Hepatol. 2004;41:935–42.
28. Parkes J, Guha IN, Roderick P, Rosenberg W. Performance of serum marker panels for liver fibrosis in chronic hepatitis C. J Hepatol. 2006;44:462–74.
29. Afdhal NH, Curry M. Technology evaluation: a critical step in the clinical utilization of novel diagnostic tests for liver fibrosis. J Hepatol. 2007;46:543–5.

30. Sebastiani G, Vario A, Guido M et al. Stepwise combination of algorithms of non-invasive markers to diagnose significant fibrosis in chronic hepatitis C. J Hepatol. 2004;44:686–93.
31. Sebastiani G, Vario A, Guido M, Alberti A. Sequential algorithms combining non-invasive markers and biopsy for the assessment of liver fibrosis in chronic hepatitis B. World J Gastroenterol. 2007;13:525–31.
32. Leroy V, Hilleret MN, Sturm N et al. Prospective comparison of six non-invasive scores for the diagnosis of liver fibrosis in chronic hepatitis C. J Hepatol. 2007;46:775–82.
33. Lackner C, Struber G, Liegl B et al. Comparison and validation of simple non-invasive tests for prediction of fibrosis in chronic hepatitis C. Hepatology. 2005;41:1376–82.
34. Lackner C, Struber G, Bankuti C, Bauer B, Stauber RE. Non-invasive diagnosis of cirrhosis in chronic hepatitis C based on standard laboratory tests. Hepatology. 2006;42:378–9.
35. Sandrin L, Tanter M, Gennisson JL, Catheline S, Fink M. Shear elasticity probe for soft tissues with 1-D transient elastography. IEEE Trans Ultrason Ferroelectr Freq Control. 2002;49:436–46.
36. Castera L, Vergniol J, Foucher J et al. Prospective comparison of transient elastography, Fibrotest, APRI, and liver biopsy for the assessment of fibrosis in chronic hepatitis C. Gastroenterology. 2005;128:343–50.
37. Carrion JA, Navasa M, Bosch J, Bruguera M, Gilabert R, Forns X. Transient elastography for diagnosis of advanced fibrosis and portal hypertension in patients with hepatitis C recurrence after liver transplantation. Liver Transplant. 2006;12:1791–8.
38. Foucher J, Chanteloup E, Vergniol J et al. Diagnosis of cirrhosis by transient elastography (FibroScan): a prospective study. Gut. 2006;55:403–8.
39. Gomez-Dominguez E, Mendoza J, Rubio S, Moreno-Monteagudo JA, García-Buey L, Moreno-Otero R. Transient elastography: a valid alternative to biopsy in patients with chronic liver disease. Aliment Pharmacol Ther. 2006;24:513–18.
40. Ganne-Carrie N, Ziol M, de Ledinghen V et al. Accuracy of liver stiffness measurement for the diagnosis of cirrhosis in patients with chronic liver diseases. Hepatology. 2006;44:1511–17.
41. de Ledinghen V, Douvin C, Kettaneh A et al. Diagnosis of hepatic fibrosis and cirrhosis by transient elastography in HIV/hepatitis C virus co-infected patients. J Acquir Immune Defic Syndr. 2006;41:175–9.
42. Kim KM. Choi WB, Park SH et al. Diagnosis of hepatic steatosis and fibrosis by transient elastography in asymptomatic healthy individuals: a prospective study of living related potential liver donors. J Gastroenterol. 2007;42:382–8.
43. Yoneda M, Yoneda M, Fujita K et al. Transient elastography in patients with nonalcoholic fatty liver disease (NAFLD). Gut. 2007;56:1330–1.
44. Ziol M, Handra-Luca A, Kettaneh A et al. Noninvasive assessment of liver fibrosis by measurement of stiffness in patients with chronic hepatitis C. Hepatology. 2005;41:48–54.
45. Fraquelli M, Rigamonti C, Casazza G et al. Reproducibility of transient elastography in the evaluation of liver fibrosis in patients with chronic liver disease. Gut. 2007;56:968–73.
46. Corpechot C, El Naggar A, Poujol-Robert A et al. Assessment of biliary fibrosis by transient elastography in patients with PBC and PSC. Hepatology. 2006;43:1118–24.
47. Coco B, Oliveri F, Maina AM et al. Transient elastography: a new surrogate marker of liver fibrosis influenced by major changes of transaminases. J Viral Hepat. 2007;14:360–9.
48. Arena U, Vizzutti F, Corti G et al. Acute viral hepatitis increases liver stiffness values measured by transient elastography. Hepatology. 2008;48 (In press).
49. Vizzutti F, Arena U, Romanelli RG et al. Liver stiffness measurement predicts severe portal hypertension in patients with HCV-related cirrhosis. Hepatology. 2007;45:1290–7.
50. Foucher J, Chanteloup E, Vergniol J et al. Diagnosis of cirrhosis by transient elastography (Fibroscan): a prospective study. Gut. 2006;55:403–8.
51. Kazemi F, Kettaneh A, N'kontchou G et al. Liver stiffness measurements selects patients with cirrhosis at risk of bearing large esophageal varices. J Hepatol. 2006;45:230–5.

16
Fibrosis regression and innovative antifibrotic therapies: from bench to bedside

M.-L. BERRES, M. M. ZALDIVAR, C. TRAUTWEIN and H. E. WASMUTH

INTRODUCTION

Fibrosis *per se* is considered as the chronic response to tissue damage that can finally lead to impaired organ function. Liver tissue damage can result from various acute or chronic stimuli, including viral infections, metabolic disorders, autoimmune reactions and toxic injury. Although initially beneficial, the healing process becomes pathogenic if it continues replacing normal by connective tissue. The excessive deposition of extracellular matrix leads to the progressive destruction of the normal organ architecture, eventually resulting in liver cirrhosis and organ failure. Furthermore, liver cirrhosis has been shown to be a precancerous condition allowing the development of hepatocellular carcinoma in a considerable number of affected patients[1].

Traditionally hepatic fibrosis and cirrhosis was considered as the irreversible endpoint of chronic liver damage. However, in recent years it has become obvious that liver scar formation is, at least in part, reversible[2]. Despite great advances in the understanding of the molecular mechanisms leading to liver fibrosis, efficient antifibrotic therapies are still lacking. This is mainly explained by the complex pathophysiological mechanisms leading to the deposition of extracellular matrix in the space of Disse, which involves multiple cell types and soluble mediators (Figure 1)[3]. As a result, effective antifibrotic therapies either have to target the initial insults, i.e. the virus or toxins leading to hepatocellular damage or the cells and mediators which mediate the fibrogenic tissue reaction. The first attempt would be a *specific* antifibrotic strategy, while the second option would imply *non-specific* attempts to induce the regression of liver fibrosis.

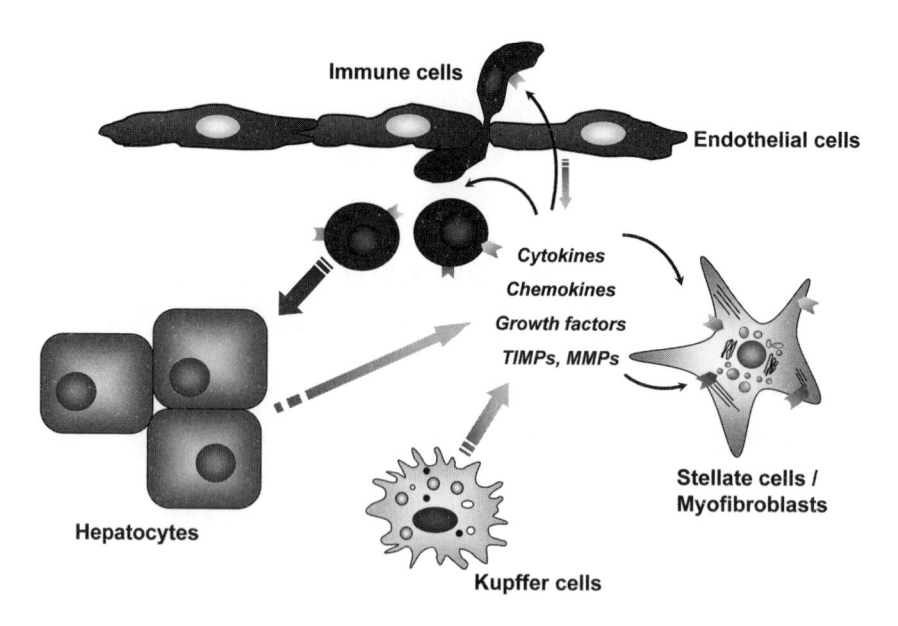

Figure 1 Major cell types involved in the pathogenesis of liver fibrosis. There is also a strong interplay between immune cells, hepatocytes, endothelial cells and hepatic stellate cells mediated by different chemokines and cytokines. Theoretically all cell types and mediators are potential targets of antifibrotic therapies. However, treatment strategies that target mediators which are involved in the regulation of different cell populations (e.g. immune cells and stellate cells) are the most promising targets

SPECIFIC ATTEMPTS TO INHIBIT LIVER FIBROSIS

Specific interventions for fibrosis regression are mainly focused on the resolution or eradication of the damaging causes. This concept was nicely proven in patients with secondary biliary fibrosis due to chronic obstruction of the common bile duct. In these patients, efficient drainage of the common bile duct leads to regression of liver fibrosis in the majority of patients after a median of 2.5 years[4]. However, biliary liver damage does not always seem to be reversible. Treatment of primary biliary cirrhosis patients with ursodeoxycholic acid (UDCA) was initially shown to be associated with a reduced progression of liver fibrosis, but no regression of established fibrosis[5]. However, these positive results have recently been questioned by a meta-analysis by the Cochrane Hepato-Biliary Group[6], and UDCA does not seem to positively influence the progression of non-biliary liver diseases, such as viral hepatitis[7] or non-alcoholic steatohepatitis (NASH)[8].

In viral hepatitis C, a sustained virological response to an interferon-based therapy has been shown to be associated with the long-term regression of histological liver damage[9,10]. However, it has to be taken into account that the presence of severe fibrosis strongly reduces the chances of sustained virological response[11], leading to a large number of patients with high stages of liver fibrosis but no response to current antiviral therapies. This underlines the need for other effective antifibrotic therapies in these HCV patients who are at considerable risk for developing end-stage liver disease and hepatocellular carcinoma.

In chronic hepatitis B, eradication of the virus is rarely possible. Nevertheless, large-scale randomized trials with nucleoside and nucleotide analogues in patients with hepatitis B have shown a reduction in histological fibrosis scores in case of an effective suppression of HBV-DNA[12–14]. In autoimmune hepatitis successful treatment with immunosuppressive therapies is also associated with a regression of extracellular matrix deposition[15], while in NASH either surgically or pharmacologically induced weight loss leads to reduced liver fibrosis in obese patients[16,17].

Taken together, these clinical trials strongly suggest that regression or even reversal of hepatic fibrosis is an achievable aim when effective therapies are initiated. Nevertheless, a significant number of patients with defined liver diseases do not respond to the currently available therapies. In these individuals, non-specific antifibrotic therapies are strongly needed in order to prevent the devastating complications of end-stage liver disease.

NON-SPECIFIC ANTIFIBROTIC INTERVENTIONS

Attempts to develop non-specific measures to inhibit the progression of liver fibrosis or induce its regression are mainly based on the current pathophysiological understanding of liver scarring. In recent years it has become clear that different intra- and extrahepatic cell populations are involved in the development of liver fibrosis. Whereas immune cells, like Kupffer cells and recruited lymphocytes, are important for the inflammatory phase of the fibrogenic response, hepatic stellate cells and portal myofibroblasts have been implicated in the later stages of fibrogenesis[18,19]. An important role of bone marrow-derived cells has been shown in animal models[20,21] and is also evolving from recent studies in humans[22]; therefore, interventions that are based on different cell populations and their soluble mediators seem to bear the highest potential as antifibrotic strategies[23].

The principal mediators which play a role during all stages of fibrogenesis are cytokines, chemokines and growth factors. These are secreted by immune cells and hepatic stellate cells, while both cell populations also respond to these molecules (Figure 1).

In experimental models of fibrosis, transforming growth factor-β (TGF-β) has been shown to play a key role in stimulating and maintaining the fibrogenic process. TGF-β stimulates the expression of extracellular matrix proteins and collagen, inhibits collagenases and promotes the activation of hepatic stellate cells[24]. It also plays an important role in the development of a tolerogenic immune response and therefore seems to be an ideal candidate for antifibrotic therapies. Interferon gamma (IFN-γ) has been shown to be a key counter-regulatory antifibrotic cytokine down-regulating the activity of TGF-β. IFN-γ inhibits the interaction of downstream proteins in the TGF-β signalling cascade. Experimental data from *in vitro* and *in vivo* studies in animals have consistently shown antifibrotic effects of IFN-γ. IFN-γ inhibits the proliferation and culture-induced activation of hepatic stellate cells leading to a significantly reduced production of extracellular matrix proteins[25] and liver fibrosis[26]. Similar findings have been described for IFN-α, another type 1 interferon, which is currently the standard treatment for chronic hepatitis C[27]. Both interferons have already been evaluated in clinical trials as antifibrotic agents. IFN-γ was first evaluated in a small pilot trial with 30 patients with chronic hepatitis C and persistently elevated alanine aminotransferase (ALT) levels. In this trial a trend towards a decreased fibrosis score was noted in IFN-γ-treated patients[28]. Therefore, a larger randomized, placebo-controlled trial was performed in almost 500 patients with advanced liver fibrosis. In this recently published study IFN-γ therapy for 1 year was not able to reverse hepatic fibrosis in patients with advanced liver disease compared to placebo treatment[29]. However, it should be taken into account that >80% of patients included in the trial had already established cirrhosis (Ishak score of 5 or 6) at baseline. In these individuals a treatment period of 1 year might just have been too short to determine a histological improvement upon liver biopsy. Another interesting finding from this study is that the interferon-inducible chemokine ITAC (CXCL11) was an independent predictor of stable or reduced Ishak scores[29]. Therefore, other downstream mediators of IFN-γ might be valuable candidates for future antifibrotic therapies. This is in line with our findings that fractalkine (CX3CL1), another Th1-associated chemokine, is involved in liver fibrosis due to chronic hepatitis C. Fractalkine down-regulates TIMP-1 mRNA expression in hepatic stellate cells, and single-nucleotide polymorphisms of its receptor CX3CR1 are strongly associated with the severity of liver fibrosis[30]. Therefore, chemokines might not only be involved in the regulation of immune cell recruitment to the damaged liver but also directly influence stellate cell function and the regulation of extracellular matrix deposition and resolution.

Compared to IFN-γ, more promising results have been published for the antifibrotic effects of IFN-α. In a randomized controlled trial with 53 patients with advanced fibrosis, 27 were kept on three times 3 MU IFN-α2b weekly for 30 months. This duration of IFN-α2b treatment was sufficient to lead to histological improvement in 80% of treated patients with a decline in the mean fibrosis score from 2.5 at baseline to 1.7 at the end of the study[31]. These results now form the basis for the evaluation of long-term IFN-α therapy in patients with chronic hepatitis C and a non-response to prior antiviral therapy (HALT-C[32], EPIC and COPILOT). No results of these long-term studies have yet been published, but the first interim analysis of data from the COPILOT study has revealed promising results in the reduction of clinical endpoints (especially variceal bleeding episodes) in patients kept on IFN-α maintenance therapy. However, more data from these trails are needed before drawing conclusions for clinical practice.

Another antifibrotic cytokine that has already evolved from bench to bedside is interleukin-10 (IL-10). IL-10 is a potent anti-inflammatory cytokine which has a strong impact on the intrahepatic immune balance and is expressed by hepatic stellate cells[33]. Stellate cells also express the IL-10 receptor, suggesting that these cells are a source and target of IL-10[34]. IL-10 inhibits both collagen production and DNA synthesis but has no effect on procollagen-alpha[1] (I) mRNA levels. Furthermore, transgenic expression of rIL-10 in mouse liver leads to reduced fibrosis after challenge of mice with tetracarbonchloride (CCl_4)[35]. The reduction in liver fibrosis in these transgenic animals was related to an attenuation of $CD8^+$ T-cell-mediated liver damage, emphasizing the close interaction between the immune system and hepatic stellate cells during liver fibrogenesis. Based on these positive *in vitro* and murine *in vivo* results, a pilot study with IL-10 in patients with hepatitis C-induced liver fibrosis was initiated. In this pilot trial IL-10 therapy was well tolerated and had no obvious antiviral effects during the treatment period of 90 days. Of note, IL-10 normalized ALT levels in 14 out of 22 patients and decreased fibrosis in 14 out of 22 treated patients[36]. These promising results were the basis for a concomitant trial of IL-10 therapy in patients with hepatitis C. In this study of 30 patients, IL-10 given for 12 months again led to a significant decrease in ALT levels and mean fibrosis score. However, in contrast to the first study, five patients developed viral loads greater than 120 M IU/ml and two of these developed an acute flare in transaminases[37]. Therefore, despite its reproducible effects on hepatic fibrosis, systemic IL-10 treatment has not yet been further tested in clinical trials.

Besides chronic viral hepatitis, liver fibrosis due to NASH has gained much interest in recent years. Mouse models for this disease include the leptin-deficient ob/ob mouse and the feeding of wild-type mice with a methionine- and choline-deficient diet. In these and other models of chonic liver damage the transcription factor NF-κB seems to play a pivotal role[38]. NF-κB is implicated in the regulation of many genes, particularly those of inflammatory responses and cell death pathways. NF-κB transcription factors are kept inactive in the cytoplasm through binding to members of the IκB family of inhibitory proteins. The IκB kinase, consisting of two catalytic subunits (IKK1 and IKK2) and a regulatory subunit (NF-κB-essential modulator, NEMO), mediates NF-κB activation in response to a variety of stimuli by phosphorylating IκB proteins[39]. These stimuli include mediators of hepatic oxidative stress such as lipoperoxides[40]. Interestingly, recent observations show that hepatocytes-specific deletion of NEMO leads to spontaneous steatohepatitis and hepatocellular carcinoma in mice. These phenotypes are associated with an increased mRNA expression of the classical NF-κB regulated genes TNF-α, IL-6, IL-1β and the CC chemokine RANTES[41]. RANTES mRNA levels are also strongly increased in mice fed the MCD diet[42]. Importantly, systemic inhibition of IKK2, on the other hand, strongly protects the liver from dietary-induced insulin resistance and progression of NASH induced by a high sucrose diet[43]. These results together strongly support a crucial role of NF-κB and its regulatory pathways in the pathophysiology of NASH.

Accordingly, pharmaceutical inhibition of NF-κB reduces the severity of MCD diet-induced steatohepatitis in mice[44]. The activation of NF-κB is also blocked by the nuclear receptor peroxisome proliferators-activated receptor-α (PPARα). Of note, agonists of this family of nuclear receptors such as glitazones have been shown to be effective in the treatment of murine[45] and human NASH-induced liver fibrosis[46,47]. However, in the latter trials only a relatively small number of individuals with defined co-morbidities were included, and members of the family of glitazones might be associated with increased cardiac mortality[48]. Therefore, long-term use of PPARγ agonists cannot be recommended on the currently available literature.

CONCLUSIONS

Until now, only specific interventions have unequivocally been shown to be able to inhibit liver fibrosis or induce its regression. Non-specific antifibrotic therapies have not yet been evolved from bench to bedside, although a number of substances have already been evaluated in clinical trials. However, it seems likely that, with increasing knowledge of the pathophysiology of liver fibrosis and the interplay of different cell types, new pathways will be explored in order to prevent the progression or even induce a regression of liver fibrosis. This will then help to reduce the increased morbidity and mortality associated with endstage liver disease.

Acknowledgements

Work by the authors regarding the genetic and molecular basis of liver fibrosis is supported by the Deutsche Forschungsgemeinschaft (DFG), the Deutsche Leberstiftung and Aachen University (START and IZKF BioMAT).

References

1. Friedman SL, Rockey DC, Bissell DM. Hepatic fibrosis 2006: report of the Third AASLD Single Topic Conference. Hepatology. 2007;45:242–9.
2. Serpaggi J, Carnot F, Nalpas B et al. Direct and indirect evidence for the reversibility of cirrhosis. Hum Pathol. 2006;37:1519–26.
3. Friedman SL, Bansal MB. Reversal of hepatic fibrosis – fact or fantasy? Hepatology. 2006;43:S82–8.
4. Hammel P, Couvelard A, O'Toole D et al. Regression of liver fibrosis after biliary drainage in patients with chronic pancreatitis and stenosis of the common bile duct. N Engl J Med. 2001;344:418–23.
5. Corpechot C, Carrat F, Bonnand AM, Poupon RE, Poupon R. The effect of ursodeoxycholic acid therapy on liver fibrosis progression in primary biliary cirrhosis. Hepatology. 2000;32:1196–9.
6. Gong Y, Huang Z, Christensen E, Gluud C. Ursodeoxycholic acid for patients with primary biliary cirrhosis: an updated systematic review and meta-analysis of randomized clinical trials using Bayesian approach as sensitivity analyses. Am J Gastroenterol. 2007;102:1799–807.
7. Chen W, Liu J, Gluud C. Bile acids for viral hepatitis. Cochrane Database Syst Rev 2003: CD003181.
8. Lindor KD, Kowdley KV, Heathcote EJ et al. Ursodeoxycholic acid for treatment of nonalcoholic steatohepatitis: results of a randomized trial. Hepatology. 2004;39:770–8.
9. Marcellin P, Boyer N, Gervais A et al. Long-term histologic improvement and loss of detectable intrahepatic HCV RNA in patients with chronic hepatitis C and sustained response to interferon-alpha therapy. Ann Intern Med. 1997;127:875–81.
10. Arif A, Levine RA, Sanderson SO et al. Regression of fibrosis in chronic hepatitis C after therapy with interferon and ribavirin. Dig Dis Sci. 2003;48:1425–30.

11. Everson GT, Hoefs JC, Seeff LB et al. Impact of disease severity on outcome of antiviral therapy for chronic hepatitis C: lessons from the HALT-C trial. Hepatology. 2006;44:1675–84.
12. Lai CL, Chien RN, Leung NW et al. A one-year trial of lamivudine for chronic hepatitis B. Asia Hepatitis Lamivudine Study Group. N Engl J Med. 1998;339:61–8.
13. Lai CL, Shouval D, Lok AS et al. Entecavir versus lamivudine for patients with HBeAg-negative chronic hepatitis B. N Engl J Med. 2006;354:1011–20.
14. Hadziyannis SJ, Tassopoulos NC, Heathcote EJ et al. Adefovir dipivoxil for the treatment of hepatitis B e antigen-negative chronic hepatitis B. N Engl J Med. 2003;348:800–7.
15. Krawitt EL. Autoimmune hepatitis. N Engl J Med. 2006;354:54–66.
16. Liu X, Lazenby AJ, Clements RH, Jhala N, Abrams GA. Resolution of nonalcoholic steatohepatits after gastric bypass surgery. Obes Surg. 2007;17:486–92.
17. Hussein O, Grosovski M, Schlesinger S, Szvalb S, Assy N. Orlistat reverses fatty infiltration and improves hepatic fibrosis in obese patients with nonalcoholic steatohepatitis (NASH). Dig Dis Sci. 2007;52:2512–19.
18. Friedman SL. Mechanisms of disease: mechanisms of hepatic fibrosis and therapeutic implications. Nat Clin Pract Gastroenterol Hepatol. 2004;1:98–105.
19. Bataller R, Brenner DA. Liver fibrosis. J Clin Invest 2005;115:209–18.
20. Kisseleva T, Uchinami H, Feirt N et al. Bone marrow-derived fibrocytes participate in pathogenesis of liver fibrosis. J Hepatol. 2006;45:429–38.
21. Russo FP, Alison MR, Bigger BW et al. The bone marrow functionally contributes to liver fibrosis. Gastroenterology. 2006;130:1807–21.
22. Terai S, Ishikawa T, Omori K et al. Improved liver function in patients with liver cirrhosis after autologous bone marrow cell infusion therapy. Stem Cells. 2006;24:2292–8.
23. Wasmuth HE, Trautwein C. CB1 cannabinoid receptor antagonism: a new strategy for the treatment of liver fibrosis. Hepatology. 2007;45:543–4.
24. Gressner AM, Weiskirchen R. Modern pathogenetic concepts of liver fibrosis suggest stellate cells and TGF-beta as major players and therapeutic targets. J Cell Mol Med. 2006;10:76–99.
25. Weng H, Mertens PR, Gressner AM, Dooley S. IFN-gamma abrogates profibrogenic TGF-beta signaling in liver by targeting expression of inhibitory and receptor Smads. J Hepatol. 2007;46:295–303.
26. Rockey DC, Chung JJ. Interferon gamma inhibits lipocyte activation and extracellular matrix mRNA expression during experimental liver injury: implications for treatment of hepatic fibrosis. J Invest Med. 1994;42:660–70.
27. Inagaki Y, Nemoto T, Kushida M et al. Interferon alfa down-regulates collagen gene transcription and suppresses experimental hepatic fibrosis in mice. Hepatology. 2003;38:890–9.
28. Saez-Royuela F, Porres JC, Moreno A et al. High doses of recombinant alpha-interferon or gamma-interferon for chronic hepatitis C: a randomized, controlled trial. Hepatology. 1991;13:327–31.
29. Pockros PJ, Jeffers L, Afdhal N et al. Final results of a double-blind, placebo-controlled trial of the antifibrotic efficacy of interferon-gamma1b in chronic hepatitis C patients with advanced fibrosis or cirrhosis. Hepatology. 2007;45:569–78.
30. Wasmuth HE, Moreno Zaldivar M, Berres M-L et al. The fractalkine receptor CX3CR1 is involved in liver fibrosis due to chronic hepatitis C infection. J Hepatol. 2008;48:208–15.
31. Shiffman ML, Hofmann CM, Contos MJ et al. A randomized, controlled trial of maintenance interferon therapy for patients with chronic hepatitis C virus and persistent viremia. Gastroenterology. 1999;117:1164–72.
32. Lee WM, Dienstag JL, Lindsay KL et al. Evolution of the HALT-C Trial: pegylated interferon as maintenance therapy for chronic hepatitis C in previous interferon nonresponders. Control Clin Trials. 2004;25:472–92.
33. Wang SC, Ohata M, Schrum L, Rippe RA, Tsukamoto H. Expression of interleukin-10 by in vitro and in vivo activated hepatic stellate cells. J Biol Chem. 1998;273:302–8.
34. Mathurin P, Xiong S, Kharbanda KK et al. IL-10 receptor and coreceptor expression in quiescent and activated hepatic stellate cells. Am J Physiol Gastrointest Liver Physio. 2002;282:G981–90.

35. Safadi R, Ohta M, Alvarez CE et al. Immune stimulation of hepatic fibrogenesis by CD8 cells and attenuation by transgenic interleukin-10 from hepatocytes. Gastroenterology. 2004;127:870–82.
36. Nelson DR, Lauwers GY, Lau JY, Davis GL. Interleukin 10 treatment reduces fibrosis in patients with chronic hepatitis C: a pilot trial of interferon nonresponders. Gastroenterology. 2000;118:655–60.
37. Nelson DR, Tu Z, Soldevila-Pico C et al. Long-term interleukin 10 therapy in chronic hepatitis C patients has a proviral and anti-inflammatory effect. Hepatology. 2003;38:859–68.
38. Elsharkawy AM, Mann DA. Nuclear factor-kappaB and the hepatic inflammation-fibrosis-cancer axis. Hepatology. 2007;46:590–7.
39. Ghosh S, Karin M. Missing pieces in the NF-kappaB puzzle. Cell. 2002;109(Suppl.):S81–96.
40. dela Pena A, Leclercq IA, Williams J, Farrell GC. NADPH oxidase is not an essential mediator of oxidative stress or liver injury in murine MCD diet-induced steatohepatitis. J Hepatol. 2007;46:304–13.
41. Luedde T, Beraza N, Kotsikoris V et al. Deletion of NEMO/IKKgamma in liver parenchymal cells causes steatohepatitis and hepatocellular carcinoma. Cancer Cell. 2007;11:119–32.
42. Scholten D, Dahl E, Beraza N et al. Functional and genetic interaction of CCL5 (RANTES) and CXCL4 (PF4) in chronic liver diseases in mice and humans. J Hepatol. 2007;46:S46.
43. Beraza N, Malato Y, Vander Broght S, Dreano M, Roskams T, Trautwein C. Systemic inhibition of IKK2 protects the liver against dietary-induced NASH. J Hepatol. 2007;46: S40.
44. Leclercq IA, Farrell GC, Sempoux C, dela Pena A, Horsmans Y. Curcumin inhibits NF-kappaB activation and reduces the severity of experimental steatohepatitis in mice. J Hepatol. 2004;41:926–34.
45. Ip E, Farrell G, Hall P, Robertson G, Leclercq I. Administration of the potent PPARalpha agonist, Wy-14,643, reverses nutritional fibrosis and steatohepatitis in mice. Hepatology. 2004;39:1286–96.
46. Promrat K, Lutchman G, Uwaifo GI et al. A pilot study of pioglitazone treatment for nonalcoholic steatohepatitis. Hepatology. 2004;39:188–96.
47. Belfort R, Harrison SA, Brown K et al. A placebo-controlled trial of pioglitazone in subjects with nonalcoholic steatohepatitis. N Engl J Med. 2006;355:2297–307.
48. Nissen SE, Wolski K. Effect of rosiglitazone on the risk of myocardial infarction and death from cardiovascular causes. N Engl J Med. 2007;356:2457–71.

Section V
Clinical management of portal hypertension: preprimary and primary prophylaxis

Chair: J HELLER and F WONG

17
Dynamic increase of intrahepatic vascular resistance in cirrhosis

A. RODRÍGUEZ-VILARRUPLA and J. C. GARCÍA-PAGÁN

INTRODUCTION

Increased resistance to portal blood flow is the primary factor in the pathophysiology of portal hypertension and may occur at any site within the portal venous system[1].

For many years it was thought that increased intrahepatic vascular resistance in the cirrhotic liver was a mechanical consequence of the disruption of the liver vascular architecture caused by fibrosis, scarring and nodule formation during the cirrhotic process. However, in recent years it has become clear that the active contraction, in response to several agonists, of different contractile cell types in the liver promotes a further increase in intrahepatic resistance[2]. It has been claimed that this dynamic and reversible component may represent up to 40% of the increased intrahepatic vascular resistance in cirrhosis. Contractile elements influencing the hepatic vascular bed can be located at sinusoidal as well as at extrasinusoidal levels. These elements include vascular smooth muscle cells of the intrahepatic vasculature (i.e. small portal venules in portal areas)[3] and activated hepatic stellate cells (HSC), that are pericyte cells located in the perisinusoidal space of Disse with extensions that wrap around the sinusoids, and reduce its caliber after contraction[4,5]. Contraction of hepatic myofibroblasts, derived either from activated HSC or from other cellular sources, by compression of venous shuntings that have been shown to be located in the fibrous septa, may also contribute to the dynamic increase in intrahepatic vascular resistance. Whatever the location in which they act, it is now clear that vasoactive mediators, either vasoconstrictors or vasodilators, may modulate intrahepatic vascular resistance either in health or liver disease.

An increased production of vasoconstrictors and an exaggerated response of the hepatic vascular bed to some of them are one of the mechanisms that have been implicated in the pathogenesis of the dynamic component of the increased intrahepatic resistance of the cirrhotic liver. In addition, the defective response of the hepatic vascular bed to endothelium-dependent vasodilators, what has been called endothelial dysfunction, also increases the intrahepatic resistance

Increased production / exaggerated response to vasoconstrictors

Endothelin
Angiotensin
Norepinephrine
Vasopressin
Leukotrienes
Thromboxane
Other?

Insufficient production of vasodilators / hyporesponse to vasodilators

Nitric oxide
Carbon monoxide
Hydrogen sulphide
Others ?

Impaired endothelial-dependent relaxation
ENDOTHELIAL DYSFUNCTION

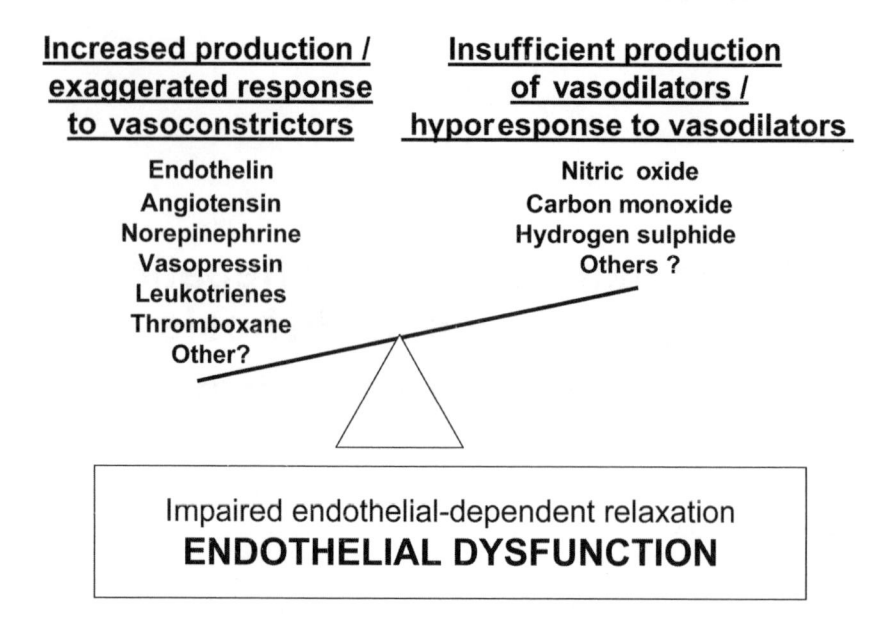

Figure 1 Factors modulating the dynamic component of increased intrahepatic resistance in cirrhosis

of the cirrhotic liver. Endothelial dysfunction is attributed to an insufficient release of hepatic vasodilators and is, at least in part, also due to an increased production of hepatic vasoconstrictors (Figure 1).

INCREASED PRODUCTION/EXAGGERATED RESPONSE OF THE HEPATIC VASCULAR BED TO VASOCONSTRICTORS

An increased activity of several endogenous vasoconstrictors such as endothelin, norepinephrine, angiotensin II, vasopressin and more recently leukotrienes and thromboxane A_2 has been demonstrated in cirrhosis. Additionally, an increased vasoconstrictive response of the hepatic vascular bed to some of these vasoconstrictors magnifies its role. This chapter will go into detail concerning the role of these pathophysiological mechanisms increasing hepatic vascular tone[6].

Adrenergic agonists

The α-adrenergic agonist norepinephrine, that is usually elevated in decompensated cirrhosis, has been shown to increase intrahepatic vascular resistance[7,8]. This increase in resistance is completely blunted by the administration of α-adrenergic antagonists such as prazosin. This agent by itself markedly reduces hepatic resistance and portal pressure in patients with cirrhosis. On the other hand, the administration of β-adrenergic agonists, such as isoproterenol, reduces intrahepatic vascular resistance in the perfused cirrhotic liver. These data suggest that adrenergic receptors may be involved in the regulation of intrahepatic resistance in cirrhosis, and that α-adrenergic receptor blockers may decrease portal pressure in cirrhosis. In addition, the hepatic vascular bed of cirrhotic livers exhibits an exaggerated response to the α-adrenergic agonist methoxamine. It has been shown that the coupling of different agonists to its membrane G-coupled receptors promotes the release of arachidonic acid from the plasma membrane, facilitating its metabolization to different vasoactive-derived metabolites, including prostaglandins (PG), thromboxanes (TX), and leukotrienes[9,10].

Thromboxane

Cyclooxygenase (COX) is the key enzyme in the biosynthetic pathway leading to PG and TX from arachidonic acid (AA)[11]. COX-1 is constitutively expressed but it can also be stimulated by factors similar to those that stimulate the constitutive isoform of NO synthase (eNOS)[12,13]. COX-2 can also be constitutively expressed in some tissues including the liver[14,15] and the mesenteric vascular bed[16]. COX-2 is an inducible isoform of cyclooxygenase that, similar to the inducible isoform of NO synthase, is usually expressed or over-expressed after stimulation with proinflammatory agents[17].

The hyper-response of the hepatic vasculature of cirrhotic livers to the vasoconstrictor methoxamine is associated with an overproduction by the isoenzyme COX-1 of thromboxane A_2 (TXA_2). This hyper-response is completely corrected by pretreating the livers either with non-selective COX blockers, with COX-1 selective blockers or with TXA_2 receptor antagonists. Thus, an increased production of TXA_2 markedly enhances the vasoconstrictive response of the cirrhotic hepatic vascular bed to methoxamine[14]. Recently it has been described that sinusoidal endothelial cells are the major contributor to this increased production of vasoconstrictors (TXA_2, and probably PGH_2) observed in cirrhotic livers[18]. Moreover, an increased PLA_2 activity may be an additional mechanism contributing to the exaggerated vasoconstrictor prostanoid formation in cirrhotic livers by increasing AA bioavailability[18]. On the other hand, it has been suggested[19] that Kupffer cell activation is also involved in the increased portal pressure of fibrotic livers via TXA_2.

Cysteinyl leukotrienes

Cysteinyl leukotrienes (CT) are a group of highly potent vasoactive substances derived from the oxygenation and dehydration of AA by 5-lipoxygenase[20,21] that increases intrahepatic vascular resistance in normal and cirrhotic rat livers. However, this response is significantly greater in cirrhotic livers that also have an increased expression of the 5-lipoxygenase mRNA and an increased production of CT. 5-Lipoxygenase inhibition produces a marked reduction in portal pressure in cirrhotic livers, which suggests that 5-lipoxygenase-derived eicosanoids also contribute to the increased hepatic vascular resistance in cirrhosis[22].

Endothelins

Endothelins are a family of homologous 21-amino acid vasoactive peptides (ET-1, ET-2, and ET-3) that also modulate hepatic vascular tone in cirrhosis[6,23]. The biological properties of endothelins are mediated essentially by two major endothelin receptors, endothelin A (ET-A) and endothelin B (ET-B) receptors. The role of a presumed type C endothelin receptor (ET_C) has not yet been clarified. The ET-A receptor shows a high affinity for ET-1, but not for ET-3, and mediates constriction; the ET-B receptor has equal affinity for ET-1 and ET-3 and is considered to mediate dilation and constriction[24]. Activation of ET-B receptors located on the vascular smooth-muscle cells promotes vasoconstriction, whereas activation of ET-B receptors located on endothelial cells promotes vasodilation, which is mediated by enhanced NO and prostacyclin production by the endothelial cell. Endothelin has also been shown to promote the closing of endothelium fenestrae in normal rat liver[25]. This may be relevant since the capillarization process and occlusion of fenestrae are thought to play a role in increasing resistance in cirrhosis.

Patients with liver cirrhosis have increased circulating plasma levels of ET-1 and ET-3[26]. A decreased clearance of ET-1 by the liver has also been demonstrated in cirrhotic rats[27]. ET-1 administration increases portal perfusion pressure by increasing intrahepatic resistance in normal and cirrhotic livers. While some experimental studies reported a slight reduction of portal pressure in cirrhotic animals after the administration of endothelin antagonists[25,28], this was not confirmed by other studies[29], so the role of endothelins in increasing the vascular tone in cirrhosis remains unsettled.

Angiotensin II

Angiotensin II (A-II) is a powerful vasoconstrictor that increases hepatic resistance in isolated cirrhotic livers. Moreover, infusion of A-II increases portal pressure and decreases hepatic blood flow in patients with cirrhosis. These effects are probably caused by the contraction of vascular smooth muscle cells as well as hepatic stellate cells[30,31].

Increased A-II is the result of the activation of the renin–angiotensin system (RAS), which is commonly observed in patients with cirrhosis. Activation of RAS may also be detrimental for portal hypertension as a result of increased liver fibrogenesis[32], which may worsen the evolution of cirrhosis.

All the above suggest that preventing the activation of RAS may have beneficial effects in decreasing portal pressure in cirrhosis. However, although A-II blockade may reduce portal pressure, it causes systemic hypotension with adverse consequences on renal function, reducing its potential as a therapeutic strategy for portal hypertension[33].

Endocannabinoids

Endogenous cannabinoids (or endocannabinoids) is a collective term describing a novel class of endogenous lipid ligands, including anandamide (arachidonyl ethanolamide). Anandamide has been reported to induce both vasodilation and vasoconstriction in cirrhotic and non-cirrhotic humans and animals. However, the effects of anandamide depend on its concentration as well as the vascular territory being examined. Therefore, it is possible that, in cirrhosis with portal hypertension, anandamide acts as a vasodilator in the peripheral circulation, since first evidence implicates cannabinoids in the hyperdynamic circulation of portal hypertension[34,35].

By contrast, recent studies suggest that anandamide serves as a vasoconstrictor involved in increased intrahepatic resistance. Cirrhotic livers may exert a hyperresponse to anandamide through an increased anandamide-related TXA_2 production in cirrhotic livers. This study pleads for a relationship between anandamide and COX, suggesting that certain actions of the cannabinoids could be explained by a mechanism involving the synthesis of eicosanoids[36].

ENDOTHELIAL DYSFUNCTION OF CIRRHOTIC LIVERS

In normal conditions the endothelium is able to generate vasodilator stimuli in response to increases in blood volume, blood pressure or vasoconstrictor agents, in an attempt to prevent or attenuate the concomitant increase in pressure. In several pathological conditions there is an impairment in this endothelium-dependent vasodilation, which has been named 'endothelial dysfunction'[37,38]. Endothelial dysfunction is considered one of the main pathological mechanisms involved in the increased vascular tone observed in several vascular disorders such as arterial hypertension[39], diabetes[40] and hypercholesterolaemia[41], and has been attributed to a diminished NO bioavailability[37,38] and to an increased production of endothelial-derived contracting factors (EDCF), such as PGH_2/TXA_2[42], endothelin[43] or anion superoxide[44]. The hepatic vascular bed of cirrhotic livers also exhibits endothelial dysfunction[45]; indeed, contrary to what happens in normal livers, the cirrhotic liver cannot accommodate the increased portal blood flow caused by the postprandial hyperaemia, which determines an abrupt postprandial increase in portal pressure[46]. In addition, in experimental models of cirrhosis, endothelial dysfunction has been further characterized by showing that the cirrhotic liver exhibits an impaired response to the endothelium-dependent vasodilator acetylcholine[15,45] (Figure 2). Endothelial dysfunction in cirrhosis has been attributed to reduced NO bioavailability and to increased vasoconstrictor COX-1-derived prostanoids.

REDUCED RELEASE OF VASODILATORS

Reduced NO bioavailability within the cirrhotic liver

NO is the natural ligand for soluble guanylate cyclase and is responsible for an increase in cyclic guanosine monophosphate (cGMP), the final agent responsible for the relaxation of the vascular wall through the extrusion of cytosolic Ca^{2+}. Endothelial NO synthase (eNOS) is responsible for most of the vascular NO produced in a reaction where L-arginine is oxidized to L-citrulline

Control Liver

Cirrhotic Liver

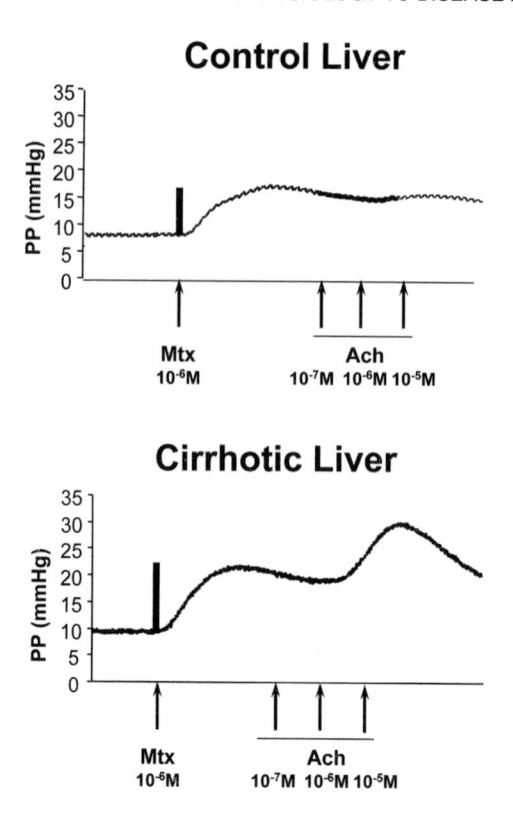

Figure 2 Representative tracings of concentration curves to acetylcholine (Ach) of control and cirrhotic perfused livers. Cirrhotic livers exhibited hyperresponse to vasoconstrictors and impaired endothelium-dependent relaxation to vasodilators (Mtx, methoxamine)

and NO[47]. In cirrhotic liver there is a reduced NO bioavailability that plays a major role increasing intrahepatic vascular resistance and thereby worsening portal hypertension. In accordance with this concept the administration of nitrates (exogenous donors of NO) has been shown to decrease portal pressure. In addition, enhancement of the expression of NO synthase in liver cells, through the portal injection of adenovirus coupled with the gene encoding NO synthase, significantly reduces portal pressure[48]. More recently, strategies aimed at increasing NO release by enhancing intrahepatic eNOS activity, based on constitutively active Akt gene transfer[49] or by simvastatin administration[50], have opened new perspectives with potential therapeutic implications.

Decreased NO production occurs despite a normal expression of eNOS mRNA and normal levels of eNOS protein[45,51] and has been attributed, at least in part, to reduced eNOS activity caused by several post-translational alterations in the regulation of the enzyme such as increased caveolin expression, or a defect of the essential cofactor of eNOS, tetrahydrobioterin (BH_4)[52,53].

Oxidative stress

As in other vascular disorders characterized by the presence of endothelial dysfunction, oxidative stress has been implicated in the increased vascular tone present in cirrhotic livers[54,55]. It is well known that superoxide is capable of reacting with NO, leading to peroxynitrite (ONOO⁻) formation[56,57], with an ongoing decrease in NO bioavailability[58–62]. Reactive oxygen species (ROS) can also affect NO biology by their capacity to oxidize, and therefore inactivate, the NO synthase cofactor, BH_4 (see ref. 39), leading to a situation that has been called eNOS uncoupling[63–65], in which the NO synthases are incapable of transferring electrons to L-arginine and start using oxygen as a substrate leading to O_2^- formation instead of NO. In that regard, further evidence sustaining a role for oxidative stress modulating NO bioavailability in the intrahepatic circulation in cirrhosis comes from a recent experimental study investigating eNOS uncoupling[66], in which it was shown that cirrhotic livers have markedly decreased levels of BH_4, due to a decreased activity and expression of the key enzyme in its synthesis, GTP cyclohydrolase. In addition, BH_4 was in a great proportion oxidized (and therefore inactivated), a fact that might cause a further deterioration in eNOS activity. In this study eNOS uncoupling was corrected by short-term BH_4 supplementation[66], suggesting that prevention of BH_4 oxidation may be another way to improve eNOS uncoupling.

Decreased SOD activity has also been reported in cirrhotic livers and associated with a significantly decreased expression of cytoplasmatic and mitochondrial SOD isoforms[54,67].

Altogether, the above findings suggest that oxidative stress may contribute to endothelial dysfunction and increased hepatic vascular tone in cirrhosis, and that antioxidant therapy may contribute to correcting this abnormality[68].

Carbon monoxide (CO)

CO is a co-product of the degradation of protohaem IX to biliverdin by haem oxygenases (HO). Similar to NO, it activates guanylyl cylcase, increasing the production of cGMP[69]. Inhibition of HO activity by protoporphyrin IX was shown to increase perfusion pressure during rat liver perfusion, an effect that was further reversed by addition of CO to the perfusate[70]. In addition, CO overproduction by induced HO-1 caused a reduction in intrahepatic vascular resistance during liver perfusion[71]. Taken together, these observations indicate that CO participates in intrahepatic vascular tone control.

Despite this, HO-1 activity in liver tissue from cirrhotic patients was shown to be higher than that in normal liver tissue, suggesting that CO production in cirrhotic livers is not impaired. It has been suggested that increased CO production could be involved in decreased production of NO in cirrhotic livers[72].

Hydrogen sulphide (H₂S)

H₂S is produced endogenously from desulphydration of cysteine by three different enzymes; cystathione-γ-lyase (CSE), cystathionine-β-synthase (CBS), or 3-mercaptosulphurtransferase[73]. Although NO and CO are the first two identified gasotransmitters, recently, different arguments have indicated H₂S as the third gasotransmitter that can modulate vascular tone[74]. Indeed, it has recently been suggested that H₂S regulates HSC contraction and that a decreased expression of CSE in HSC may be responsible for the increased intrahepatic resistance in rodent models of liver cirrhosis[75].

INCREASED PRODUCTION OF VASOCONSTRICTOR PROSTANOIDS

Endothelial dysfunction was also shown to be associated with an increased production of TXA₂ and completely prevented by selective COX-1 blockers and by TXA₂ antagonists. These results suggest that an increased production of a COX-1-derived vasoconstrictor prostanoid, probably TXA₂ is, at least in part, responsible for endothelial dysfunction[15]. All these findings suggest that in cirrhotic livers there is an overactivation of the COX-1 pathway with an increased production of their vasoconstrictor-derived compounds.

Recently it has been postulated that a possible pharmacological strategy in the treatment of portal hypertension would be to abrogate the generation of TXA₂ in combination with a replenishment of the decreased hepatic NO bioavailiability. Regarding that point it has been demonstrated that nitroflurbiprofen, an NO-releasing cyclooxygenase inhibitor, improves portal hypertension by attenuating intrahepatic vascular resistance, endothelial dysfunction and hepatic hyporeactivity to vasoconstrictors of thioacetamide-induced cirrhotic livers[76].

Acknowledgements

This study was supported by grants from the Ministerio de Educación y Ciencia (SAF:04/04783) and from the Fondo de Investigaciones Sanitarias (FIS 04/0655, 05/1285, 06/0623).

References

1. Bosch J, García-Pagán JC. Complications of cirrhosis. I. Portal hypertension. J Hepatol. 2000;32:141–56.
2. Bathal PS, Grossmann HJ. Reduction of the increased portal vascular resistance of the isolated perfused cirrhotic rat liver by vasodilators. J Hepatol. 1985;1:325–9.
3. Kaneda K, Ekataksin W, Sogawa M, Matsumura A, Cho A, Kawada N. Endothelin-1-induced vasoconstriction causes a significant increase in portal pressure of rat liver: localized constrictive effect on the distal segment of preterminal portal venules as revealed by light and electron microscopy and serial reconstruction. Hepatology. 1998;27:735–47.
4. Zhang JX, Pegoli W, Clemens MG. Endothelin-1 induces direct constriction of hepatic sinusoids. Am J Physiol. 1994;266:G624–32.

5. Kawada N, Tran-Thi TA, Klein H, Decker K. The contraction of hepatic stellate (Ito) cells stimulated with vasoactive substances. Possible involvement of endothelin 1 and nitric oxide in the regulation of the sinusoidal tonus. Eur J Biochem. 1993;213:815–23.
6. García-Pagán JC, Bosch J, Rodes J. The role of vasoactive mediators in portal hypertension. Semin Gastrointest Dis. 1995;6:140–7.
7. Ballet F, Chretien Y, Rey C, Poupon R. Differential response of normal and cirrhotic liver to vasoactive agents – a study in the isolated perfused rat liver. J Pharmacol Exp Ther. 1988;244:283–9.
8. Lautt WW, Greenway CV, Legare DJ. Effect of hepatic nerves, norepinephrine, angiotensin, and elevated central venous-pressure on post-sinusoidal resistance sites and intrahepatic pressures in cats. Microvasc Res. 1987;33:50–61.
9. Xing M, Insel PA. Protein kinase C-dependent activation of cytosolic phospholipase A2 and mitogen-activated protein kinase by alpha 1-adrenergic receptors in Madin–Darby canine kidney cells. J Clin Invest. 1996;97:1302–10.
10. Athari A, Hanecke K, Jungermann K. Prostaglandin F2 alpha and D2 release from primary Ito cell cultures after stimulation with noradrenaline and ATP but not adenosine. Hepatology. 1994;20:142–8.
11. Miyamoto T, Ogino N, Yamamoto S, Hayaishi O. Purification of prostaglandin endoperoxide synthetase from bovine vesicular gland microsomes. J Biol Chem. 1976;251:2629–36.
12. Smith WL. Prostanoid biosynthesis and mechanisms of action. Am J Physiol. 1992;263: F181–91.
13. Smith WL, Garavito RM, DeWitt DL. Prostaglandin endoperoxide H synthases (cyclooxygenases)-1 and -2. J Biol Chem. 1996;271:33157–60.
14. Graupera M, García-Pagán JC, Abraldes JG et al. Cyclooxygenase-derived products modulate the increased intrahepatic resistance of cirrhotic rat livers. Hepatology. 2003;37:172–81.
15. Graupera M, García-Pagán JC, Pares M et al. Cyclooxyenase-1 inhibition corrects endothelial dysfunction in cirrhotic rat livers. J Hepatol. 2003;39:515–21.
16. Potenza MA, Botrugno OA, De Salvia MA et al. Endothelial COX-1 and -2 differentially affect reactivity of MVB in portal hypertensive rats. Am J Physiol Gastrointest Liver Physiol. 2002;283:G587–94.
17. Smith WL, Langenbach R. Why there are two cyclooxygenase isozymes. J Clin Invest. 2001;107:1491–5.
18. Gracia-Sancho J, Lavina B, Rodriguez-Vilarrupla A, Garcia-Caldero H, Bosch J, García-Pagán JC. Enhanced vasoconstrictor prostanoid production by sinusoidal endothelial cells increases portal perfusion pressure in cirrhotic rat livers. J Hepatol. 2007;47:220–7.
19. Steib CJ, Gerbes AL, Bystron M et al. Kupffer cell activation in normal and fibrotic livers increases portal pressure via thromboxane A(2). J Hepatol. 2007;47:228–38.
20. Samuelsson B, Dahlen SE, Lindgren JA, Rouzer CA, Serhan CN. Leukotrienes and lipoxins: structures, biosynthesis, and biological effects. Science. 1987;237:1171–6.
21. Keppler D. Leukotrienes: biosynthesis, transport, inactivation, and analysis. Rev Physiol Biochem Pharmacol. 1992;121:1–30.
22. Graupera M, García-Pagán JC, Titos E et al. 5-Lipoxygenase inhibition reduces intrahepatic vascular resistance of cirrhotic rat livers: a possible role of cysteinyl-leukotrienes. Gastroenterology. 2002;122:387–93.
23. Angus PW. Role of endothelin in systemic and portal resistance in cirrhosis. Gut. 2006;55:1230–2.
24. Clozel M, Gray GA, Breu V, Loffler BM, Osterwalder R. The endothelin ETB receptor mediates both vasodilation and vasoconstriction *in vivo*. Biochem Biophys Res Commun. 1992;186:867–73.
25. Reichen J, Gerbes AL, Steiner MJ, Sagesser H, Clozel M. The effect of endothelin and its antagonist Bosentan on hemodynamics and microvascular exchange in cirrhotic rat liver. J Hepatol. 1998;28:1020–30.
26. Moller S, Gulberg V, Henriksen JH, Gerbes AL. Endothelin-1 and endothelin-3 in cirrhosis: relations to systemic and splanchnic haemodynamics. J Hepatol. 1995;23:135–44.
27. Gandhi CR, Sproat LA, Subbotin VM. Increased hepatic endothelin-1 levels and endothelin receptor density in cirrhotic rats. Life Sci. 1996;58:55–62.

28. Rockey DC, Weisiger RA. Endothelin induced contractility of stellate cells from normal and cirrhotic rat liver: implications for regulation of portal pressure and resistance. Hepatology. 1996;24:233–40.
29. Poo JL, Jimenez W, Maria MR et al. Chronic blockade of endothelin receptors in cirrhotic rats: hepatic and hemodynamic effects. Gastroenterology. 1999;116:161–7.
30. Bataller R, Gines P, Nicolas JM et al. Angiotensin II induces contraction and proliferation of human hepatic stellate cells. Gastroenterology. 2000;118:1149–56.
31. Bataller R, Sancho-Bru P, Gines P et al. Activated human hepatic stellate cells express the renin-angiotensin system and synthesize angiotensin II. Gastroenterology. 2003;125:117–25.
32. Rockey DC. Vasoactive agents in intrahepatic portal hypertension and fibrogenesis: implications for therapy. Gastroenterology. 2000;118:1261–5.
33. Gonzalez-Abraldes J, Albillos A, Banares R et al. Randomized comparison of long-term losartan versus propranolol in lowering portal pressure in cirrhosis. Gastroenterology. 2001;121:382–8.
34. Batkai S, Jarai Z, Wagner JA et al. Endocannabinoids acting at vascular CB1 receptors mediate the vasodilated state in advanced liver cirrhosis. Nat Med. 2001;7:827–32.
35. Ros J, Claria J, To-Figueras J et al. Endogenous cannabinoids: a new system involved in the homeostasis of arterial pressure in experimental cirrhosis in the rat. Gastroenterology. 2002;122:85–93.
36. Yang YY, Lin HC, Huang YT et al. Roles of anandamide in the hepatic microcirculation in cirrhotic rats. Am J Physiol Gastrointest Liver Physiol. 2006;290:G328–34.
37. Harrison DG. Cellular and molecular mechanisms of endothelial cell dysfunction. J Clin Invest. 1997;100:2153–7.
38. Harrison DG. Endothelial function and oxidant stress. Clin Cardiol. 1997;20:II–7.
39. Landmesser U, Dikalov S, Price SR et al. Oxidation of tetrahydrobiopterin leads to uncoupling of endothelial cell nitric oxide synthase in hypertension. J Clin Invest. 2003;111:1201–9.
40. Dixon LJ, Hughes SM, Rooney K et al. Increased superoxide production in hypertensive patients with diabetes mellitus: role of nitric oxide synthase. Am J Hypertens. 2005;18:839–43.
41. Ohara Y, Peterson TE, Harrison DG. Hypercholesterolemia increases endothelial superoxide anion production. J Clin Invest. 1993;91:2546–51.
42. Ge T, Hughes H, Junquero DC, Wu KK, Vanhoutte PM, Boulanger CM. Endothelium-dependent contractions are associated with both augmented expression of prostaglandin H synthase-1 and hypersensitivity to prostaglandin H2 in the SHR aorta. Circ Res. 1995;76:1003–10.
43. Lerman A, Holmes DR Jr, Bell MR, Garratt KN, Nishimura RA, Burnett JC Jr. Endothelin in coronary endothelial dysfunction and early atherosclerosis in humans. Circulation. 1995;92:2426–31.
44. Tagawa H, Tomoike H, Nakamura M. Putative mechanisms of the impairment of endothelium-dependent relaxation of the aorta with atheromatous plaque in heritable hyperlipidemic rabbits. Circ Res. 1991;68:330–7.
45. Gupta TK, Toruner M, Chung MK, Groszmann RJ. Endothelial dysfunction and decreased production of nitric oxide in the intrahepatic microcirculation of cirrhotic rats. Hepatology. 1998;28:926–31.
46. Bellis L, Berzigotti A, Abraldes JG et al. Low doses of isosorbide mononitrate attenuate the postprandial increase in portal pressure in patients with cirrhosis. Hepatology. 2003;37:378–84.
47. Moncada S, Higgs A. The L-arginine-nitric oxide pathway. N Engl J Med. 1993;329:2002–12.
48. Fevery J, Roskams T, Van de CM et al. NO synthase in the liver: prospects of *in vivo* gene transfer. Digestion. 1998;59:58–9.
49. Morales-Ruiz M, Cejudo-Martn P, Fernandez-Varo G et al. Transduction of the liver with activated Akt normalizes portal pressure in cirrhotic rats. Gastroenterology. 2003;125:522–31.
50. Zafra C, Abraldes JG, Turnes J et al. Simvastatin enhances hepatic nitric oxide production and decreases the hepatic vascular tone in patients with cirrhosis. Gastroenterology. 2004;126:749–55.

51. Mittal MK, Gupta TK, Lee FY, Sieber CC, Groszmann RJ. Nitric oxide modulates hepatic vascular tone in normal rat liver. Am J Physiol. 1994;267:G416–22.
52. Miller DR, Collier JM, Billings RE. Protein tyrosine kinase activity regulates nitric oxide synthase induction in rat hepatocytes. Am J Physiol. 1997;272:G207–14.
53. Shah V, Toruner M, Haddad F et al. Impaired endothelial nitric oxide synthase activity associated with enhanced caveolin binding in experimental cirrhosis in the rat. Gastroenterology. 1999;117:1222–8.
54. Gracia-Sancho J, Laviña B, Rodriguez-Vilarrupla A, Garcia H, Bosch J, García-Pagán JC. Oxidative stress reduces nitric oxide biodisponibility and may contribute to endothelial dysfunction of cirrhotic livers. J Hepatol. 2006;44:S75.
55. Rodriguez-Vilarrupla A, Bosch J, García-Pagán JC. Potential role of antioxidants in the treatment of portal hypertension. J Hepatol. 2007;46:193–7.
56. Huie RE, Padmaja S. The reaction of NO with superoxide. Free Radic Res Commun. 1993;18:195–9.
57. Fridovich I. Superoxide radical: an endogenous toxicant. Annu Rev Pharmacol Toxicol. 1983;23:239–57.
58. Cai H, Harrison DG. Endothelial dysfunction in cardiovascular diseases: the role of oxidant stress. Circ Res. 2000;87:840–4.
59. Madamanchi NR, Vendrov A, Runge MS. Oxidative stress and vascular disease. Arterioscler Thromb Vasc Biol. 2005;25:29–38.
60. Lum H, Roebuck KA. Oxidant stress and endothelial cell dysfunction. Am J Physiol Cell Physiol. 2001;280:C719–41.
61. Jay D, Hitomi H, Griendling KK. Oxidative stress and diabetic cardiovascular complications. Free Radic Biol Med. 2006;40:183–92.
62. Heistad DD. Oxidative stress and vascular disease: 2005 Duff Lecture. Arterioscler Thromb Vasc Biol. 2006;26:689–95.
63. Vasquez-Vivar J, Kalyanaraman B, Martasek P et al. Superoxide generation by endothelial nitric oxide synthase: the influence of cofactors. Proc Natl Acad Sci USA. 1998;95:9220–5.
64. Kuzkaya N, Weissmann N, Harrison DG, Dikalov S. Interactions of peroxynitrite, tetrahydrobiopterin, ascorbic acid, and thiols: implications for uncoupling endothelial nitric-oxide synthase. J Biol Chem. 2003;278:22546–54.
65. Stroes E, Hijmering M, van Zandvoort M, Wever R, Rabelink TJ, van Faassen EE. Origin of superoxide production by endothelial nitric oxide synthase. FEBS Lett. 1998;438:161–4.
66. Matei V, Rodriguez-Vilarrupla A, Deulofeu R et al. The eNOS cofactor tetrahydrobiopterin improves endothelial dysfunction in livers of rats with CCl4 cirrhosis. Hepatology. 2006;44:44–52.
67. Van de CM, Van Pelt JF, Nevens F, Fevery J, Reichen J. Low NO bioavailability in CCl_4 cirrhotic rat livers might result from low NO synthesis combined with decreased superoxide dismutase activity allowing superoxide-mediated NO breakdown: a comparison of two portal hypertensive rat models with healthy controls. Comp Hepatol. 2003;2:2.
68. Hernandez-Guerra M, García-Pagán JC, Turnes J et al. Ascorbic acid improves the intrahepatic endothelial dysfunction of patients with cirrhosis and portal hypertension. Hepatology. 2006;43:485–91.
69. Maines MD. Heme oxygenase – function, multiplicity, regulatory mechanisms, and clinical applications. FASEB J. 1988;2:2557–68.
70. Suematsu M, Kashiwagi S, Sano T, Goda N, Shinoda Y, Ishimura Y. Carbon monoxide as an endogenous modulator of hepatic vascular perfusion. Biochem Biophys Res Commun. 1994;205:1333–7.
71. Wakabayashi Y, Takamiya R, Mizuki A et al. Carbon monoxide overproduced by heme oxygenase-1 causes a reduction of vascular resistance in perfused rat liver. Am J Physiol. 1999;277:G1088–96.
72. Makino N, Suematsu M, Sugiura Y et al. Altered expression of heme oxygenase-1 in the livers of patients with portal hypertensive diseases. Hepatology. 2001;33:32–42.
73. Stipanuk MH, Beck PW. Characterization of the enzymic capacity for cysteine desulfhydration in liver and kidney of the rat. Biochem J. 1982;206:267–77.
74. Wang R. Two's company, three's a crowd: can H2S be the third endogenous gaseous transmitter? FASEB J. 2002;16:1792–8.

75. Fiorucci S, Antonelli E, Mencarelli A et al. The third gas: H2S regulates perfusion pressure in both the isolated and perfused normal rat liver and in cirrhosis. Hepatology. 2005;42:539–48.
76. Laleman W, Van Landeghem L, Van der Elst I, Zeegers M, Fevery J, Nevens F. Nitroflurbiprofen, a nitric oxide-releasing cyclooxygenase inhibitor, improves cirrhotic portal hypertension in rats. Gastroenterology. 2007;132:709–19.

18
Remodelling portal hypertension: preprimary prophylaxis

G. GARCIA-TSAO

INTRODUCTION

Portal hypertension is the main complication of cirrhosis, regardless of its aetiology. Gastro-oesophageal varices are a direct consequence of portal hypertension and develop after a minimal portal pressure of 10–12 mmHg is reached[1,2].

PATHOPHYSIOLOGY OF PORTAL HYPERTENSION IN CIRRHOSIS

In cirrhosis, portal pressure increases initially as a consequence of an increased resistance to flow, mostly due to an architectural distortion of the liver secondary to fibrous tissue and regenerative nodules. In addition to this structural resistance to blood flow, there is an active intrahepatic vasoconstriction that accounts for 20–30% of the increased intrahepatic resistance[3], and that is mostly due to a decrease in the endogenous production of nitric oxide[4,5]. Portal hypertension leads to the formation of portosystemic collaterals that would theoretically decompress the system. However, portal hypertension persists despite the development of collaterals, partly because they are insufficient to decompress the portal system[6]. More importantly, the portal hypertensive state is maintained because, concomitant with the formation of collaterals, there is an increase in portal venous inflow that results from splanchnic arteriolar vasodilation[7,8]. Vasodilation occurs not only in the splanchnic circulation but also in the systemic circulation, and is the main pathogenic event that leads to the hyperdynamic circulatory state in cirrhosis that in turn leads to variceal growth and other complications of cirrhosis such as ascites, the hepatorenal syndrome and the hepatopulmonary syndrome. Splanchnic and peripheral vasodilation is mostly due to an increase in nitric oxide[5].

Therefore, portal hypertension results from both an increase in resistance to portal flow (intrahepatic and collateral) and an increase in portal blood inflow.

NATURAL HISTORY OF VARICES

Gastro-oesophageal varices are present in approximately 50% of patients with cirrhosis, with a higher prevalence in patients with more severe liver disease[9]. Patients with primary biliary cirrhosis may develop varices and variceal haemorrhage early in the course of the disease, even in the absence of established cirrhosis[10]. It has also been shown that 16% of patients with hepatitis C and bridging fibrosis have oesophageal varices[11].

Patients without varices develop them at a rate of ~8% per year[12] and, as shown below, independent predictors of variceal development are the degree of portal hypertension and aspartate aminotransferase serum levels[13].

Patients with small varices develop large varices also at a rate of ~8% per year and independent predictors of variceal growth are decompensated cirrhosis, i.e. a Child–Turcotte–Pugh (CTP) class B or C and the presence of red signs on varices[12].

Patients with varices develop variceal haemorrhage at a rate of ~12% per year and the strongest independent predictor of haemorrhage is a large variceal size[14]. However, other independent predictors of haemorrhage are decompensated cirrhosis (CT class B or C) and the endoscopic presence of red wale marks[14]. Therefore, the risk of bleeding in a patient with small varices who has decompensated cirrhosis, or whose varices have red signs, is the same as that of a patient with large varices.

Although bleeding from oesophageal varices ceases spontaneously in up to 40% of patients, and despite improvements in therapy over the past decade, variceal haemorrhage is still associated with a mortality of at least 20% at 6 weeks[15–17]. In a large cohort of untreated patients with cirrhosis followed prospectively, the highest 1-year mortality was observed in patients with variceal haemorrhage: 57% compared to 20% in patients with ascites but without variceal haemorrhage[18]. In this same study the presence of varices in a subgroup of patients with compensated cirrhosis was associated with a significantly poorer prognosis (1-year mortality of 3%) compared with patients with compensated cirrhosis who had not yet developed varices (1-year mortality of 1%).

The natural history of portal hypertension evolves from a patient with cirrhosis and portal hypertension who has not yet developed varices, to a patient who develops small varices that, as flow increases through them, grow in size and may eventually rupture, leading to variceal haemorrhage (Figure 1).

BASES OF PROPHYLACTIC THERAPY IN PORTAL HYPERTENSION

Patients who have bled from varices have a risk of rebleeding of ~60% in the first 1–2 years after the index variceal haemorrhage. In these patients, preventing recurrent haemorrhage is the goal of therapy and is termed secondary prophylaxis (Figure 1). As the risk of bleeding is the greatest in this group of patients, one is more willing to risk the development of side-effects and therefore combination therapies (with a higher rate of adverse events) are more commonly used.

```
┌─────────────┐     ┌─────────────┐  ⎫
│  No varices │ ──▶ │ Prevention  │  ⎪
│             │     │  of varices │  ⎬  Pre-primary
└─────────────┘     └─────────────┘  ⎪  Prophylaxis
       │                             ⎪
       ▼                             ⎪
┌─────────────┐     ┌─────────────┐  ⎪
│Small varices│ ──▶ │ Prevention  │  ⎪
│No haemorrhage│    │  of growth  │  ⎭
└─────────────┘     └─────────────┘
       │
       ▼
┌─────────────┐     ┌─────────────┐  ⎫
│Large or high-│ ──▶│Prevention of│  ⎬  Primary
│ risk small   │    │1st haemorrhage│ ⎪  Prophylaxis
│varices No    │    │             │  ⎭
│haemorrhage   │    └─────────────┘
└─────────────┘
       │
       ▼
┌─────────────┐     ┌─────────────┐  ⎫
│  Variceal   │ ──▶ │Prevention of│  ⎬  Secondary
│haemorrhage  │     │ recurrence  │  ⎭  Prophylaxis
└─────────────┘     └─────────────┘
```

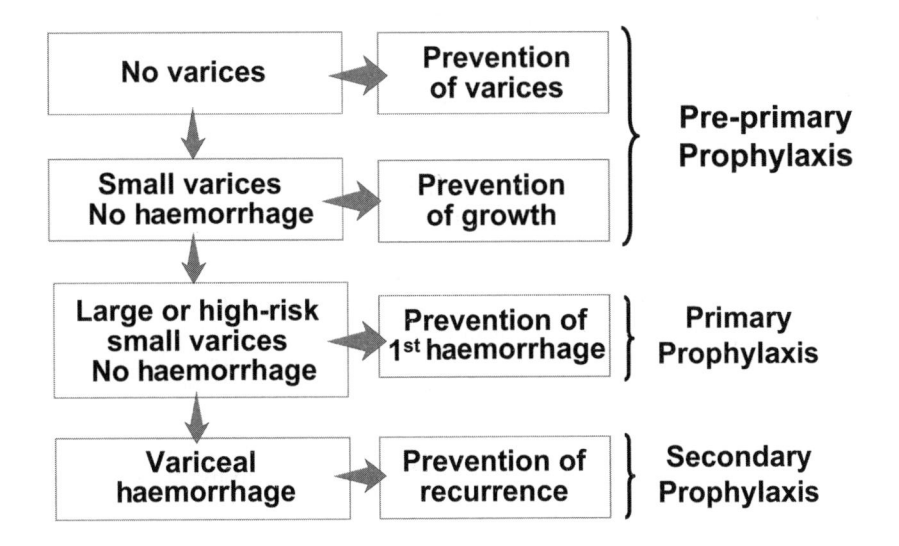

Figure 1 Natural history of varices in the context of the different prophylactic strategies. From the bottom, secondary prophylaxis refers to prevention of recurrent variceal haemorrhage in patients who have bled from varices. Primary prophylaxis refers to preventing the first episode of variceal haemorrhage in patients with high-risk varices who have never bled. Therefore, pre-primary prophylaxis refers to prevention of varices (in patients with cirrhosis who have not yet developed them) or prevention of growth of varices (in patients with small varices that are not at a high risk of haemorrhage)

Patients with large varices who have never bled from them (or a patient with high-risk small varices, i.e. those with red signs or those present in a CTP class B or C patient) have a risk of developing a first episode of variceal haemorrhage of $\sim 30\%$ in the first 2 years after being diagnosed. In these patients, preventing the first variceal haemorrhage is the goal of therapy and this is called primary prophylaxis (Figure 1). As the risk of bleeding is significantly lower than for rebleeding, single therapy (with a consequent lower rate of adverse events) is recommended.

Pre-primary prophylaxis refers to prevention of development of varices (in patients with cirrhosis who have no varices) and prevention of the growth of varices (in patients with small, low-risk, varices) (Figure 1). As mentioned previously, the risk of developing an outcome in these patients is $\sim 8\%$ in the first year after diagnosis. In these patients the least invasive therapy, i.e. pharmacological therapy, has been investigated in both settings and is described below.

NON-SELECTIVE β-ADRENERGIC BLOCKERS IN PORTAL HYPERTENSION

Non-selective β-adrenergic blockers (propranolol, nadolol, timolol) reduce portal pressure through a reduction in portal venous inflow. This effect is the result of both a decrease in cardiac output (β_1-blocking effect) and from splanchnic arteriolar vasoconstriction secondary to blockade of β_2-receptor-mediated splanchnic vasodilation[19] (Figure 2).

Data derived from studies of primary and secondary prophylaxis of variceal haemorrhage have shown that pharmacological reduction in portal pressure (as determined by the hepatic venous pressure gradient or HVPG) in patients with cirrhosis has been shown to significantly decrease first and recurrent variceal haemorrhage. Patients in whom the HVPG decreases below 12 mmHg are essentially protected from bleeding, and those in whom the HVPG decreases by more than 20% from baseline have a significantly lower rate of recurrent haemorrhage[20,21]. This reduction in HVPG has also been associated with a reduction in the incidence of other complications of portal hypertension such as ascites, spontaneous bacterial peritonitis and encephalopathy[21–23]. Importantly, HVPG 'responders' (i.e. patients in whom HVPG decreases below 12 mmHg or by more than 20% from baseline) have a lower mortality[20].

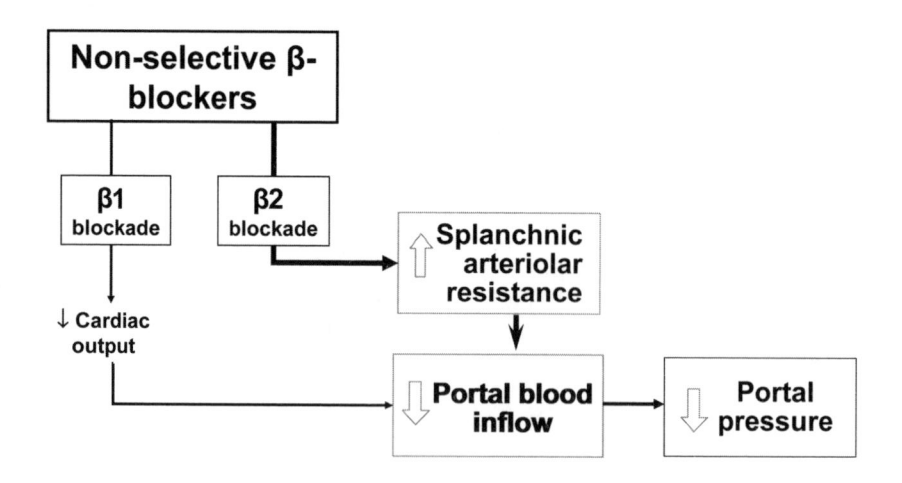

Figure 2 Non-selective β-adrenergic blockers reduce portal pressure by decreasing portal blood inflow. The β_2 blocking effect (leading to splanchnic vasoconstriction) is more important than the β_1 blocking effect (leading to a decrease in cardiac output) and therefore selective β_1-adrenergic blockers are not recommended in the treatment of portal hypertension

PREVENTION OF VARICES

In experimental portal hypertension the reduction in portal pressure and portal venous inflow induced by β-adrenergic blockers prevented the development of portosystemic collaterals. In a study performed in mice with schistosomiasis, the early administration of propranolol led to a significantly lower portal pressure (7.9 vs 10.8 mmHg), a lower portal-systemic shunting (2.5% vs 12.2%) and a lower portal venous inflow (2.50 vs 4.00 ml/min). These results demonstrate that, in chronic liver disease induced by schistosomiasis, the development of portal-systemic shunting could be decreased or prevented by a propranolol-induced reduction of flow and pressure in the portal system[24].

By decreasing portal pressure at earlier stages it may be possible to prevent or ameliorate not only the development of gastro-oesophageal varices but also the detrimental hepatic and systemic metabolic effects due to portal-systemic shunting and the development of ascites, thereby improving the survival of patients with cirrhosis and portal hypertension.

With this hypothesis a large multicentre randomized placebo-controlled trial was performed with the objectives of evaluating the efficacy of a non-selective β-adrenergic blocker, timolol, in preventing the development of gastro-oesophageal varices and to assess the usefulness of baseline and sequential measurements of HVPG in predicting the development of varices and other complications of cirrhosis[13].

In this trial 213 patients with cirrhosis without varices but with portal hypertension (HVPG of at least 6 mmHg) were randomly assigned, 108 to the timolol group and 105 to the placebo group. Every year an upper endoscopy, abdominal ultrasound and HVPG measurements were performed. The primary endpoints were development of varices or variceal haemorrhage. In a median follow-up of 54.9 months, 84 (39%) patients developed a primary endpoint, 42 in the timolol group (35 small varices, four large varices, two variceal haemorrhage, one bleeding from gastropathy) and 42 in the placebo group (35 small varices, four large varices, three variceal haemorrhage) (n.s.). No differences in development of ascites, encephalopathy, liver transplants or death were found between groups. More patients in the timolol group developed serious adverse events leading to withdrawal of study medication (18% vs 6%, $p = 0.006$), with the most common being symptomatic bradycardia, severe fatigue and wheezing/shortness of breath.

On Cox multivariate regression analysis two parameters were independently predictive of a primary endpoint: HVPG > 10 mmHg ($p = 0.005$) and aspartate aminotransferase ($p = 0.007$).

Furthermore, primary endpoints developed at a significantly lower rate in patients who had a reduction in HVPG >10% at 1 year (19/69 or 28%) compared to those in whom the reduction was ⩽10% (44/85 or 52%) ($p = 0.003$). Notably, 53% patients randomized to timolol had a reduction in HVPG >10% while this reduction occurred in only 38% of patients in the placebo group ($p = 0.04$). As expected, patients with a baseline HVPG <10 mmHg who additionally had a 1-year reduction >10% from baseline, were essentially free from developing varices throughout the study[25]. Conversely, primary endpoints developed at a significantly higher rate in patients who had an increase in

HVPG >10% at 1 year (27/37 or 73%) compared to patients in whom the increase was ⩽10% (36/117 or 31%) ($p<0.001$)[25]. There was no difference in the proportion of patients in either study group regarding the increase in HVPG.

A follow-up study in this patient cohort aimed at identifying predictors of clinical decompensation (defined as the development of ascites, variceal haemorrhage or hepatic encephalopathy) showed that, in a median follow-up time of 51.1 months, 62/213 patients (29%) developed decompensation: 46 (21.6%) ascites, 17 (8%) encephalopathy and six (3%) variceal haemorrhage. On multivariable analysis, three predictors of decompensation were identified: HVPG, Model for End-stage Liver Disease (MELD) score and albumin. Diagnostic capacity of HVPG was greater than for MELD or CTP score. An HVPG of 10 mmHg distinguished two populations with a different rate of incidence of decompensation with a negative predictive value of 90%[26]; that is, compensated patients with a HVPG value below 10 mmHg have a 90% chance of not having any clinical decompensation in a median follow-up of 4 years.

Therefore, non-selective β-adrenergic blockers are not effective in preventing the development of varices and are associated with a significant rate of adverse events. They are therefore not recommended in compensated cirrhotic patients without varices (Figure 3). However, even in this very compensated patient population, the importance of baseline HVPG levels and of reductions in HVPG >10% from baseline in predicting the development of both varices and clinical decompensation is demonstrated. Therefore future trials of prevention of varices should ideally include patients with an HVPG >10 mmHg and the therapeutic goal that should be achieved through the use of β-blockers or other drugs should be a reduction in HVPG >10%.

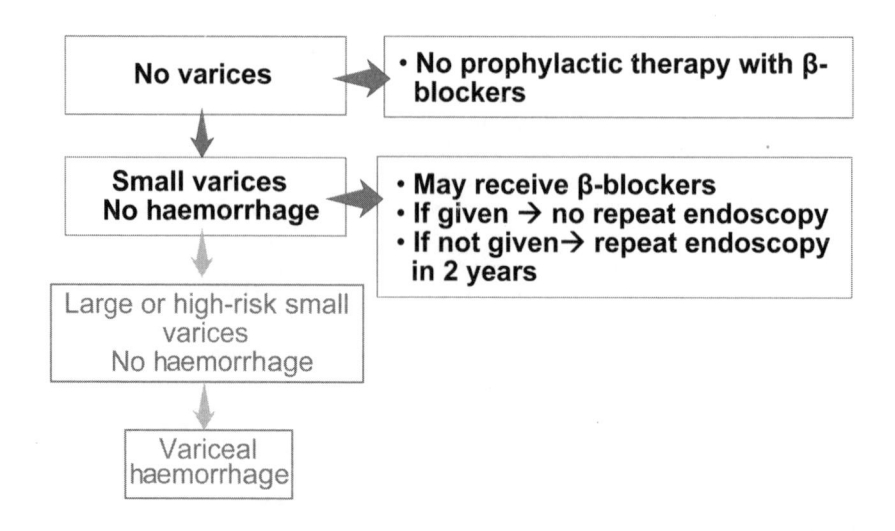

Figure 3 Current recommendations for the pre-primary prophylaxis of portal hypertension

PREVENTION OF GROWTH OF SMALL VARICES

Small varices progress to moderate/large varices and non-selective β-adrenergic blockers may delay their growth. Two randomized controlled trials have investigated the efficacy of non-selective β-adrenergic blockers in preventing the enlargement of small varices, with contradictory results. In one of them[27], that included both patients with no and small varices, development of large varices at 2 years occurred in a larger proportion of patients in the propranolol group (31%) compared to patients in the placebo group (14%); however, differences were no longer significant at 3 years and there were no significant differences in variceal group when the subgroup of patients with small varices was analysed. Notably, over a third of the patients in this study were lost to follow-up and characteristics of those with small varices were not specified (e.g. small vs high-risk small varices). The other study, a large multicentre randomized controlled trial (RCT), showed that patients with small varices with a low risk of haemorrhage (i.e. those occurring in a patient with CTP class B or C, or who had red signs) treated with nadolol had a significantly slower progression to large varices compared to patients on placebo (11% vs 37% at 3 years), with no differences in survival[28]. Additionally, the risk of bleeding was lower in the nadolol group (2% vs 11%) consistent with results of a meta-analysis of three trials of primary prophylaxis (2% vs 9%)[29]. Similar to the study on prevention of varices, a higher percentage of patients on β-blockers had to be withdrawn from the study because of adverse events (11%) compared to patients on placebo (1%).

Based on these results, and on a recent AASLD/EASL consensus conference among experts, current guidelines recommend that patients with small varices who are not at high risk of bleeding can receive β-blockers to prevent variceal growth, although their long-term benefit has not been well established[30]. In those who choose not to take β-blockers, expert consensus panels have determined that surveillance endoscopies should be performed every 2 years, and annually in the setting of decompensation.

CONCLUSION

1. Compensated cirrhotic patients without varices should not receive therapy with non-selective β-adrenergic blockers as they are not effective in preventing the development of varices and are associated with a significant rate of adverse events (Figure 3).

2. Patients with small varices at a low risk of first variceal haemorrhage can receive β-blockers. If β-blockers are given, repeat screening endoscopy is not necessary. If β-blockers are not given, endoscopy should be repeated in 2 years (Figure 3).

3. Although it is unlikely that additional trials using β-blockers in the prevention of varices will be performed, if another trial with a more effective pharmacological therapy is planned, it should include only patients with a baseline HVPG > 10 mmHg.

4. Although it is also unlikely that additional trials using β-blockers in preventing the growth of small (low-risk) varices will be performed, future trials combining endpoints such as an increase in HVPG and clinical decompensation in addition to variceal growth may be more appropriate.

References

1. Lebrec D, De Fleury P, Rueff B, Nahum H, Benhamou JP. Portal hypertension, size of esophageal varices, and risk of gastrointestinal bleeding in alcoholic cirrhosis. Gastroenterology. 1980;79:1139–44.
2. Garcia-Tsao G, Groszmann RJ, Fisher RL, Conn HO, Atterbury CE, Glickman M. Portal pressure, presence of gastroesophageal varices and variceal bleeding. Hepatology. 1985;5:419–24.
3. Bhathal PS, Grossman HJ. Reduction of the increased portal vascular resistance of the isolated perfused cirrhotic rat liver by vasodilators. J Hepatol. 1985;1:325–37.
4. Gupta TK, Chung MK, Toruner M, Groszmann RJ. Endothelial dysfunction in the intrahepatic microcirculation of the cirrhotic rat. Hepatology. 1998;28:926–31.
5. Wiest R, Groszmann RJ. Nitric oxide and portal hypertension: its role in the regulation of intrahepatic and splanchnic vascular resistance. Semin Liver Dis. 2000;19:411–26.
6. Sikuler E, Groszmann RJ. Interaction of flow and resistance in maintenance of portal hypertension in a rat model. Am J Physiol. 1986;250:G205–12.
7. Vorobioff J, Bredfeldt JE, Groszmann RJ. Increased blood flow through the portal system in cirrhotic rats. Gastroenterology. 1984;87:1120–6.
8. Sikuler E, Kravetz D, Groszmann RJ. Evolution of portal hypertension and mechanisms involved in its maintenance in a rat model. Am J Physiol. 1985;248:G618–25.
9. Pagliaro L, D'Amico G, Pasta L et al. Portal hypertension in cirrhosis: natural history. In: Bosch J, Groszmann RJ, editors. Portal Hypertension: Pathophysiology and Treatment. Oxford: Blackwell, 1994:72–92.
10. Navasa M, Pares A, Bruguera M, Caballeria J, Bosch J, Rodes J. Portal hypertension in primary biliary cirrhosis. Relationship with histological features. J Hepatol. 1987;5:292–8.
11. Sanyal AJ, Fontana RJ, DiBisceglie AM et al. The prevalence and risk factors associated with esophageal varices in subjects with hepatitis C and advanced fibrosis. Gastrointest Endosc. 2006;64:855–64.
12. Merli M, Nicolini G, Angeloni S et al. Incidence and natural history of small esophageal varices in cirrhotic patients. J Hepatol. 2003;38:266–72.
13. Groszmann RJ, Garcia-Tsao G, Bosch J et al. Beta-blockers to prevent gastroesophageal varices in patients with cirrhosis. N Engl J Med. 2005;353:2254–61.
14. North Italian Endoscopic Club for the Study and Treatment of Esophageal Varices. Prediction of the first variceal hemorrhage in patients with cirrhosis of the liver and esophageal varices. A prospective multicenter study. N Engl J Med. 1988;319:983–9.
15. El-Serag HB, Everhart JE. Improved survival after variceal hemorrhage over an 11-year period in the Department of Veterans Affairs. Am J Gastroenterol. 2000;95:3566–73.
16. D'Amico G, de Franchis R. Upper digestive bleeding in cirrhosis. Post-therapeutic outcome and prognostic indicators. Hepatology. 2003;38:599–612.
17. Carbonell N, Pauwels A, Serfaty L, Fourdan O, Levy VG, Poupon R. Improved survival after variceal bleeding in patients with cirrhosis over the past two decades. Hepatology. 2004;40:652–9.
18. D'Amico G, Garcia-Tsao G, Pagliaro L. Natural history and prognostic indicators of survival in cirrhosis. A systematic review of 118 studies. J Hepatol. 2006;44:217–31.
19. Kroeger RJ, Groszmann RJ. Effect of selective blockade of beta-2 adrenergic receptors on portal and systemic hemodynamics in a portal hypertensive rat model. Gastroenterology. 1985;88:896–900.
20. D'Amico G, Garcia-Pagan JC, Luca A, Bosch J. HVPG reduction and prevention of variceal bleeding in cirrhosis. A systematic review. Gastroenterology. 2006;131:1624.
21. Bosch J, Garcia-Pagan JC. Prevention of variceal rebleeding. Lancet. 2003;361:952–4.

22. Turnes J, Garcia-Pagan JC, Abraldes JG, Hernandez-Guerra M, Dell'era A, Bosch J. Pharmacological reduction of portal pressure and long-term risk of first variceal bleeding in patients with cirrhosis. Am J Gastroenterol. 2006;101:506–12.
23. Abraldes JG, Tarantino I, Turnes J, Garcia-Pagan JC, Rodes J, Bosch J. Hemodynamic response to pharmacological treatment of portal hypertension and long-term prognosis of cirrhosis. Hepatology. 2003;37:902–8.
24. Sarin SK, Groszmann RJ, Mosca PG et al. Propranolol ameliorates the development of portal-systemic shunting in a chronic murine schistosomiasis model of portal hypertension. J Clin Invest. 1991;87:1032–6.
25. Gao H, Groszmann RJ, Garcia-Tsao G et al. Changes in portal pressure are associated with the development of gastroesophageal varices in compensated cirrhotic patients. Hepatology. 2005;42(Suppl. 1):235A.
26. Ripoll C, Groszmann R, Garcia-Tsao G et al. Hepatic venous pressure gradient predicts clinical decompensation in patients with compensated cirrhosis. Gastroenterology. 2007; 133:481–8.
27. Cales P, Oberti F, Payen JL et al. Lack of effect of propranolol in the prevention of large oesophageal varices in patients with cirrhosis: a randomized trial. French-Speaking Club for the Study of Portal Hypertension. Eur J Gastroenterol Hepatol. 1999;11:741–5.
28. Merkel C, Marin R, Angeli P et al. A placebo-controlled clinical trial of nadolol in the prophylaxis of growth of small esophageal varices in cirrhosis. Gastroenterology. 2004;127: 476–84.
29. D'Amico G, Pagliaro L, Bosch J. Pharmacological treatment of portal hypertension: an evidence-based approach. Semin Liver Dis. 1999;19:475–505.
30. Garcia-Tsao G, Sanyal AJ, Grace ND, Carey W. Prevention and management of gastroesophageal varices and variceal hemorrhage in cirrhosis. Hepatology. 2007;46:922–38 and Am J Gastroenterol. 2007;102:2086–212.

19
When and how to scope in portal hypertension

R. DE FRANCHIS, A. DELL'ERA and M. PRIMIGNANI

INTRODUCTION

Portal hypertension (PH) plays a crucial role in the transition from the preclinical to the clinical phase of cirrhosis. PH is a contributing factor for the development of ascites and hepatic encephalopathy and a direct cause of variceal haemorrhage and of bleeding-related death. The increase of portal pressure leads to the development of a collateral circulation, of which oesophago-gastric varices are the most important feature from a clinical standpoint. Varices tend to increase in size in parallel with the increase in portal pressure, and rupture when variceal wall tension exceeds a critical level. Bleeding from oesophagogastric varices is the most important complication of cirrhosis, marking the progression of decompensation of the disease to a stage with an extremely high risk of death[1]. It should be noted that, despite the advances achieved in recent decades in its treatment, variceal bleeding still carries a mortality of around 20% within 6 weeks of the bleeding episode[2].

Portal pressure can be measured only by invasive methods; the most widely used method is measurement of the hepatic vein pressure gradient (HVPG), which is an indirect but precise measure of portal pressure[3]. The upper limit of normal for the HVPG is 5 mmHg[4]. Any value in excess of this limit marks the existence of portal hypertension.

Portal hypertension is defined as clinically significant (CSPH) when the level of portal pressure is such that the patient is at risk of developing complications: patients with CSPH should undergo treatment to prevent such complications. Several cross-sectional[5-7] and longitudinal[8-14] studies have shown that varices neither develop nor bleed when the HVPG is below the threshold value of 10–12 mmHg. In addition, it has recently been shown that patients with a HVPG < 10 mmHg have a 90% probability of not developing clinical decompensation of cirrhosis[15]. As a consequence the following definition of CSPH has been given at a recent international consensus development workshop on portal hypertension[16]: 'CSPH is defined by the increase of the HVPG above a threshold value of about 10 mmHg. The presence of oesophagogastric varices, of variceal bleeding and/or ascites indicates the presence of CSPH'. Hence, the strategy of identifying and surveying patients with portal hypertension should be mainly focused on patients with CSPH.

WHY TO SCOPE

HVPG measurement is an accurate and reproducible method: when it is done correctly the coefficient of variation of the technique is $2.6\pm2.6\%$[6]. However, at present, HVPG measurement cannot be done routinely; therefore alternative methods must be used.

Complete endoscopic examination of the oesophagus, stomach and duodenum, which is far more widely available than HVPG measurement, is an appropriate method, since the size of varices is clearly related to the risk of bleeding[17]: using this technique a good degree of inter-observer agreement for the assessment of variceal size can be achieved[17,18], together with a good accuracy for the diagnosis of cirrhosis[19]. In addition, endoscopy allows the identification of other potentially bleeding lesions related to portal hypertension, such as portal hypertensive gastropathy and gastric antral vascular ectasia. As a consequence, upper gastrointestinal endoscopy has become the method of choice for the routine evaluation of cirrhotic patients for the detection and surveillance of oesophageal varices.

WHEN TO SCOPE

Identification of patients with varices

Varices eventually develop in all cirrhotic patients[20], and once they have developed, they tend to increase in size and to bleed[21]. The prevalence of varices is higher in decompensated than in compensated cirrhosis[21], and large varices have a higher propensity to bleed than small ones[17,22]. However, at a given point in time a variable proportion of patients will not have varices; the reported prevalence of oesophageal varices is variable[23], ranging in different series between 24% and 80%. Thus, screening all cirrhotic patients with upper gastrointestinal endoscopy to detect the presence of varices implies a number of unnecessary endoscopies, which increase the workload of endoscopy units. Predicting the presence of oesophageal varices by non-invasive means would restrict the performance of endoscopy to those patients with a high probability of having varices. Until recently, scanty data were available on this matter[24,25]; however, in recent years a number of studies[26-37] have addressed the issue of identifying patients with varices by non-invasive, non-endoscopic means, with the aim of avoiding endoscopy in those at low risk of having varices. The majority of these studies have assessed the potential of biochemical, clinical and ultrasound parameters, of blood markers of fibrosis and of transient elastography. However, so far, none of the proposed methods has been shown to be precise enough to allow avoiding endoscopy in selected cases. As a consequence the conclusions of the most recent Baveno Consensus Workshop on Portal Hypertension[38] were that there are no satisfactory non-endoscopic indicators of the presence of varices and, while further studies are awaited, endoscopic screening is still the best practice to detect varices.

By doing so, three different categories of patients are identified: those with no varices, those with small varices (occupying up to a third of the radius of the oesophagus)[18] and those with medium–large varices. The latter must be treated prophylactically to prevent variceal bleeding, while patients in the other two categories should undergo periodic surveillance endoscopy to detect the 'de novo' appearance of varices or the growth of small varices to large, respectively[16].

Development of 'new' oesophageal varices

Knowledge of the rate of development and growth of varices would be important, since it would help in defining the optimal intervals for surveillance endoscopy, with the aim of identifying varices at risk of bleeding before they bleed, in order to start prophylactic treatment. Too-short intervals would unnecessarily increase the workload of endoscopic units, while too-long intervals would increase the risk of bleeding of patients between surveillance endoscopies.

Several studies[20,21,24,39-45] have evaluated the incidence of 'new' oesophageal varices (Table 1). The reported annual incidence varies between 3% and 23%. However, in all studies but one such incidence is in the order of 3–10%. The exception is the study by Calès et al.[40], who, in 41 cirrhotic patients of alcoholic aetiology with a relatively large proportion of Child B and C patients, observed a 1-year incidence of varices of 23%. A possible explanation of this discrepancy is that in the other studies the proportions of alcoholic cirrhosis and of patients with advanced liver disease were much lower than in the Calès study. Concerning the identification of predictors of the 'de novo' appearance of oesophageal varices, the results of the above studies are inconsistent. Interestingly, Groszmann et al.[44] showed that a baseline HVPG value ≥ 10 mmHg was the single most powerful predictor of variceal formation.

Table 1 One-year incidence and progression of oesophageal varices in various studies

Reference	Yearly incidence of varices (%)	Yearly rate of progression of varices (%)
Christensen et al., 1981[20]	8	
D'Amico et al., 1986[39]	7	
Calès et al., 1990[40]	23	31
Pagliaro et al., 1994[24]	8	8
Gentilini et al., 1997[41]	11.7	
Primignani et al., 1998[42]	5	
Calès et al., 1999[45]		30*
Zoli et al., 2000[47]		10
Merli et al., 2003[43]	9	12
Merkel et al., 2004[46]		12
Groszmann et al., 2005[44]	3	

* 2 years.

Progression of varices from small to large

Reported figures on the yearly rate of increase of the size of varices from small to large range between 8% and 31%[24,40,43,45–47], with most values in the order of 10–12%. Again, the Calès et al.[40] study is the exception, with a 31% yearly rate of progression. As far as predictors of variceal progression are concerned, the only factors identified in more than one study are the Child–Pugh class at baseline[40,43], or its worsening during follow-up[43,46]. In patients undergoing yearly surveillance endoscopy to detect the '*de novo*' appearance of varices, the proportion of patients with medium-sized or large varices at first detection ranged between 2.7% and 7%[24,42,43].

Timing of follow-up endoscopies

As far as deciding the timing of follow-up endoscopy is concerned, we must first decide which level of risk (i.e. what proportion of patients bleeding before starting prophylactic treatment) we are willing to accept. If we set this level at 10%, then patients with no varices at baseline can be re-endoscoped at 3-year intervals. The rate of development of large varices and the rate of bleeding in these patients are both below the 10% threshold[24,40,43]. For patients with small varices at baseline the picture is much more complicated, since the reported incidences of bleeding range between 4% at 16 months[46] and 24% at 2 years[40]. Accordingly, the current recommendations[16] are that follow-up endoscopy should be performed at 1–2-year intervals in compensated patients with small varices, adopting the shorter interval for patients with alcoholic cirrhosis[40,43], with more severe impairment of liver function[24,40,43] and with endoscopic risk signs[17,43].

Once large varices have developed there is no need for further follow-up endoscopy, since at this stage the patients should be treated to prevent bleeding.

HOW TO SCOPE

The systematic application of these recommendations generates a considerable burden for endoscopy units. In addition, the adherence of patients to screening programmes may be hampered by the need to repeatedly undergo a procedure that is perceived as unpleasant, requires conscious sedation in most cases, may lead to decreased work productivity, and has a small but not-insignificant risk of complications[48].

The oesophageal videocapsule endoscopy system (PillCam ESO, Given imaging ltd, Yoqneam, Israel) provides a less invasive approach to visualizing the oesophagus. Advantages include the elimination of the need for conscious sedation, the minimally invasive nature of the test, and the ability to pursue normal daily activities following the procedure. Furthermore, capsule endoscopy is likely to be more readily accepted by patients as compared to standard upper gastrointestinal endoscopy (EGD).

Three pilot studies[49–51] carried out with this capsule showed a very good degree of correlation between the capsule and standard EGD in the detection of varices. More recently, a large international multicentre trial has been presented[52], including 288 patients with portal hypertension. Using conventional EGD as the gold standard, capsule endoscopy had a sensitivity of 84% and a specificity of 88% for the detection of varices. The LR ratios were: LR +: 7.0; LR –: 0.18. For the discrimination between medium–large varices and small–no varices, the corresponding figures were: sensitivity 78%, specificity 96%; LR +: 19.5; LR –: 0.2. A questionnaire evaluating pre-test patients' perception and post-test patients satisfaction showed that the capsule was preferred over EGD. These data show that capsule endoscopy is somewhat inferior to conventional EGD in diagnosing the presence and grading the size of varices. However, it appears to be more patient-friendly, and this might increase patients' adherence to screening programmes. For the time being capsule endoscopy appears to be a suitable alternative to EGD for diagnosing and grading oesophageal varices in patients unable or unwilling to undergo conventional endoscopy. Whether capsule endoscopy will ultimately replace conventional endoscopy as the first-line tool to detect and grade varices will depend on the results of appropriately designed cost-effectiveness analyses.

PRACTICE POINTS

- All cirrhotic patients should undergo upper gastrointestinal endoscopy at the time of diagnosis of cirrhosis.

- Patients with compensated disease and without varices at screening endoscopy should undergo surveillance endoscopy at 2–3-year intervals.

- Patients with small varices at screening endoscopy should undergo surveillance endoscopy at 1–2-year intervals; the interval should be 1 year for patients with alcoholic cirrhosis, with more severe impairment of liver function and with endoscopic risk signs.

- At the present time capsule endoscopy can be proposed as an alternative to EGD for patients unable or unwilling to undergo upper gastrointestinal endoscopy.

References

1. D'Amico G, Garcia-Tsao G, Pagliaro L. Natural history and prognostic indicators of survival in cirrhosis: a systematic review of 118 studies. J Hepatol. 2006;1:217–31.
2. D'Amico G, de Franchis R. Upper digestive bleeding in cirrhosis. Post-therapeutic outcome and prognostic indicators. Hepatology. 2003;3:599–612.
3. Groszmann RJ, Wongcharatrawee S. The hepatic venous pressure gradient: anything worth doing should be done right. Hepatology. 2004;39:280–2.
4. Bosch J, Garcia-Pagan JC. Pathophysiology of portal hypertension and its complications. In: Bircher J, Benhamou JP, McIntire N, Rizzetto M, Rodes J, editors. Textbook of Clinical Hepatology. Oxford: Oxford University Press, 1999:653–9.

5. Lebrec D, Fleury P, Rueff B, Nahum M, Benhamou JP. Portal hypertension, size of esophageal varices, and risk of gastrointestinal bleeding in alcoholic cirrhosis. Gastroenterology. 1980;79:1139.
6. Garcia-Tsao G, Groszmann R, Fisher R, Conn HO, Atterbury CE, Glickman M. Portal pressure, presence of gastroesophageal varices and variceal bleeding. Hepatology. 1985;5:419.
7. Viallet A, Marleau MH, Huet M et al. Hemodynamic evaluation of patients with intrahepatic portal hypertension: relationship between bleeding varices and the portohepatic gradient. Gastroenterology. 1975;69:1297.
8. Groszmann R, Bosch J, Grace N et al. Hemodynamic events in a prospective randomized trial of propranolol versus placebo in the prevention of a first variceal hemorrhage. Gastroenterology. 1990; 99:1401.
9. Vorobioff J, Groszmann RJ, Picabea E et al. Prognostic value of hepatic venous pressure gradient measurement in alcoholic cirrhosis. Gastroenterology. 1996;111:701–9.
10. Vinel JP, Cassigneul J, Levade M, Voigt JJ, Pascal JP. Assessment of short-term prognosis after variceal bleeding in patients with alcoholic cirrhosis by early measurement of portohepatic gradient. Hepatology. 1986;6:116–17.
11. Gluud C, Henriksen JH, Nielsen G, and the Copenhagen Study Group for Liver Disease. Prognostic indicators in alcoholic cirrhotic men. Hepatology. 1988;8:222–7.
12. Garcia-Pagan JC, Feu F, Bosch J, Rodes J. Propranolol compared with propranolol plus isosorbide-5-mononitrate for portal hypertension in cirrhosis. A randomized controlled study. Ann Intern Med. 1991;114:869–73.
13. Villanueva C, Balanzo J, Novella MT et al. Nadolol plus isosorbide mononitrate compared with sclerotherapy for the prevention of variceal rebleeding. N Engl J Med. 1996;334:1624–9.
14. Moitinho E, Escorsell A, Bandi JC et al. Prognostic value of early measurements of portal pressure in acute variceal bleeding. Gastroenterology. 1999;117:626–31.
15. Ripoll C, Groszmann RJ, Garcia-Tsao G et al. Hepatic venous pressure gradient (HVPG) predicts clinical decompensation (CD) in patients (pts) with compensated cirrhosis. Gastroenterology. 2007;133:481–8.
16. de Franchis R. Updating consensus in portal hypertension: report of the Baveno III consensus workshop on definitions, methodology and therapeutic strategies in portal hypertension. J Hepatol. 2000;33:846–52.
17. North-Italian Endoscopic Club for the Study and Treatment of Esophageal Varices. Prediction of the first variceal hemorrhage in patients with cirrhosis of the liver and esophageal varices. N Engl J Med. 1988;319:983–9.
18. Italian Liver Cirrhosis Project. Reliability of endoscopy in the assessment of variceal features. J Hepatol. 1987:4:93–8.
19. D'Amico G, Garcia-Tsao G, Calès P et al. Diagnosis of portal hypertension: how and when. In: de Franchis R, editor. Portal Hypertension III: Proceedings of the Third Baveno International Consensus Workshop on Definitions, Methodology and Therapeutic Strategies. Oxford: Blackwell, 2000:36–64.
20. Christensen E, Fauerholdt L, Schlichting P, Juhl E, Poulsen H, Tygstrup N. Aspects of natural history of gastrointestinal bleeding in cirrhosis and the effect of prednisone. Gastroenterology. 1981;81:944–52.
21. D'Amico G, Luca A. Natural history. Clinical–haemodynamic correlations. Prediction of the risk of bleeding. Bailliere's Clin Gastroenterol. 1997;11:243–56.
22. D'Amico G, Pagliaro L, Bosch J. Pharmacologic treatment of portal hypertension: an evidence-based approach. Semin Liver Dis. 1999;19:475–505.
23. Pascal JP, Calès P, Desmorat H. Natural history of esophageal varices. In: Bosch J, Rodès J, editors. Recent Advances in the Pathophysiology and Treatment of Portal Hypertension. Rome: Serono Symposia review no. 22; 1989:127–42.
24. Pagliaro L, D'Amico G, Pasta L et al. Portal hypertension in cirrhosis: natural history. In: Bosch J, Groszmann RJ, editors. Portal Hypertension, Pathophysiology and Treatment. Oxford: Blackwell, 1994:72–92.
25. Cottone M, D'Amico G, Maringhini A et al. Predictive value of ultrasonography in the screening of non-ascitic cirrhotic patients with large varices. J Ultrasound Med. 1986;5:189–92.

26. Ng FH, Wong SY, Loo CK, Lam KM, Lai CW, Cheng CS. Prediction of oesophagogastric varices in patients with liver cirrhosis. J Gastroenterol Hepatol. 1999;14:785–90.
27. Pilette C, Oberti F, Aube C et al. Non-invasive diagnosis of esophageal varices in chronic liver diseases. J Hepatol. 1999;31:867–73.
28. Chalasani N, Imperiale TF, Ismail A et al. Predictors of large esophageal varices in cirrhosis. Am J Gastroenterol. 1999;94:3103–5.
29. Schepis F, Cammà C, Niceforo D et al. Which patients should undergo endoscopic screening for esophageal varices detection? Hepatology. 2001;33:333–8.
30. Zaman A, Becker T, Lapidus J, Benner K Risk factors for the presence of varices in cirrhotic patients without history of variceal hemorrhage. Arch Intern Med. 2001;161:2564–70.
31. Madhotra R, Mulcahy HE, Willner I, Reuben A. Prediction of esophageal varices in patients with cirrhosis. J Clin Gastroenterol. 2002;34:81–5.
32. Thomopoulos KC, Labropoulou-Karatza C, Mimidis KP, Katsakoulis EC, Iconomou G, Nikolopoulou VN. Non-invasive predictors of the presence of large oesophageal varices in patients with cirrhosis. Dig Liver Dis. 2003;35:473–8.
33. Zein CO, Lindor KD, Angulo P. Prevalence and predictors of esophageal varices in patients with primary sclerosing cholangitis. Hepatology. 2004;39:204–10.
34. Giannini E, Botta F, Borro P et al. Platelet count/spleen diameter ratio: proposal and validation of a non-invasive parameter to predict the presence of esophageal varices in patients with liver cirrhosis. Gu. 2003;52:1200–5.
35. Giannini E, Zaman A, Kreil A et al. Platelet count/spleen diameter ratio for the non invasive diagnosis of esophageal varices. Results of a multicenter, prospective, validation study. Am J Gastroenterol. 2006;101:2511–19.
36. Thabut D, Trabut JB, Massard J et al. Non-invasive diagnosis of large oesophageal varices by fibrotest in patents with cirrhosis: a preliminary retrospective study. Liver Int. 2006;26:271–8.
37. Kazemi F, Kettaneh A, N'Kontchou G et al. Liver stiffness measurement selects patients with cirrhosis at risk of bearing large oesophageal varices. J Hepatol. 2006;45:230–5.
38. de Franchis R. Evolving consensus in portal hypertension. Report of the Baveno IV Consensus Workshop on Methodology of Diagnosis and Therapy in Portal Hypertension. J Hepatol. 2005;43:167–76.
39. D'Amico G, Morabito A, Pagliaro L, Marubini E. Survival and prognostic indicators in compensated and decompensated cirrhosis. Dig Dis Sci. 1986;31:468–75.
40. Calès P, Desmorat H, Vinel JP et al. Incidence of large oesophageal varices in patients with cirrhosis: application to prophylaxis of first bleeding. Gut. 1990;31:1298–302.
41. Gentilini P, Laffi G, La Villa G et al. Long course and prognostic factors of virus-induced cirrhosis of the liver. Am J Gastroenterol. 1997;92:66–72.
42. Primignani M, Albè R, Preatoni P et al. 'De novo' development of esophageal varices in patients with a recent histologic diagnosis of liver cirrhosis. Gastroenterology. 1998;114: A1324 (Abstract).
43. Merli M, Nicolini G, Angeloni S et al. Incidence and natural history of small oesophageal varices in cirrhotic patients. J Hepatol. 2003;38:266–72.
44. Groszmann RJ, Garcia-Tsao G, Bosch J et al. Beta-blockers to prevent gastroesophageal varices in patients with cirrhosis. N Engl J Med. 2005;353:2254–61.
45. Calès P, Oberti F, Payen JL et al. Lack of effect of propranolol in the prevention of large esophageal varices in patients with cirrhosis. Eur J Gastroenterol Hepatol. 1999;11:741–5.
46. Merkel C, Marin R, Angeli P et al. A placebo-controlled clinical trial of nadolol in the prophylaxis of growth of small esophageal varices in cirrhosis. Gastroenterology. 2004;2:476–84.
47. Zoli M, Merkel C, Magalotti D et al. Natural history of cirrhotic patients with small esophageal varices: a prospective study. Am J Gastroenterol. 2000;2:503–8.
48. Eisen G, Baron TH, Dominitz J; American Society for Gastrointestinal Endoscopy. Complications of upper GI endoscopy. Gastrointest Endosc. 2002;55:784–93.
49. Eisen G, Eliakim R, Zaman A et al. The accuracy of PillCam ESO capsule endoscopy versus conventional upper endoscopy for the diagnosis of esophageal varices: a prospective three-center pilot study. Endoscopy. 2006;38:31–5.

50. Lapalus MG, Dumortier J, Fumex F et al. Esophageal capsule endoscopy versus esophagogastroduodenoscopy for evaluating portal hypertension: a prospective comparative study of performance and tolerance. Endoscopy. 2006:38:36–41.
51. Groce JR, Raju GS, Sood GK, Snyder N. A prospective blinded comparative trial of capsule esophagoscopy vs. traditional EGD for variceal screening. Gastroenterology. 2007;132(Suppl. 2):A802.
52. de Franchis R, Eisen GM, Eliakim R et al. Esophageal capsule endoscopy (PillCam ESO) is comparable to traditional endoscopy for detection of esophageal varices – an international multicenter study. Endoscopy. 2007;65 (DDW abstract issue): AB107.

20
Prevention of first variceal bleeding

P. CALÈS, N. DIB and F. OBERTI

INTRODUCTION

Our team has had the privilege to conduct the first randomized studies in primary[1], and pre-primary prevention, which is a clinical setting closely related[2] to variceal bleeding due to portal hypertension. Over a period of 20 years several studies and consensus statements or guidelines have been published. Nevertheless, several recent surveys have shown that these guidelines were not applied in a substantial proportion of patients, or that practical conditions, such as the dose regimen of β-adrenergic blockers (BB) were poorly known. This chapter presents recent data as well as practical conditions in the light of recent guidelines. Special attention has been paid to failures of therapy.

NATURAL HISTORY OF PORTAL HYPERTENSION

Four clinical stages of increasing severity are identified: stage 1: no ascites, no varices; stage 2: varices, no ascites; stage 3: ascites ± varices; stage 4: bleeding ± ascites[3,4].

Oesophageal varices are present in about 55% of patients at initial diagnosis of cirrhosis[3]. During monitoring the expected incidence of new varices is about 5% per year[3] and the growth of varices occurs with a rate ranging from 5% to 12% per year [3]. Severity of liver dysfunction, assessed by Child–Pugh score – a reflection of liver severity – seems to be a predictor of variceal enlargement[5,6]. Variceal bleeding occurs in about 7% at 2 years in patients with small varices at the date of diagnosis and 30% at 2 years in those with medium or large varices[7]. The main predictive factors related to the risk of variceal bleeding are variceal size, presence of red wale marks on the varices and Child–Pugh score[8]. The current mortality rate of variceal bleeding is about 20% at 6 weeks (vs 50% in the 1970s) despite advances in treatment[4,9,10]; and 5–8% of patients die within 48 h from uncontrolled bleeding[7,11].

PREVENTION OF FIRST VARICEAL BLEEDING

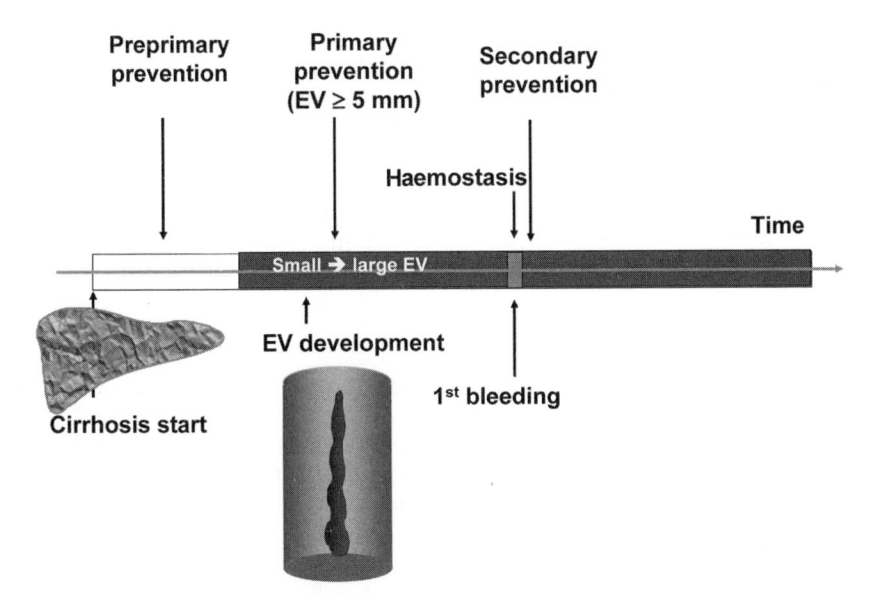

Figure 1 Prophylaxis of variceal bleeding. Prophylaxis of variceal bleeding consists of: (1) preprimary prophylaxis, i.e. prevention of the development of varices; (2) primary prophylaxis or the prevention of a first variceal bleeding episode; (3) secondary prophylaxis or the prevention of rebleeding (EV = oesophageal varices)

The prevention of variceal bleeding is mainly divided into the prevention of first bleeding and rebleeding (Figure 1): primary prevention is the prevention of first bleeding in patients with large varices; secondary prevention is the prevention of rebleeding.

METHODS

Pharmacological therapy

β-Adrenergic blockers

BB reduce portal pressure by reducing portal blood flow as a consequence of a decrease in cardiac output (β_1 receptor blockade) and arteriolar splanchnic vasoconstriction by an unopposed α-vasoconstrictive effect (β_2 receptor blockade)[12]. Non-selective BB such as propranolol, nadolol and timolol are more effective in reducing hepatic venous pressure gradient (HVPG) than selective β_1-adrenergic blockers[13,14]. The median reduction of HVPG by non-selective β-adrenergic blockers is approximately 15%[13,15–18]. Propranolol also prevents the increase in portal pressure related to physical exercise in patients with cirrhosis[19]. Non-selective BB induce a reduction in variceal pressure[20] and in azygos blood flow[21–23] even in patients who do not exhibit a marked decrease in HVPG (propranolol non-responders)[22,24]. Furthermore, propranolol reduces postprandial peak in portal pressure, but this effect is debatable[25], and decreases the rates of bacterial translocation[26]. Carvedilol is a non-selective vasodilating BB with weak α_1-receptor antagonism[27]. Carvedilol has a greater portal hypotensive effect than propranolol in patients with cirrhosis[28]; however, its clinical applicability may be limited by its systemic hypotensive effects[28]. A recent randomized trial has shown that carvedilol was responsible for the first study to demonstrate lower bleeding rates with BB therapy for primary prophylaxis compared with endoscopic band ligation (EBL)[29].

Nitrates

The mechanism of nitrates' vasodilatory effects, i.e. vascular tone reduction and decreased intrahepatic resistance, is not completely established. The mechanism probably involves nitric oxide release. Isosorbide mononitrate is the only nitrate that has been tested in randomized trials. Its use reduces HVPG[30] and enhances the splanchnic haemodynamic effect of propranolol[31]; however, its systemic effects can lead to deleterious arterial hypotension.

Endoscopy: screening and treatment

At present there is no satisfactory non-endoscopic indicator to detect the presence of oesophageal varices[4,32], but this research area is very active. Endoscopic screening is the best technique to detect varices[32,33]. Endoscopy is also useful in treating bleeding oesophagogastric varices. Three endoscopic techniques are currently used: EBL, endoscopic sclerotherapy (ES) and variceal obturation using glue.

Endoscopic sclerotherapy

Several sclerosant agents can be used (polidocanol, ethanolamine, ethanol, tetradecylsulphate and sodium morrhuate) with similar results. ES consists of intravariceal or paravariceal injections of the sclerosant, injecting a total volume of 10–30 ml per treatment session. ES is performed at 1–3-week intervals until the varices have been eradicated[34]. Given that the recurrence of varices ranges between 50% and 70%[35] surveillance endoscopy every 3–6 months is required[35,36]. Frequent complications of ES are retrosternal pain, dysphagia or postsclerotherapy bleeding ulcers. More severe complications such as oesophageal perforation or stricture are reported[34].

Endoscopic band ligation

At the present time EBL is the first-choice endoscopic treatment for oesophageal varices. EBL consists of placing an elastic band on a varix, allowing its aspiration in a cylinder attached to an endoscope. A maximum of five to eight elastic bands should be used per session (multiband). During eradication treatment, EBL sessions should be performed every 2–3 weeks until variceal obliteration or until varices have become so small that ligation is impossible[37]. Complications of EBL are fewer than those with ES. Generally, bleeding from post-ligation ulcer is moderate[34]. A recent meta-analysis has shown that EBL was superior to BB in preventing the first variceal bleed, with fewer adverse events resulting in treatment discontinuation. Careful attention to technique and patient selection are important to minimize iatrogenic complications with EBL[38]. If only cost per life year is considered, then EBL is not cost-effective compared to BB therapy; however, if quality of life is considered, then EBL is cost-effective[39].

Variceal obturation with glue

This treatment is especially useful for gastric variceal bleeding and has never been tested in primary prevention. It consists of the embolization of a varix by locally injecting tissue glue (n-butyl-2-cyanoacrylate), which polymerizes in contact with blood. One millilitre of tissue glue is injected at a time with a maximum of three injections per treatment session. The most serious risk associated with this procedure is embolization of the lung, spleen, or brain[40].

Transjugular intrahepatic portosystemic shunt (TIPS)

This has not been evaluated in primary prevention.

INDICATIONS (Table 1)

Endoscopic screening for the presence of oesophageal varices should be done in all patients at the diagnosis of cirrhosis[4,37]. Endoscopic follow-up should then relate to the initial oesophageal varix size (Figure 2). Endoscopy should be repeated every 3 years in patients without varices and every 2 years in those with small varices[37] (Figure 2). In case of large varices, primary prophylaxis by non-selective BB (propranolol, nadolol) should be begun and endoscopic

Table 1 Recommendations for primary prophylaxis of variceal bleeding based on the Baveno[4] and the French[37] consensus on portal hypertension

- All patients with cirrhosis should be screened by endoscopy for the presence of varices (at diagnosis with follow-up adapted according to the initial size of varices and to the degree of liver failure)[4,37].

- Patients with medium-sized or large varices should be treated with non-selective β-adrenergic blockers initially[37]. Treatment should be continued indefinitely[37].

- Patients with medium-sized or large varices with contraindications or intolerance to β-adrenergic blockers should benefit from endoscopic band ligation of varices[4,37].

- In case of small varices, patients with red signs or of Child–Pugh C class may benefit from non-selective β-adrenergic blockers[4].

- Usual dose is 80–160 mg/day for propranolol and 80 mg/day for nadolol[37].

- Doses of non-selective β-adrenergic blockers should be adjusted to obtain a 20–25% reduction in heart rate or a heart rate of less than 55 beats/min[37].

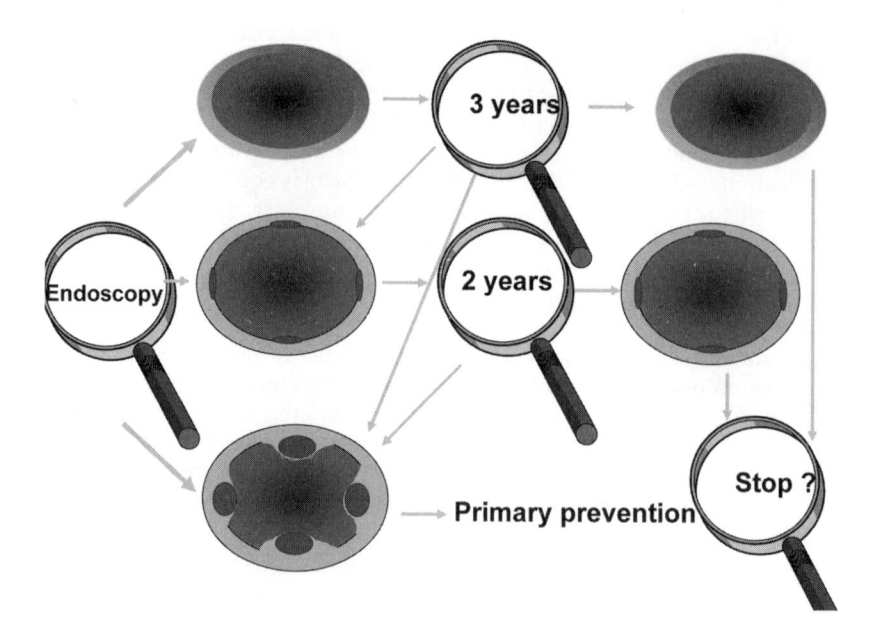

Figure 2 Endoscopic screening for the presence of oesophageal varices with respect to primary prevention. The stop rule was suggested in the French consensus when oesophageal varices stage was unchanged in non-progressive cirrhosis

follow-up is not necessary[37]. EBL is also useful in preventing variceal bleeding in patients with medium or large oesophageal varices; however, the long-term benefit of EBL requires further research[4] and is currently proposed in primary prophylaxis when there are contraindications to, or side-effects of, non-selective BB.

Non-selective BB are effective in reducing the risk of first bleeding from oesophageal varices in patients with medium or large varices[1,4,41–44]. The chronic administration consists of a singly daily oral intake of long-acting propranolol at a dose of 80 or 160 mg, whatever the available dosage is in the relevant country[45,46]. Propranolol is effective for a few days in cirrhotic patients[47]. Another empirical approach consists of b.i.d. administration and a titration of the oral dose according to patient tolerance and treatment objectives[48,49]. In all cases, doses should be adjusted to obtain a 20–25% reduction in heart rate or a heart rate of less than 55 beats/min[37]. β-Blockade therapy is maintained indefinitely[37] as late withdrawal can be deleterious on survival despite the lack of an increased bleeding risk[50]. In patients with intolerance or contraindications to BB, EBL is recommended[4,37] (Figure 3). Nitrates (isosorbide mononitrate) are ineffective in preventing variceal bleeding if used alone[51,52], and their use in primary prophylaxis is not recommended[4,37]. No combination of drugs or drug + EBL has been shown to be effective in primary prevention.

PREVENTION OF FIRST VARICEAL BLEEDING

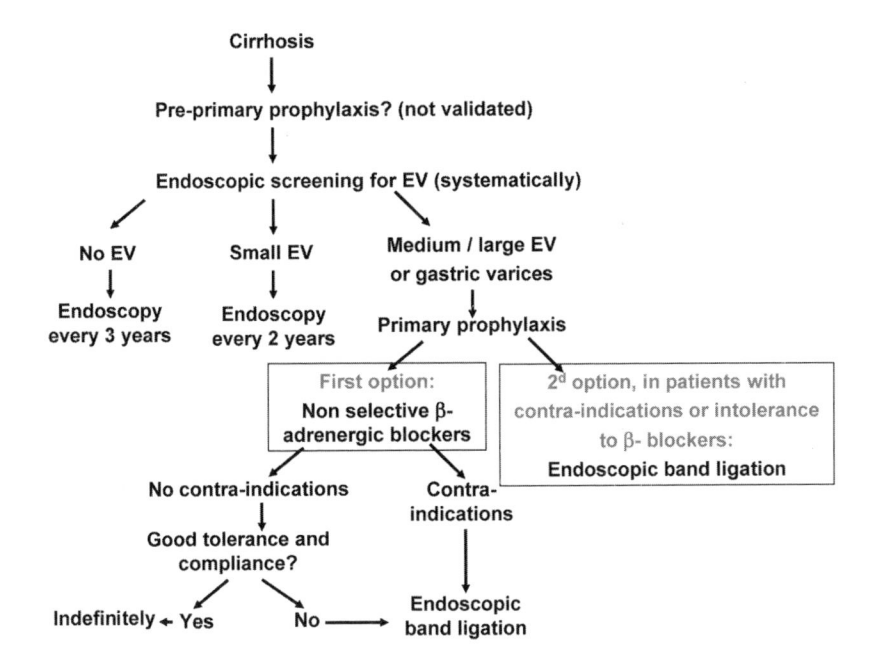

Figure 3 Algorithm of primary prophylaxis of variceal bleeding in cirrhosis. According to the French and Baveno consensus, and 2007 AASLD guidelines (EV = oesophageal varices)

GUIDELINES

Three consensus conferences were recently published on portal hypertension[4,37,53] with a special ensuing report in paediatrics[54], as well the AASLD guidelines[55,56]. As with other practice guidelines, these guidelines are not intended to replace clinical judgement but rather to provide general guidelines applicable to the majority of patients. They are intended to be flexible, in contrast to standards of care, which are inflexible policies designed to be followed in every case. They are summarized in Tables 1 and 2.

WHAT TO DO WHEN STANDARD THERAPY FAILS?

With improved prognosis of variceal bleeding and cirrhosis therapeutic failures in variceal bleeding are more frequent. Thus, the failure of prevention occurs in around 50% of cases both in primary and secondary preventions. Therapeutic failures in variceal bleeding have not been clearly evaluated in trials; thus most of the proposals are provided here through expert opinions. Medicine and clinical practice have a common approach to clinical problems: the use of decision analysis. In both settings the main criteria are: efficacy, cost-effectiveness analysis and quality of life. The study of portal hypertension has

Table 2 Recommendations of 2007 AASLD practice guidelines on prevention and management of gastroesophageal varices and variceal hemorrhage in cirrhosis[55,56]

Diagnosis of varices and variceal haemorrhage

1. Screening esophagogastroduodenoscopy (EGD) for the diagnosis of oesophageal and gastric varices is recommended when the diagnosis of cirrhosis is made.

2. On EGD, oesophageal varices should be graded as small or large (>5 mm) with the latter classification encompassing medium-sized varices when three grades are used (small, medium, large). The presence or absence of red signs (red wale marks or red spots) on varices should be noted.

Management recommendations

A. Patients with cirrhosis and no varices

3. In patients with cirrhosis who do not have varices, non-selective β-blockers cannot be recommended to prevent their development.

4. In patients who have compensated cirrhosis and no varices on the initial EGD, it should be repeated in 3 years. If there is evidence of hepatic decompensation, EGD should be done at that time and repeated annually.

B. Patients with cirrhosis and small varices that have not bled

5. In patients with cirrhosis and small varices that have not bled but have criteria for increased risk of haemorrhage (Child B/C or presence of red wale marks on varices), non-selective β-blockers should be used for the prevention of first variceal haemorrhage.

6. In patients with cirrhosis and small varices that have not bled and have no criteria for increased risk of bleeding, β-blockers can be used, although their long-term benefit has not been established.

7. In patients with small varices that have not bled and who are not receiving β-blockers, EGD should be repeated in 2 years. If there is evidence of hepatic decompensation, EGD should be done at that time and repeated annually. In patients with small varices who receive? b-blockers, a follow-up EGD is not necessary.

C. Patients with cirrhosis and medium/large varices that have not bled

8. In patients with medium/large varices that have not bled but have a high risk of haemorrhage (Child B/C or variceal red wale markings on endoscopy), non-selective β-blockers (propranolol or nadolol) or EBL may be recommended for the prevention of first variceal haemorrhage.

9. In patients with medium/large varices that have not bled and are not at the highest risk of haemorrhage (Child A patients and no red signs), non-selective β-blockers (propranolol, nadolol) are preferred and EBL should be considered in patients with contraindications or intolerance or non-compliance to β-blockers.

10. If a patient is placed on a non-selective β-blocker, it should be adjusted to the maximal tolerated dose; follow-up surveillance EGD is unnecessary. If a patient is treated with EBL, it should be repeated every 1–2 weeks until obliteration with the first surveillance EGD performed 1–3 months after obliteration and then every 6–12 months to check for variceal recurrence.

11. Nitrates (either alone or in combination with β-blockers), shunt therapy, or sclerotherapy should not be used in the primary prophylaxis of variceal haemorrhage.

investigated therapeutic efficacy in numerous clinical trials. Cost-effectiveness is an emerging issue that analyses the conclusions of clinical trails from another point of view.

This chapter investigates only the treatment of oesophageal varices with special attention to decision analyses. It should always be remembered that, when failure occurs in a patient with advanced liver disease, liver transplantation is always an option to be considered. In order to have a coherent presentation, all types of prevention are described here.

How to prevent different types of variceal bleeding?

First, to describe the types of prevention, we have to distinguish the prevention of variceal development and that of variceal bleeding. The prevention of variceal development can be divided into:

1. The prevention of occurrence, which is called pre-prevention: this concerns mainly the first occurrence which is called *pre-primary prevention*. Pre-primary prevention is thus the prevention of the occurrence of large varices, i.e. varices with a risk of rupture.

2. The prevention of recurrence that might be called *post-prevention*: this post-prevention can concern both primary and secondary preventions.

The prevention of variceal bleeding is mainly divided into the prevention of first bleeding, *primary prevention*, and rebleeding, *secondary prevention*. However, certain events are not included in these definitions: in particular the prevention of the first and second rebleeding must be distinguished since the respective therapeutic options are different. This could be called *secondary* and *tertiary prevention*, respectively.

Other events include: the prevention of recurrence of oesophageal varices (e.g. after endoscopic eradication) that could be called post-prevention, i.e. post-primary prevention or post-secondary prevention.

What is the standard treatment?

When discussing treatment, three points must be considered:

1. Whether a patient has been previously treated for the prevention of portal hypertension: *naive* patient or not?

2. *Intention* rank: the first-intention treatment is proposed first, and the second-intention treatment is proposed if there is a contraindication or refusal of the first-intention treatment.

3. *Line* rank: the first-line treatment is the first treatment that the patient undergoes. A second-line treatment can be administered after a first-line treatment without clinical failure if the first-line treatment is stopped for withdrawal due to side-effect, non-compliance or non-response. Two examples are presented in Figures 4 and 5. In this section we will discuss only the first-line treatment in naive patients.

Naive patient: no previous tt

β-blocker (BB) ? → Contraindication → Ligation (EBL)

1st intention tt   2nd intention tt

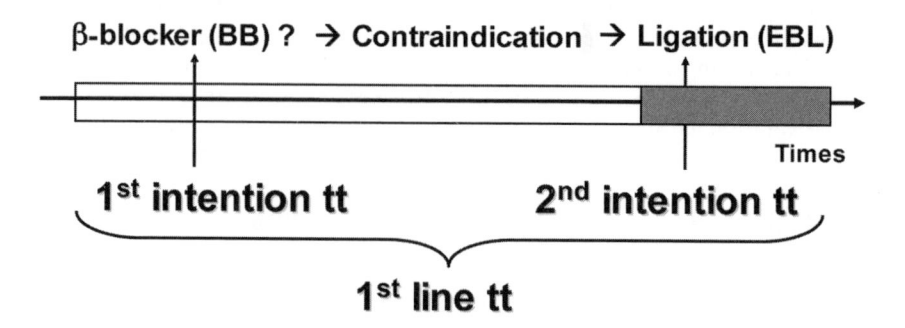

1st line tt

Figure 4 Definition of standard treatment (tt): example 1

Naive patient: no previous tt

β-blocker (BB)   → Side-effect   → Ligation

1st line tt   2nd line tt

Primary prevention

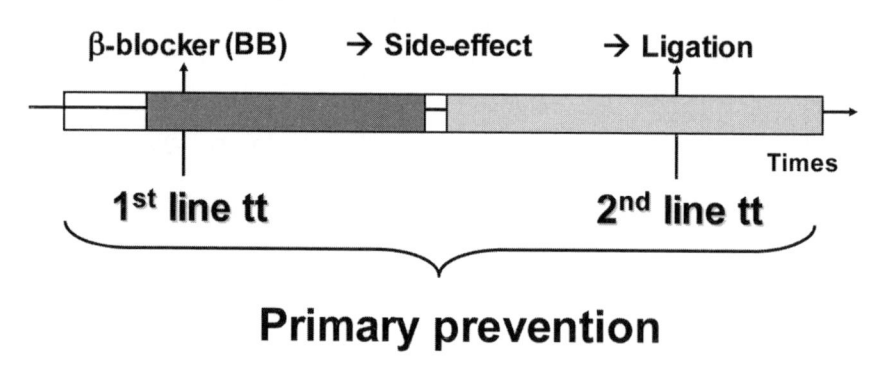

Figure 5 Definition of standard treatment (tt): example 2

The recommendations were agreed upon in the consensus meetings of Paris[37] and Baveno[4] that were recently updated in the 2007 AASLD guidelines[55].

In pre-primary prevention no demonstration of effective treatment has been confirmed. Indeed, the results of randomized controlled trials (RCT) with BB are contradictory.

In primary prevention the first-intention treatment is BB in all conferences. In patients with contraindications, intolerance or non-compliance to BB, EBL in these patients is a second-intention (or line) treatment.

In secondary prevention the first-intention treatment is either BB or EBL[37,57]. In tertiary prevention the first-intention treatment is mainly TIPS[37,57].

What is a therapeutic failure?

Therapeutic failure is based on two events:

1. A *clinical failure* when bleeding occurs after treatment has begun. The definition of bleeding must be precise. Usually this refers to significant bleeding requiring transfusion of at least two blood units (packed red cells). The definition of clinical failure has to be more precise: a significant therapeutic failure is defined by a bleeding that leads to change of treatment by introducing a new therapeutic method, that is a conversion or combination. In clinical practice the decision has also to take into account: (a) the severity, the number, and the cause of bleeding; (b) the severity of liver and associated diseases; (c) regarding treatment, we have to consider its duration, especially for endoscopic treatment and the predictors of failure such as severe dysfunction. The main clinical failure is a bleeding under treatment. The two main preventions where we are faced with a clinical failure are: secondary prevention in non-naive patients and tertiary prevention. The occurrence of large oesophageal varices in pre-primary prevention can also be a clinical failure.

2. A *non-response*: the physiopathological target of treatment is not reached. The definition of a non-response depends on the treatment used. The response to pharmacological treatment in prevention of variceal bleeding is (arbitrarily) defined in relation to baseline haemodynamic characteristics: a decrease in portal pressure $<20\%$ or to below the absolute value of 12 mmHg. With that definition the bleeding rate at 3 years is $<10\%$ in responders and $>50\%$ in non-responders. It has recently been suggested that the objective could be a decrease of $\geqslant 10\%$ in primary prevention[58]. The definition of response to endoscopic treatment is the eradication of oesophageal varices that depends on the endoscopic method used: disappearance of oesophageal varices after sclerotherapy or non-treatable oesophageal varices with EBL.

Prevention of failure

Before describing the therapeutic options (second-line treatment) of failure to a first-line treatment, we must discuss and attempt to prevent failure, for several reasons:

1. Variceal bleeding remains a life-threatening event with a death rate of around 15% at 42 days with recent treatments[59]. However, this figure should be interpreted with caution since this is an in-hospital mortality. The true death rate of variceal bleeding is not well known, as recent data suggest that patients might die at home[60].

2. Variceal bleeding can lead to other complications of portal hypertension and requires costly hospitalization.

3. In real conditions this failure will result in treatment conversion, whereas the first-line treatment is sometimes administered under bad or unadapted conditions.

The prevention of therapeutic failure is based on several approaches:

Prevention of non-use

This might seem trivial but it is striking that, in a US study, half of the patients on the waiting list for liver transplantation had not been screened for primary prevention[61]. Thus, physicians must be educated to apply guidelines in real life. A checklist should be used for the follow-up of cirrhotic patients.

Prediction of therapeutic failure

As mentioned earlier, we must distinguish predictors of clinical failure and those of non-response. Understanding these predictors helps the practitioner to choose methods that are the most adapted for a patient, e.g. a cirrhotic patient with large oesophageal varices and red signs with hepatocellular carcinoma being treated by chemoembolization should be offered EBL rather than BB for primary prevention.

Response measurement

This mainly concerns pharmacodynamic treatments whose response is evaluated by measurement of portal pressure. However, the applicability of portal pressure measurement is questionable and the efficacy of 'à-la-carte' treatment has to be confirmed[45]. Moreover, non-invasive means must be developed.

Treatment optimization

The indications of treatment are partially known in clinical practice and the modalities of these treatments are not well known. For example, BB are very popular; however, there are several limitations to their use. The clinical target is normally a reduction of heart rate of 25% but in RCT this mean is 22%. It has been suggested that the dose should be fractionated, and that the bedtime dose is important[62]; however, this contradicts the pharmacodynamics of BB in cirrhosis[47]. We recommend prescribing a single daily dose of 160 mg long-acting propranolol[47].

Prevention of side bleeding

This means proceeding with caution in endoscopic treatment since it can induce bleeding ulcers or aggravate associated gastric varices.

Other characteristics

These include the applicability of treatment to local conditions and to the individual patient, the therapeutic education, and compliance management (measurement, optimization).

What to do?

Principles

We have several options: we can optimize the administration of BB by underlying the need for a strict compliance to intake, and we recommend prescribing a single daily dose of 160 mg long-acting propranolol provided there is no suspicion of side-effect occurrence. We can optimize the technique of endoscopy, e.g. by increasing the number of bands or adding sclerotherapy at the end of eradication to prevent recurrence (see below). An important principle is the *conversion* or *combination* principle. Usually this means a conversion or a combination of BB to EBL.

What is the factual basis for conversion and combination?

Regarding conversion there is only one trial in which a true second-line treatment has been evaluated, but it was a non-randomized trial and the number of patients was low: a clinical failure to EBL was observed in 88% of patients who were previously non-responders to drug[45]. Importantly, this could mean that the non-responders are the same patients in both these first- and second-line treatments that are BB and EBL. This setting is called a *selective* treatment in opposition to a *universal* treatment that is given without screening.

Concerning drugs, combinations were tested only as first-line treatment or universal treatment. It appears that combination of drugs does not provide any advantage in both preventions with the actual data. Note that advantage here means a decrease in bleeding incidence. Regarding the combination of drugs or drug + EBL: preliminary data suggest equivalence in primary prevention whereas there might be an advantage of pharmaco-endoscopic treatment in secondary prevention.

In the setting of combination of endoscopic techniques there are many data in first-line treatment. The meta-analyses indicate that the simultaneous combination of banding and sclerotherapy provides no advantage, and even induces more side-effects compared to EBL. However, several small RCT show that adding another endoscopic treatment such as sclerotherapy or argon plasma coagulation (APC) at the end of a banding programme is able to significantly prevent the recurrence of oesophageal varices.

In summary, we can state that data are insufficient in primary prevention. Whereas the combination could be effective in secondary prevention where (a) the interest of drug combination has to be confirmed; (b) the combination EBL + BB could be effective. Finally, the prevention of the recurrence of oesophageal varices at the end of EBL by another endoscopic technique seems promising.

When a non-response occurs

Pre-primary prevention

Even if preprimary prevention was recommended in certain patients with small oesophageal varices, there seems to be no need to monitor response (e.g. haemodynamics) in pre-primary prevention since the clinical failure is a non-morbid event.

Primary prevention

We consider the case of patients naive to BB. The opposite case has been discussed in the previous paragraph.

The Baveno conference stated that 'it is not mandatory to check the HVPG response'[57]. One RCT suggested that 'à-la-carte' treatment by adding nitrates could be effective[45], but this should be confirmed. Moreover, the cost-effectiveness of the measurement of haemodynamic response is controversial[63,64]. Theoretically, a non-response to BB in primary prevention could lead to a combination (drugs such as nitrates or EBL) or to a conversion to EBL. However, these combinations have mainly been tested as first-line treatment: the combination of BB with nitrates was generally ineffective in RCT and the combination of EBL with BB has not been tested vs BB alone[65]. The conversion to EBL has been evaluated in one RCT with null results[66]. Theoretically, a non-response to EBL (which is a rare event) cannot lead to a conversion or addition to BB since they are contraindicated when EBL is indicated. It should be noted that a preliminary RCT suggested that the combination of EBL + BB was better than EBL in terms of variceal bleeding. Other pharmacological treatments have not been tested.

Secondary prevention

Theoretically, a non-response to BB in secondary prevention could lead to a combination (drugs such as nitrates or EBL) or to a conversion to EBL. However, these combinations have mainly been tested as first-line treatment: the results of RCT on the combination of BB with nitrates were heterogeneous and the combination of EBL with BB has not been tested vs BB alone. The conversion to EBL has not been evaluated. Theoretically, a non-response to EBL (which is a rare event) can lead to a conversion or addition to BB. In summary, the conversion has not been tested and the combination has only been evaluated as first-line treatment.

When a clinical failure occurs

Pre-primary prevention

There is no recommended treatment at present; however, this must be discussed since BB might be used under certain circumstances such as inpatients with small oesophageal varices and viral cirrhosis[67]. Finally, the recent AASLD guidelines have brought about a split in pre-primary prevention[55] by suggesting treating patients with small oesophageal varices with criteria for increased risk of haemorrhage (Child B/C or presence of red wale marks on varices). Moreover, BB can be used for indications other than portal hypertension.

Unlike in primary prevention, patients being treated for pre-primary prevention might need follow-up endoscopy to detect the occurrence of large oesophageal varices. Indeed, this event is a clinical failure although non-morbid. This could be an argument for a therapeutic conversion; however, it should be noted that a non-response to BB during pre-primary prevention does not necessarily imply the same in primary prevention. Thus, in our RCT of pre-primary prevention, patients with the occurrence of large oesophageal varices subsequently treated by BB for primary prevention had no variceal bleeding when they had been previously treated by BB, unlike those treated by placebo in pre-primary prevention[2]. Finally, the need for endoscopic follow-up in pre-primary prevention is open to discussion.

Primary prevention

If there is treatment failure in a patient who survives and is not treated with TIPS for variceal bleeding, secondary prevention must be started. In naive patients this secondary prevention is the standard treatment (see above). The recent French conference has specifically addressed these issues in non-naive patients according to two situations:

1. Primary prevention with BB: this can be subdivided according to optimization of BB: (a) BB treatment was not optimal (low dose): EBL or BB (at appropriate doses) can be proposed as in naive patients. BB can also be proposed in poorly compliant patients since the level of compliance cannot be determined from the previous step; moreover, the level of compliance increases in relation to the degree of morbidity. (b) BB treatment was optimal: EBL is offered. It should be noted that one RCT on the combination of EBL + BB vs EBL showed no advantage of combination. However, this cannot support the discontinuation of BB in case of conversion to EBL since this specific setting has not been evaluated.

2. Primary prevention with EBL. As EBL was used in patients without indication of BB, a TIPS is the first option. If TIPS is not possible the second option is to try to optimize endoscopic treatment. We would add that a non-clinically significant bleeding attributable to EBL should not be considered as a EBL failure.

Secondary prevention

This can be called tertiary prevention. This concerns patients failing first-line therapy of secondary prevention. Consensus conferences recommend TIPS in that setting[37,57]. In addition, the Baveno conference offers the possibility of surgical shunt in low-risk patients[57].

Table 3 Summary of therapeutic options for treatment failures in the prevention of variceal bleeding. Each grey cell is the treatment proposal in case of treatment failure to the previous step (located on the grey cell on the left hand). Thus for example (4th line of grey cells), if BB failed in primary prevention due to a non optimal dosage (e.g. 40 mg/d), the patient might again receive BB but with an optimal dosage (e.g. 160 mg/d, footnote #3). If BB failed again in the same patient, then a TIPS could be proposed (consensus) or EBL (author's opinion). Tertiary prevention has been divided into the consensus opinion and the author's opinion

	Prevention		
Primary	Secondary	Tertiary	
		Consensus	Authors
Naïve patients:			
-	BB	TIPS[1]	Conversion or combination[2]
-	EBL		
Non-naïve patients:			
BB	EBL	TIPS	TIPS
	BB[3]		EBL
EBL	TIPS[4]	?	Revision or combination

BB: beta-blockers, EBL: endoscopic band ligation, TIPS: transjugular porto-systemic shunt

---
[1] Or surgical shunt in low risk patients (Baveno conference)
[2] Conversion or combination to the other previous option (BB or EBL)
[3] if BB were not optimal in primary prevention
[4] French consensus conference

However, we think that tertiary prevention has been only partially addressed in previous consensus conferences. When secondary prevention fails in a previously naive patient, TIPS as a second-line treatment seems to us a somewhat rapid option, especially when TIPS is poorly available (i.e. in most countries) or when TIPS was already used in secondary prevention in a patient failing primary prevention with EBL. So the combination or conversion concept (CCC) could be applied, and other first-line treatment could be proposed as an alternative or a combination, e.g. a patient failing BB could receive EBL or EBL + BB. In non-naive patients with non-optimal BB, BB can be an option as previously depicted. A BB failure in secondary prevention could also lead to the CCC principle as an alternative to TIPS.

Finally, the case of TIPS failure has not been addressed in consensus conferences. This can be treated by stent revision or combined therapy (BB or EBL).

Synthesis

We can summarize the therapeutic options here. In case of treatment failure for primary prevention naive patients, that is without previous prevention, will be offered standard treatment of secondary prevention either BB or EBL. In non-naive patients that is true therapeutic failure; those previously treated by BB will be proposed for EBL or sometimes optimized BB if BB was not optimal. In those previously treated by EBL a significant failure indicates TIPS. In secondary prevention TIPS is the main option but several alternatives are available.

In recent years the management of treatment failure for the prevention of variceal bleeding has improved. Management steps are summarized in Table 3; however, most of these recommendations rely on expert opinion. Although additional RCT, for example studies testing treatment combinations, could help confirm these recommendations, this may not be possible, because a certain number of these RCT will be difficult to perform. The principles of recommendations are based on the combination or conversion concept. The usual chronological order of conversion is: BB→EBL→TIPS. The main possible combination is BB + EBL.

CONCLUSIONS

Primary prevention is an important step in patient care of cirrhosis. It relies on an early and active diagnosis of cirrhosis which is now facilitated by non-invasive tests[68], then an endoscopic screening since the non-invasive diagnosis of oesophageal varices is not sufficiently effective nowadays[69]. In cases of large oesophageal varices, the first-line option is BB and the second-line, if side-effects or poor compliance are thereafter detected, or second intention first-line option, whether contraindication is already present, is EBL. Combination of drugs or BB + EBL is not recommended as first-line option in primary prevention. New drugs, such as carvedilol, seem promising. Therapeutic failures without event are managed according to the principle of conversion, although debated as second-line or second-intention option[66], whereas combination has never been evaluated as second-line option in primary prevention. The results of RCT cannot easily be extrapolated to clinical therapeutic failure since we have clearly to distinguish naive and non-naive patients; indeed the non-responders to a first-line treatment, such as BB, could be also non-responders to a second-line treatment, such as EBL. Therefore, specific RCT should be conducted in non-naive patients.

References

1. Pascal JP, Cales P. Propranolol in the prevention of first upper gastrointestinal tract hemorrhage in patients with cirrhosis of the liver and esophageal varices. N Engl J Med. 1987;317:856–61.
2. Cales P, Oberti F, Payen JL et al. Lack of effect of propranolol in the prevention of large oesophageal varices in patients with cirrhosis: a randomized trial. French-Speaking Club for the Study of Portal Hypertension. Eur J Gastroenterol Hepatol. 1999;11:741–5.
3. D'Amico G. Esophageal varices: from appearance to rupture; natural history and prognostic indicators. In: Grozmann RJ, Bosh J, editors. Portal Hypertension in the 21st Century. Dordrecht: Kluwer; 2004:147–54.
4. de Franchis R. Evolving consensus in portal hypertension. Report of the Baveno IV consensus workshop on methodology of diagnosis and therapy in portal hypertension. J Hepatol. 2005;43:167–76.

5. Cales P, Desmorat H, Vinel JP et al. Incidence of large oesophageal varices in patients with cirrhosis: application to prophylaxis of first bleeding. Gut. 1990;31:1298–302.
6. Zoli M, Merkel C, Magalotti D et al. Natural history of cirrhotic patients with small esophageal varices: a prospective study. Am J Gastroenterol. 2000;95:503–8.
7. de Franchis R, Primignani M. Natural history of portal hypertension in patients with cirrhosis. Clin Liver Dis. 2001;5:645–63.
8. Prediction of the first variceal hemorrhage in patients with cirrhosis of the liver and esophageal varices. A prospective multicenter study. North Italian Endoscopic Club for the Study and Treatment of Esophageal Varices. N Engl J Med. 1988;319:983–9.
9. D'Amico G, De Franchis R. Upper digestive bleeding in cirrhosis. Post-therapeutic outcome and prognostic indicators. Hepatology. 2003;38:599–612.
10. McCormick PA, O'Keefe C. Improving prognosis following a first variceal haemorrhage over four decades. Gut. 2001;49:682–5.
11. D'Amico G, Luca A. Natural history. Clinical–haemodynamic correlations. Prediction of the risk of bleeding. Baillieres Clin Gastroenterol. 1997;11:243–56.
12. Garcia-Tsao G. Current management of the complications of cirrhosis and portal hypertension: variceal hemorrhage, ascites, and spontaneous bacterial peritonitis. Gastroenterology. 2001;120:726–48.
13. Hillon P, Lebrec D, Munoz C, Jungers M, Goldfarb G, Benhamou JP. Comparison of the effects of a cardioselective and a nonselective beta-blocker on portal hypertension in patients with cirrhosis. Hepatology. 1982;2:528–31.
14. Mills PR, Rae AP, Farah DA, Russell RI, Lorimer AR, Carter DC. Comparison of three adrenoreceptor blocking agents in patients with cirrhosis and portal hypertension. Gut. 1984;25:73–8.
15. Groszmann RJ, Bosch J, Grace ND et al. Hemodynamic events in a prospective randomized trial of propranolol versus placebo in the prevention of a first variceal hemorrhage. Gastroenterology. 1990;99:1401–7.
16. Lebrec D, Hillon P, Munoz C, Goldfarb G, Nouel O, Benhamou JP. The effect of propranolol on portal hypertension in patients with cirrhosis: a hemodynamic study. Hepatology. 1982;2:523–7.
17. Garcia-Tsao G, Grace ND, Groszmann RJ et al. Short-term effects of propranolol on portal venous pressure. Hepatology. 1986;6:101–6.
18. Vorobioff J, Picabea E, Gamen M et al. Propranolol compared with propranolol plus isosorbide dinitrate in portal-hypertensive patients: long-term hemodynamic and renal effects. Hepatology. 1993;18:477–84.
19. Bandi JC, Garcia-Pagan JC, Escorsell A et al. Effects of propranolol on the hepatic hemodynamic response to physical exercise in patients with cirrhosis. Hepatology. 1998;28:677–82.
20. Feu F, Bordas JM, Garcia-Pagan JC, Bosch J, Rodes J. Double-blind investigation of the effects of propranolol and placebo on the pressure of esophageal varices in patients with portal hypertension. Hepatology. 1991;13:917–22.
21. Bosch J, Groszmann RJ. Measurement of azygos venous blood flow by a continuous thermal dilution technique: an index of blood flow through gastroesophageal collaterals in cirrhosis. Hepatology. 1984;4:424–9.
22. Cales P, Braillon A, Jiron MI, Lebrec D. Superior portosystemic collateral circulation estimated by azygos blood flow in patients with cirrhosis. Lack of correlation with oesophageal varices and gastrointestinal bleeding. Effect of propranolol. J Hepatol. 1985;1:37–46.
23. Bosch J, Masti R, Kravetz D et al. Effects of propranolol on azygos venous blood flow and hepatic and systemic hemodynamics in cirrhosis. Hepatology. 1984;4:1200–5.
24. Feu F, Bordas JM, Luca A et al. Reduction of variceal pressure by propranolol: comparison of the effects on portal pressure and azygos blood flow in patients with cirrhosis. Hepatology. 1993;18:1082–9.
25. Vorobioff JD, Gamen M, Kravetz D et al. Effects of long-term propranolol and octreotide on postprandial hemodynamics in cirrhosis: a randomized, controlled trial. Gastroenterology. 2002;122:916–22.
26. Perez-Paramo M, Munoz J, Albillos A et al. Effect of propranolol on the factors promoting bacterial translocation in cirrhotic rats with ascites. Hepatology. 2000;31:43–8.

27. Tripathi D, Therapondos G, Lui HF, Stanley AJ, Hayes PC. Haemodynamic effects of acute and chronic administration of low-dose carvedilol, a vasodilating beta-blocker, in patients with cirrhosis and portal hypertension. Aliment Pharmacol Ther. 2002;16:373–80.
28. Banares R, Moitinho E, Matilla A et al. Randomized comparison of long-term carvedilol and propranolol administration in the treatment of portal hypertension in cirrhosis. Hepatology. 2002;36:1367–73.
29. Tripathi D, Ferguson J, Kochar N et al. Multicenter randomized controlled trial of carvedilol versus variceal band ligation for the prevention of the first variceal bleed. Hepatology. 2007;46:269A.
30. Navasa M, Chesta J, Bosch J, Rodes J. Reduction of portal pressure by isosorbide-5-mononitrate in patients with cirrhosis. Effects on splanchnic and systemic hemodynamics and liver function. Gastroenterology. 1989;96:1110–18.
31. Garcia-Pagan JC, Navasa M, Bosch J, Bru C, Pizcueta P, Rodes J. Enhancement of portal pressure reduction by the association of isosorbide-5-mononitrate to propranolol administration in patients with cirrhosis. Hepatology. 1990;11:230–8.
32. Dib N, Konate A, Oberti F, Cales P. Non-invasive diagnosis of portal hypertension in cirrhosis. Application to the primary prevention of varices. Gastroenterol Clin Biol. 2005;29:957–87.
33. Cales P, Oberti F, Bernard-Chabert B, Payen JL. Evaluation of Baveno recommendations for grading esophageal varices. J Hepatol. 2003;39:657–9.
34. Luketic VA. Management of portal hypertension after variceal hemorrhage. Clin Liver Dis. 2001;5:677–707, ix.
35. Waked I, Korula J. Analysis of long-term endoscopic surveillance during follow-up after variceal sclerotherapy from a 13-year experience. Am J Med. 1997;102:192–9.
36. Westaby D, Macdougall BR, Williams R. Improved survival following injection sclerotherapy for esophageal varices: final analysis of a controlled trial. Hepatology. 1985;5:827–30.
37. Lebrec D, Vinel JP, Dupas JL. Complications of portal hypertension in adults: a French consensus. Eur J Gastroenterol Hepatol. 2005;17:403–10.
38. Tripathi D, Graham C, Hayes PC. Variceal band ligation versus beta-blockers for primary prevention of variceal bleeding: a meta-analysis. Eur J Gastroenterol Hepatol. 2007;19:835–45.
39. Imperiale TF, Klein RW, Chalasani N. Cost-effectiveness analysis of variceal ligation vs. beta-blockers for primary prevention of variceal bleeding. Hepatology. 2007;45:870–8.
40. Seewald S, Sriram PV, Naga M et al. Cyanoacrylate glue in gastric variceal bleeding. Endoscopy. 2002;34:926–32.
41. Italian Multicenter Project for Propranolol in Prevention of Bleeding. Propranolol prevents first gastrointestinal bleeding in non-ascitic cirrhotic patients. Final report of a multicenter randomized trial. J Hepatol. 1989;9:75–83.
42. Conn HO. Propranolol-induced reduction in recurrent variceal hemorrhage in schistosomiasis. Hepatology. 1990;11:1090–2.
43. Lebrec D, Poynard T, Capron JP et al. Nadolol for prophylaxis of gastrointestinal bleeding in patients with cirrhosis. A randomized trial. J Hepatol. 1988;7:118–25.
44. Talwalkar JA, Kamath PS. An evidence-based medicine approach to beta-blocker therapy in patients with cirrhosis. Am J Med. 2004;116:759–66.
45. Bureau C, Peron JM, Alric L et al. 'A la carte' treatment of portal hypertension: adapting medical therapy to hemodynamic response for the prevention of bleeding. Hepatology. 2002;36:1361–6.
46. Cales P. Optimal use of propranolol in portal hypertension. Gastroenterol Clin Biol. 2005;29:207–8.
47. Cales P, Grasset D, Ravaud A et al. Pharmacodynamic and pharmacokinetic study of propranolol in patients with cirrhosis and portal hypertension. Br J Clin Pharmacol. 1989;27:763–70.
48. Bosch J, Garcia-Pagan JC. Complications of cirrhosis. I. Portal hypertension. J Hepatol. 2000;32:141–56.
49. Bosch J, Garcia-Pagan JC. Prevention of variceal rebleeding. Lancet. 2003;361:952–4.
50. Abraczinskas DR, Ookubo R, Grace ND et al. Propranolol for the prevention of first esophageal variceal hemorrhage: a lifetime commitment? Hepatology. 2001;34:1096–102.

51. Angelico M, Carli L, Piat C, Gentile S, Capocaccia L. Effects of isosorbide-5-mononitrate compared with propranolol on first bleeding and long-term survival in cirrhosis. Gastroenterology. 1997;113:1632–9.
52. Garcia-Pagan JC, Villanueva C, Vila MC et al. Isosorbide mononitrate in the prevention of first variceal bleed in patients who cannot receive beta-blockers. Gastroenterology. 2001;121:908–14.
53. Peck-Radosavljevic M, Trauner M, Schreiber F. Austrian consensus on the definition and treatment of portal hypertension and its complications. Endoscopy. 2005;37:667–73.
54. Shneider B, Emre S, Groszmann R et al. Expert pediatric opinion on the report of the Baveno IV consensus workshop on methodology of diagnosis and therapy in portal hypertension. Pediatr Transplant. 2006;10:893–907.
55. Garcia-Tsao G, Sanyal AJ, Grace ND, Carey W. Prevention and management of gastroesophageal varices and variceal hemorrhage in cirrhosis. Hepatology. 2007;46:922–38.
56. Garcia-Tsao G, Sanyal AJ, Grace ND, Carey WD. Prevention and management of gastroesophageal varices and variceal hemorrhage in cirrhosis. Am J Gastroenterol. 2007;102:2086–102.
57. de Franchis R. Updating consensus in portal hypertension: report of the Baveno III Consensus Workshop on definitions, methodology and therapeutic strategies in portal hypertension. J Hepatol. 2000;33:846–52.
58. Villanueva C, Lopez-Balaguer JM, Aracil C et al. Maintenance of hemodynamic response to treatment for portal hypertension and influence on complications of cirrhosis. J Hepatol. 2004;40:757–65.
59. Cales P, Masliah C, Bernard B et al. Early administration of vapreotide for variceal bleeding in patients with cirrhosis. French Club for the Study of Portal Hypertension. N Engl J Med. 2001;344:23–8.
60. Tsokos M, Turk EE. Esophageal variceal hemorrhage presenting as sudden death in outpatients. Arch Pathol Lab Med. 2002;126:1197–200.
61. Arguedas MR, McGuire BM, Fallon MB, Abrams GA. The use of screening and preventive therapies for gastroesophageal varices in patients referred for evaluation of orthotopic liver transplantation. Am J Gastroenterol. 2001;96:833–7.
62. Mann NS, Leung JW. Circadian variation in portal pressure: appropriate use of non-selective beta blockers in the prevention of variceal bleed. Med Hypotheses. 2001;57:423–5.
63. Hicken BL, Sharara AI, Abrams GA, Eloubeidi M, Fallon MB, Arguedas MR. Hepatic venous pressure gradient measurements to assess response to primary prophylaxis in patients with cirrhosis: a decision analytical study. Aliment Pharmacol Ther. 2003;17:145–53.
64. Imperiale TF, Chalasani N, Klein RW. Measuring the hemodynamic response to primary pharmacoprophylaxis of variceal bleeding: a cost-effectiveness analysis. Am J Gastroenterol. 2003;98:2742–50.
65. Barriere E, Cales P. [How to prevent the first variceal bleeding?]. Gastroenterol Clin Biol. 2004;28(Spec. No. 2):B208–17.
66. Triantos C, Vlachogiannakos J, Armonis A et al. Primary prophylaxis of variceal bleeding in cirrhotics unable to take beta-blockers: a randomized trial of ligation. Aliment Pharmacol Ther. 2005;21:1435–43.
67. Merkel C, Marin R, Angeli P et al. A placebo-controlled clinical trial of nadolol in the prophylaxis of growth of small esophageal varices in cirrhosis. Gastroenterology. 2004;127:476–84.
68. Oberti F, Valsesia E, Pilette C et al. Noninvasive diagnosis of hepatic fibrosis or cirrhosis. Gastroenterology. 1997;113:1609–16.
69. Dib N, Konate A, Oberti F, Cales P. [Non-invasive diagnosis of portal hypertension in cirrhosis. Application to the primary prevention of varices]. Gastroenterol Clin Biol. 2005;29:975–87.

Section VI
Clinical management of portal hypertension: complications of cirrhosis

Chair: J BOSCH and R WIEST

21
Therapy of acute variceal bleeding

C. K. TRIANTOS and A. K. BURROUGHS

INTRODUCTION

Portal hypertension is a major complication of chronic liver disease, leading to the development of portosystemic collaterals of which the most clinically significant are those that form gastro-oesophageal varices. Variceal haemorrhage is the most serious complication of portal hypertension and is associated with a high mortality rate which ranges from 30% to 50%[1], although recently it has been well established that there has been a significant reduction in mortality from bleeding over the past 40 years[2,3]. Although overall survival may be improving, mortality is still closely related to failure to control haemorrhage or early rebleeding, and occurs in high rates in the first days to 6 weeks after admission[4,5].

Several factors have been validated for the prediction of the outcome of an acute variceal bleeding. Active bleeding at endoscopy, severity of liver disease, encephalopathy, platelet count, history of alcoholism, Child–Pugh grade C, shock at admission and the use of antibiotics have been associated with failure to control bleeding[5–12]. Regarding mortality, prognostic factors include: presentation with haematemesis, failure to control bleeding within 5 days, raised bilirubin, encephalopathy, shorter interval to admission to hospital, plasma urea, bleeding starting in hospital, prothrombin time <40%, recent use of steroid drugs within 7 days of bleeding, age >60 years, hepatic venous pressure gradient (HVPG), concomitant hepatocellular cancer and transfusion need[13–17].

Several new therapeutic approaches have been introduced for the prevention and treatment of variceal bleeding. The therapeutic armamentarium for portal hypertensive bleeding is now considerably expanded by the use of various drugs, including antibiotics and vasoactive agents, the endoscopic sclerotherapy or ligation of oesophageal varices and transjugular intrahepatic portosystemic shunts (TIPS). Recently the use of a self-expanding covered oesophageal stent has shown promise as a substitute for balloon tamponade[18]. The most important therapeutic manoeuvre in terms of increasing survival seems to be the use of prophylactic antibiotics[19], oral quinolones (and recently cephalosporins which have been shown to be superior in one study[20]). The relative risk of mortality is reduced to 0.39 (95% CI 0.32–0.48), which is a greater reduction than that seen with specific vasoactive drugs. Prophylactic antibiotics also reduce the incidence of early rebleeding, supporting the hypothesis of infection as a trigger for bleeding[9,11].

HVPG

The measurement of HVPG, in acute variceal bleeding, provides prognostic information on the evolution of the bleeding episode[17,21,22]. Moitinho et al.[23] evaluated 65 cirrhotics with acute variceal bleeding: the only independent variable associated with the outcome was HVPG, which was higher in patients with a poor evolution ($p<0.0004$). An initial HVPG of $\geqslant 20$ mmHg was associated with a significantly longer stay in an intensive-care unit, longer hospital stay, greater transfusion requirements, and a worse actuarial probability of survival (1-year mortality 64% vs 20%; $p<0.002$). Recently Abraldes et al.[13] evaluated a cohort of 117 cirrhotics concluding that HVPG independently predicted short-term prognosis in patients with acute variceal bleeding treated with pharmacological and endoscopic therapy. However, they showed that similar predictive accuracy can be achieved using only simple clinical variables that have universal applicability, i.e. that Child grade C patients are the difficult patients for control of bleeding and at greater risk of death. The authors confirm what was already known clinically about these patients with difficult bleeding[24], with the added data that this is associated with a higher HVPG. This gives the basis for the rationale of using portal pressure-lowering agents as soon as possible before admission[25] and/or before endoscopy.

The applicability of measuring HVPG in this setting, and its use in everyday clinical practice, is clearly a difficult issue, and in our opinion is not currently feasible outside of a research setting[26].

BACTERIAL INFECTION

Bacterial infections are frequently associated with upper gastrointestinal bleeding in cirrhotic patients[9,19,27]. Goulis et al.[9] showed in a prospective study that independent prognostic factors of failure to control bleeding were proven bacterial infection ($p<0.0001$) or antibiotic use ($p<0.003$), as well as active bleeding at endoscopy ($p<0.001$) and Child–Pugh score ($p<0.02$). In another report (1037 cirrhotics) the 297 with infection had a 4-fold increase in the incidence of gastrointestinal bleeding ($p<0.001$) compared to 346 without infection[28]. In addition others report that the presence of bacterial infection in bleeding cirrhotic patients is independently associated with early mortality and failure to control bleeding[29,30]. These data from different parts of the world confirm the original study which prospectively set out to assess the association of infection with bleeding[9].

A recent meta-analysis confirmed that antibiotic prophylaxis prevents infections in cirrhotic patients with gastrointestinal bleeding and significantly increases the short-term survival rate[19].

In a randomized trial[11] cirrhotics with variceal bleeding but without evidence of bacterial infection were randomized to receive prophylactic antibiotics (ofloxacin 200 mg intravenously q 12 h for 2 days followed by oral ofloxacin 200 mg q 12 h for 5 days) or receive antibiotics only when infection became evident (on-demand group). Antibiotic prophylaxis decreased infections ($p < 0.002$). The actuarial probability of rebleeding was higher in patients without prophylactic antibiotics ($p = 0.0029$). Bacterial infection and association with hepatocellular carcinoma were independent factors predictive of rebleeding. There was no difference in survival between the two groups. These data support the original hypothesis[10] supporting the role of bacterial infection in the initiation of variceal bleeding. Jun et al.[12] compared prophylactic third-generation cephalosporins with on-demand antibiotics for the prevention of gastro-oesophageal variceal rebleeding. The authors concluded that antibiotic prophylaxis using third-generation cephalosporins can prevent bacterial infection and early rebleeding in patients with the first acute gastro-oesophageal variceal bleeding.

Intravenous third-generation cephalosporins, compared to oral quinolones, are a good option for prophylaxis in upper gastrointestinal bleeding in cirrhosis[20], being active against Gram-negative bacteria and non-enterococcal streptococci. In addition many cirrhotics already receive quinolones as prophylaxis for spontaneous bacterial peritonitis. Current trials have started antibiotics after endoscopic diagnosis. Possibly the administration should be started at admission before endoscopy, with the potential to increase therapeutic benefit.

An additional issue surrounding infection is that it is known that severe sepsis is associated with a subnormal adrenal response, also in cirrhosis, and that steroid therapy improves survival[20,31]. Studies should be performed in patients who bled, to assess whether adrenal insufficiency is present with bleeding *per se*, and/or only in the presence of infection, mild or severe.

GENERAL MEASURES

Effective resuscitation, protection of the airway, particularly with severe bleeding and disturbed conscious level, especially during endoscopy, are initial priorities. Sedation may be required during endoscopy and endotracheal intubation is needed if there is concern about the safety of the airway. As well as assessment of vital signs, measurement of central venous pressure is usually necessary and preferred, and cardiac function by echocardiography may be needed. Preferably access to the circulation should be both peripheral and central. The presence of coagulopathy and thrombocytopenia is not a contraindication to central venous access. The infusion of plasma or a colloidal preparation depends on the degree of hypovolaemia. Blood should be transfused to achieve a haemoglobin level of 8 g/dl. Overtransfusion should be avoided as it may exacerbate increases in portal and variceal pressure. In animal models this provokes continued bleeding due to a portal pressure increase, but in humans the balance should be towards establishing an effective circulating volume to maintain renal function. A normal central venous pressure should be maintained, taking into account the severity of ascites, if present, in order to reduce the likelihood of renal failure. Clotting and platelet deficiencies may be ameliorated with fresh-frozen plasma and platelet transfusions, but there is no formal study assessing whether this helps to treat bleeding and/or improve outcome. Lastly rapid imaging should include a chest X-ray and the use of ultrasound/Doppler to establish the patency of portal vein and exclusion of hepatocellular carcinoma.

TREATMENT STRATEGIES

The following treatment strategies have been compared in acute variceal bleeding: (a) vasoactive drugs (±tamponade) vs vasoactive drugs (±tamponade) + sclerotherapy; (b) vasoactive drugs vs sclerotherapy; (c) vasoactive drugs + therapeutic endoscopy vs therapeutic endoscopy; (d) sclerotherapy vs ligation; and (e) recombinant factor VII + therapeutic endoscopy vs placebo + therapeutic endoscopy.

The vasoactive drugs currently used in the management of acute variceal bleeding are terlipressin, somatostatin and octreotide. Data favour the use of terlipressin, as mortality is reduced[32,33], and it may have an added role in maintaining renal function. Starting vasoactive therapy before diagnostic endoscopy is supported by trials, and prolonged therapy up to 5 days has been used, as this is the period of greatest risk of early rebleeding[5,34,35].

Moitinho et al.[36] evaluated a total of 174 patients with acute variceal bleeding who were randomized to receive somatostatin for 48 h: (a) one 250 µg bolus + 250 µg/h infusion; (b) three 250 µg boluses + 250 µg/h infusion; (c) three 250 µg boluses + 500 µg/h infusion. The 500 µg/h infusion dose achieved a higher rate of control of bleeding (82 vs 60%, $p<0.05$), less transfusions (3.7 ±2.7 vs 2.5±2.3 UU, $p = 0.07$) and better survival (93 vs 70%, $p<0.05$) than schedules (a) and (b). Others have confirmed the above results using somatostatin 500 µg/h[37,38]. Lastly octreotide has been reported to cause a reduction in portal pressure, but others have not confirmed these data. In a recent trial octreotide only transiently reduced portal pressure and flow, whereas the effects of terlipressin were sustained, suggesting that terlipressin may have more sustained haemodynamic effects in patients with bleeding varices[39].

In a recent meta-analysis[35] we have evaluated sclerotherapy in randomized trials: (a) combined with vasoconstrictors versus these alone, (b) versus vasoconstrictors alone, (c) versus combination of vasoconstrictors and sclerotherapy, (d) versus ligation. The efficacy of acute sclerotherapy was highest versus ligation at 95%, with a small advantage for ligation 2.5% (95% CI 0.4%–4.6%) ($p = 0.018$), but no survival difference. The efficacy combined with vasoconstrictors versus these alone was 86%, whereas it was 83% versus vasoconstrictors alone. In both these groups sclerotherapy was superior for control of bleeding, respectively 16.3% (95% CI 8.7%–23.9% ($p = 0.0001$) and 5.9% (95% CI 1.5%–10.3%) ($p = 0.008$), with increased survival in the latter. In the combination group of sclerotherapy with vasoconstrictors the efficacy of sclerotherapy alone was 69%, with the combination superior in controlling bleeding: 13.2% (95% CI 8.4%–18.1%) ($p < 0.0001$)) but with no survival difference. This comparison of sclerotherapy across trials demonstrates a problem in defining its real efficacy. Our data support the conclusion that sclerotherapy remains the 'gold standard' in acute variceal bleeding.

In a recent trial published after the meta-analysis favouring ligation[40] endoscopy was performed within 6 h and those with oesophageal variceal bleeding were randomized to receive either sclerotherapy ($n = 89$) or ligation ($n = 90$). Failure to control bleeding occurred in 15% vs 4%, respectively ($p = 0.02$). Six-week survival probability without therapeutic failure was better with ligation ($p = 0.01$); however, in those with active bleeding or Child Grade C, who are the patients with the most likelihood of having difficulty in controlling bleeding, there was no difference between ligation and sclerotherapy[41].

The early effects of endoscopic injection sclerotherapy (EIS) and endoscopic band ligation (EBL) on HVPG during acute bleeding have also been investigated[42]. In 50 cirrhotic patients HVPG measurements were performed before and immediately after endoscopic treatment, and every 24 h for a 5-day period. In both groups a significant increase was observed in mean portal pressure immediately after treatment as compared with pretreatment ($p < 0.0001$); however, in the EBL group HVPG returned to baseline values within 48 h after treatment, while in the EIS group it remained high during the 120-h study period ($p < 0.0001$). Thus during acute variceal bleeding EIS, but not EBL, was associated with a sustained increase in HVPG. During the 42-day follow-up period the rebleeding rate over time was lower in the EBL group compared with the EIS group ($p = 0.024$) confirming previous studies of repeated endoscopic therapy. The mechanism of the increased HVPG with endotherapy, and why portal pressure returned to baseline values within 48 h of banding but not EIS, is not clear. In addition Vlachogiannakos et al.[43] showed that somatostatin, but not octreotide, effectively prevents the post-endoscopic increase of HVPG.

Recombinant coagulation factor VIIa (rFVIIa) has been shown to correct the prolonged prothrombin time in patients with cirrhosis and UGIB (upper gastrointestinal bleeding). Bosch et al.[44] aimed to determine efficacy and safety of rFVIIa in cirrhotic patients with variceal and non-variceal UGIB; 245 cirrhotics (Child–Pugh < 13; Child–Pugh A = 20%, B = 52%, C = 28%) with UGIB (variceal = 66%, non-variceal = 29%, bleeding source unknown = 5%) were randomized equally to receive eight doses of 100 µg/kg rFVIIa or placebo in addition to pharmacological and endoscopic treatment. rFVIIa significantly decreased the number of failures ($p = 0.03$) and the 24-h bleeding control endpoint ($p = 0.01$) in the subgroup of Child–Pugh B and C variceal bleeders. There were no significant differences between rFVIIa and placebo groups in mortality (5- or 42-day). More recently the same group, in a randomized trial[45], aimed to determine the efficacy and safety of rFVIIa in patients with advanced cirrhosis and active (oozing/spurting) variceal bleeding. There were no significant differences between the groups (placebo, 600 µg/kg and 30 µg/kg), in terms of bleeding; however, treatment with 600 µg/kg significantly reduced 42-day mortality, which cannot be explained by a control of bleeding. Adverse events were comparable between groups.

UNCONTROLLED VARICEAL BLEEDING

The definition of uncontrolled variceal bleeding includes the continued/early variceal rebleeding (within 5 days) despite two sessions of therapeutic endoscopy, continued variceal bleeding despite balloon tamponade and continued/early gastric or ectopic variceal bleeding despite vasoconstrictor therapy.

Balloon tamponade has most often been used to arrest life-threatening haemorrhage or if other measures fail. It has also been used in the absence of a definite diagnosis, but if bleeding from varices is strongly suspected. The usual tube is a modified four-lumen Sengstaken–Blakemore tube (SBT). The airway should be protected by an endotracheal tube under a short general anaesthetic, as the risk of aspiration is very high, particularly in unskilled hands[46]. If blood is still coming up the gastric aspiration lumen, then varices are less likely to be the cause of blood loss, although gastric fundal varices are not always controlled by tamponade. Whenever this occurs, if the position of the SBT has been checked and adequate traction applied, the diagnosis of variceal bleeding should be questioned, and emergency angiography performed.

In a recent report[18] the use of self-expandable metallic stents was evaluated to arrest uncontrollable acute variceal bleeding (20 patients, mean age 52, eight Child–Pugh C). The patients had not been successfully managed with prior pharmacological or endoscopic therapy. The stents were successfully placed in all of the patients and were left in place for 2–14 days. Bleeding from the oesophageal varices ceased immediately after implantation of the stent in all cases. No recurrent bleeding, morbidity, or mortality occurred during treatment with the oesophageal stent. All of the stents were extracted without any complications after definitive treatment had been started.

TIPS stops bleeding in a significant percentage[47]. In uncontrolled studies TIPS is effective in stopping variceal haemorrhage[48–52], but presents high mortality[53]. Monescillo et al.[17] evaluated variceal bleeders with HVPG $\geqslant 20$ mmHg, and they were randomly allocated to receiving TIPS (HR-TIPS group, $n = 26$) within the first 24 h after admission or not (HR-non-TIPS group). The HR-non-TIPS group had more treatment failures ($p = 0.0001$). Early TIPS placement reduced treatment failure ($p = 0.003$), in-hospital and 1-year mortality ($p < 0.05$). Overall TIPS remains a good choice as a rescue therapy, although when it is not available staple transection of the oesophagus could be considered[54].

New diagnostic and treatment algorithms of acute variceal bleeding are needed using known predictive factors of failure to control bleeding and mortality in order to identify the group of bleeders with poor outcome. In this group more effective vasoactive regimens, early TIPS after diagnostic endoscopy, and the use of self-expanding covered oesophageal stent could be considered[26].

GASTRIC VARICES

In active bleeding from gastric varices the use of sclerotherapy and ligation is not effective with high early rebleeding rates[55]. Glues[55] and TIPS[52] are effective. The consensus at Baveno IV was to use endoscopic therapy with tissue adhesive (e.g. N-butyl-cyanoacrylate)[24]. In a recent trial[56] TIPS proved more effective than glue injection in preventing rebleeding from gastric varices, with similar survival and frequency of complications.

IN THE FUTURE

Potential areas of further clinical study in acute variceal bleeding are: (1) prophylactic antibiotics given at admission, not after diagnosis; (2) in patients with high risk of failure to control bleeding the use of glue or TIPS or oesophageal stent as first-line therapy; (3) assessment of the risks of double intubation (diagnostic endoscopy and then band ligation); (4) routine endotracheal intubation in high-risk patients (to prevent aspiration pneumonia); and (5) steroids in infected patients.

The number of randomized clinical trials dealing with the treatment of portal hypertension is ever-increasing; however, in our opinion any new treatment strategy needs careful interpretation[4,57] because, despite the consensus meetings of Baveno, trials often use heterogeneous criteria for the definition of their main endpoints, lack adequate statistical power, and unfortunately are not comparable to one another.

References

1. D'Amico G, Pagliaro L, Bosch J. The treatment of portal hypertension: a meta-analytic review. Hepatology. 1995;22:332–54.
2. McCormick PA, O'Keefe C. Improving prognosis following a first variceal haemorrhage over four decades. Gut. 2001;49:682–5.
3. Carbonell N, Pauwels A, Serfaty L, Fourdan O, Levy VG, Poupon R. Improved survival after variceal bleeding in patients with cirrhosis over the past two decades. Hepatology. 2004;40:652–9.
4. Burroughs AK, Mezzanotte G, Phillips A, McCormick PA, McIntyre N. Cirrhotics with variceal hemorrhage: the importance of the time interval between admission and the start of analysis for survival and rebleeding rates. Hepatology. 1989;9:801–7.
5. Ben Ari Z, Cardin F, McCormick AP, Wannamethee G, Burroughs AK. A predictive model for failure to control bleeding during acute variceal haemorrhage. J Hepatol. 1999;31:443–50.
6. Lo GH, Chen WC, Chen MH et al. The characteristics and the prognosis for patients presenting with actively bleeding esophageal varices at endoscopy. Gastrointest Endosc. 2004;60:714–20.
7. Thomopoulos K, Theocharis G, Mimidis K, Lampropoulou-Karatza C, Alexandridis E, Nikolopoulou V. Improved survival of patients presenting with acute variceal bleeding. Prognostic indicators of short- and long-term mortality. Dig Liver Dis. 2006;38:899–904.
8. Bernard B, Grange JD, Khac EN, Amiot X, Opolon P, Poynard T. Antibiotic prophylaxis for the prevention of bacterial infections in cirrhotic patients with gastrointestinal bleeding: a meta-analysis. Hepatology. 1999;29:1655–61.
9. Goulis J, Armonis A, Patch D, Sabin C, Greenslade L, Burroughs AK. Bacterial infection is independently associated with failure to control bleeding in cirrhotic patients with gastrointestinal hemorrhage. Hepatology. 1998;27:1207–12.

10. Goulis J, Patch D, Burroughs AK. Bacterial infection in the pathogenesis of variceal bleeding. Lancet. 1999;353:139–42.
11. Hou MC, Lin HC, Liu TT et al. Antibiotic prophylaxis after endoscopic therapy prevents rebleeding in acute variceal hemorrhage: a randomized trial. Hepatology. 2004;39:746–53.
12. Jun CH, Park CH, Lee WS et al. Antibiotic prophylaxis using third generation cephalosporins can reduce the risk of early rebleeding in the first acute gastroesophageal variceal hemorrhage: a prospective randomized study. J Korean Med Sci. 2006;21:883–90.
13. Abraldes JG, Villanueva C, Benares R et al. Hepatic venous pressure gradient and prognosis in patients with acute variceal bleeding treated with pharmacologic and endoscopic therapy. J Hepatol. 2008;48:229–36.
14. Amitrano L, Guardascione MA, Bennato R, Manguso F, Balzano A. MELD score and hepatocellular carcinoma identify patients at different risk of short-term mortality among cirrhotics bleeding from esophageal varices. J Hepatol. 2005;42:820–5.
15. Lang BH, Poon RT, Fan ST, Wong J. Outcomes of patients with hepatocellular carcinoma presenting with variceal bleeding. Am J Gastroenterol. 2004;99:2158–65.
16. Lecleire S, Di Fiore F, Merle V et al. Acute upper gastrointestinal bleeding in patients with liver cirrhosis and in noncirrhotic patients: epidemiology and predictive factors of mortality in a prospective multicenter population-based study. J Clin Gastroenterol. 2005;39:321–7.
17. Monescillo A, Martinez-Lagares F, Ruiz-Del-Arbol L et al. Influence of portal hypertension and its early decompression by TIPS placement on the outcome of variceal bleeding. Hepatology. 2004;40:793.
18. Hubmann R, Bodlaj G, Czompo M et al. The use of self-expanding metal stents to treat acute esophageal variceal bleeding. Endoscopy. 2006;38:896–901.
19. Soares-Weiser K, Brezis M, Tur-Kaspa R, Paul M, Yahav J, Leibovici L. Antibiotic prophylaxis of bacterial infections in cirrhotic inpatients: a meta-analysis of randomized controlled trials. Scand J Gastroenterol. 2003;38:193–200.
20. Fernandez J, Escorsell A, Zabalza M et al. Adrenal insufficiency in patients with cirrhosis and septic shock: effect of treatment with hydrocortisone on survival. Hepatology. 2006;44:1288–95.
21. Ready JB, Robertson AD, Goff JS, Rector WG Jr. Assessment of the risk of bleeding from esophageal varices by continuous monitoring of portal pressure. Gastroenterology. 1991;100:1403–10.
22. Vinel JP, Cassigneul J, Levade M, Voigt JJ, Pascal JP. Assessment of short-term prognosis after variceal bleeding in patients with alcoholic cirrhosis by early measurement of portohepatic gradient. Hepatology. 1986;6:116–17.
23. Moitinho E, Escorsell A, Bandi JC et al. Prognostic value of early measurements of portal pressure in acute variceal bleeding. Gastroenterology. 1999;117:626–31.
24. de Franchis R. Evolving consensus in portal hypertension. Report of the Baveno IV consensus workshop on methodology of diagnosis and therapy in portal hypertension. J Hepatol. 2005;43:167–76.
25. Levacher S, Letoumelin P, Pateron D, Blaise M, Lapandry C, Pourriat JL. Early administration of terlipressin plus glyceryl trinitrate to control active upper gastrointestinal bleeding in cirrhotic patients. Lancet. 1995;346:865–8.
26. Burroughs AK, Triantos CK. Predicting failure to control bleeding and mortality in acute variceal bleeding. J Hepatol. 2008;48:185–8.
27. Thalheimer U, Triantos CK, Samonakis DN, Patch D, Burroughs AK. Infection, coagulation, and variceal bleeding in cirrhosis. Gut. 2005;54:556–63.
28. Benavides J, Fernadez N, Colombato L et al. Further evidence linking bacterial infection and upper GI bleeding in cirrhosis. Results from a large multicentre prospective survey in Argentina. J Hepatol. 2003;38(Suppl. 2):A176.
29. Vivas S, Rodriguez M, Palacio MA, Linares A, Alonso JL, Rodrigo L. Presence of bacterial infection in bleeding cirrhotic patients is independently associated with early mortality and failure to control bleeding. Dig Dis Sci. 2001;46:2752–7.
30. Pohl J, Pollmann K, Sauer P, Ring A, Stremmel W, Schlenker T. Antibiotic prophylaxis after variceal hemorrhage reduces incidence of early rebleeding. Hepatogastroenterology. 2004;51:541–6.
31. Tsai MH, Peng YS, Chen YC et al. Adrenal insufficiency in patients with cirrhosis, severe sepsis and septic shock. Hepatology. 2006;43:673–81.

32. Gotzsche PC. Somatostatin analogues for acute bleeding oesophageal varices. Cochrane Database Syst Rev 2002;(1):CD000193.
33. Ioannou G, Doust J, Rockey DC. Terlipressin for acute esophageal variceal hemorrhage. Cochrane Database Syst Rev 2003;(1):CD002147.
34. D'Amico G, Pietrosi G, Tarantino I, Pagliaro L. Emergency sclerotherapy versus vasoactive drugs for variceal bleeding in cirrhosis: a Cochrane meta-analysis. Gastroenterology. 2003;124:1277–91.
35. Triantos CK, Goulis J, Patch D et al. An evaluation of emergency sclerotherapy of varices in randomized trials: looking the needle in the eye. Endoscopy. 2006;38:797–807.
36. Moitinho E, Planas R, Banares R et al. Multicenter randomized controlled trial comparing different schedules of somatostatin in the treatment of acute variceal bleeding. J Hepatol. 2001;35:712–18.
37. Palazon JM, Such J, Sanchez-Paya J et al. A comparison of two different dosages of somatostatin combined with sclerotherapy for the treatment of acute esophageal variceal bleeding: a prospective randomized trial. Rev Esp Enferm Dig. 2006;98:249–54.
38. Villanueva C, Planella M, Aracil C et al. Hemodynamic effects of terlipressin and high somatostatin dose during acute variceal bleeding in nonresponders to the usual somatostatin dose. Am J Gastroenterol. 2005;100:624–30.
39. Baik SK, Jeong PH, Ji SW et al. Acute hemodynamic effects of octreotide and terlipressin in patients with cirrhosis: a randomized comparison. Am J Gastroenterol. 2005;100:631–5.
40. Villanueva C, Piqueras M, Aracil C et al. A randomized controlled trial comparing ligation and sclerotherapy as emergency endoscopic treatment added to somatostatin in acute variceal bleeding. J Hepatol. 2006;45:560–7.
41. Triantos C, Goulis J, Patch D et al. Reply to Dr. Krag et al. Endoscopy. 2007;39:374.
42. Avgerinos A, Armonis A, Stefanidis G et al. Sustained rise of portal pressure after sclerotherapy, but not band ligation, in acute variceal bleeding in cirrhosis. Hepatology. 2004;39:1623–30.
43. Vlachogiannakos J, Kougioumtzan A, Triantos C et al. The effect of somatostatin versus octreotide in preventing the post-endoscopic increase of HVPG in cirrhotics with bleeding varices. Aliment Pharmacol Ther. 2007;26:1479–87.
44. Bosch J, Thabut D, Bendtsen F et al. Recombinant factor VIIa for upper gastrointestinal bleeding in patients with cirrhosis: a randomized, double-blind trial. Gastroenterology. 2004;127:1123–30.
45. Bosch J, Thabut D, Albillos A et al. Recombinant factor VIIA (RFVIIA) for active variceal bleeding in patients with advanced cirrhosis: a multi-centre randomized double-blind placebo-controlled trial. J Hepatol. 2007;46(Suppl. 1):295.
46. Vlavianos P, Gimson AE, Westaby D, Williams R. Balloon tamponade in variceal bleeding: use and misuse. Br Med J. 1989;298:1158.
47. Vangeli M, Patch D, Burroughs AK. Salvage tips for uncontrolled variceal bleeding. J Hepatol. 2002;37:703–4.
48. McCormick PA, Dick R, Panagou EB et al. Emergency transjugular intrahepatic portasystemic stent shunting as salvage treatment for uncontrolled variceal bleeding. Br J Surg. 1994;81:1324–7.
49. Sanyal AJ, Freedman AM, Luketic VA et al. Transjugular intrahepatic portosystemic shunts for patients with active variceal hemorrhage unresponsive to sclerotherapy. Gastroenterology. 1996;111:138–46.
50. Gerbes AL, Gulberg V, Waggershauser T, Holl J, Reiser M. Transjugular intrahepatic portosystemic shunt (TIPS) for variceal bleeding in portal hypertension: comparison of emergency and elective interventions. Dig Dis Sci. 1998;43:2463–9.
51. Chau TN, Patch D, Chan YW, Nagral A, Dick R, Burroughs AK. 'Salvage' transjugular intrahepatic portosystemic shunts: gastric fundal compared with esophageal variceal bleeding. Gastroenterology. 1998;114(5):981–7.
52. Azoulay D, Castaing D, Majno P et al. Salvage transjugular intrahepatic portosystemic shunt for uncontrolled variceal bleeding in patients with decompensated cirrhosis. J Hepatol. 2001;35:590–7.
53. Patch D, Nikolopoulou V, McCormick A et al. Factors related to early mortality after transjugular intrahepatic portosystemic shunt for failed endoscopic therapy in acute variceal bleeding. J Hepatol. 1998;28:454–60.

54. Samonakis DN, Triantos CK, Thalheimer U, Patch DW, Burroughs AK. Management of portal hypertension. Postgrad Med J. 2004;80:634–41.
55. Tan PC, Hou MC, Lin HC et al. A randomized trial of endoscopic treatment of acute gastric variceal hemorrhage: N-butyl-2-cyanoacrylate injection versus band ligation. Hepatology. 2006;43:690–7.
56. Lo GH, Liang HL, Chen WC et al. A prospective, randomized controlled trial of transjugular intrahepatic portosystemic shunt versus cyanoacrylate injection in the prevention of gastric variceal rebleeding. Endoscopy. 2007;39:679–85.
57. Burroughs AK, Patch D. Therapeutic benefit of vaso-active drugs for acute variceal bleeding: a real pharmacological effect, or a side-effect of definitions in trials? Hepatology. 1996;24:737–9.

22
Prevention of variceal rebleeding

D. LEBREC

INTRODUCTION

In patients who bleed from oesophageal haemorrhage and do not receive any prevention for rebleeding, the risk of recurrent gastrointestinal bleeding is approximately 75% at 2 years[1]. The risk of rebleeding is especially elevated in the first 6 weeks after bleeding. The severity of initial haemorrhage and the severity of cirrhosis are the main predictive factors of rebleeding. Considering the risk of recurrent haemorrhage and its associated mortality, treatment for the prevention of rebleeding should be begun after bleeding.

The aim of this chapter is to summarize and discuss treatments to prevent recurrent variceal bleeding. Different types of treatment for the prevention of rebleeding exist, in particular pharmacological, endoscopic, radiological and surgical. Surgical treatments, in particular portosystemic shunts, are very effective in preventing variceal rebleeding but significantly increase the risk of hepatic encephalopathy and have no beneficial effect on survival. Thus, surgical shunts have been abandoned in many centres. In addition, a negative relationship has been shown between treatment efficacy and the invasiveness of the method for the pharmacological, endoscopic and radiological treatments. For example, transjugular intrahepatic portosystemic shunts (TIPS) are more effective than pharmacological and endoscopic treatments, but more invasive and thus accompanied by more side-effects. Finally, all types of treatments are better than no treatment or a placebo for preventing bleeding, and all treatments improve survival rate, but no significant difference exists in the mortality rate for the different treatments.

PHARMACOLOGICAL THERAPY

Since it has been demonstrated that non-cardioselective beta-adrenergic blockers significantly decrease portal pressure in patients with portal hypertension[2], several trials, performed with a large number of patients, have been published comparing beta-blockers and other treatments.

Beta-blockers versus no treatment

Twelve randomized, placebo-controlled trials and two meta-analyses have shown that non-cardioselective beta-blocker administration (propranolol or nadolol) significantly reduces the rebleeding rate by approximately 40% and increases the survival rate by 20% at 2 years[3,4]. These beneficial effects were observed in patients with or without ascites and in patients with non-cirrhotic portal hypertension. Certain factors were shown to be associated with the risk of rebleeding in patients treated with beta-blockers: lack of compliance and lack of persistent decrease in heart rate[5]. The relationship between the decrease in the hepatic venous pressure gradient (HVPG) and the risk of rebleeding has been demonstrated but remains controversial, indicating that further haemodynamic studies are needed[6].

Beta-blockers versus endoscopic sclerotherapy

In patients with cirrhosis, sclerotherapy reduces the risk of rebleeding from 65% to 35% but it does not appear to significantly reduce overall mortality[7].

Ten controlled trials have compared the efficacy of beta-blockers and endoscopic sclerotherapy in the prevention of rebleeding. The results of two meta-analyses comparing beta-blockers and sclerotherapy showed that endoscopic treatment was more effective than pharmacological treatment for the prevention of rebleeding but the incidence of side-effects was significantly higher in the sclerotherapy group[3,8]. There was, however, no difference in the survival rate between the two treatments.

The results of the comparison between beta-blockers alone and the combination of beta-blockers and endoscopic sclerotherapy are controversial. The risk of rebleeding was lower in patients receiving combined treatment than in patients treated with sclerotherapy alone; there was no difference in survival rate between the two groups.

Beta-blockers versus beta-blockers plus isosorbide mononitrate

The addition of nitrate to beta-blockers appears to enhance the haemodynamic effects of beta-blockers alone, but this effect remains controversial.

Three controlled trials have compared beta-blockers and combination of beta-blockers and isosorbide mononitrate[9-11]. Two were published only in abstract form. In one trial the rebleeding rate was lower in patients receiving combination therapy, but the difference was not significant. Mortality was also not significantly different between the two groups. In a second trial the rebleeding rate was higher in patients receiving the combination therapy but, again, the difference was not significant. However, the mortality rate was significantly higher in the combination group than in the beta-blocker group. The adverse event rate was significantly higher in patients treated with nitrate and beta-blockers than in patients treated with beta-blockers alone in both trials. The third study found no significant difference between the two groups.

Thus, the combination of beta-blockers and nitrate cannot be recommended for the prevention of recurrent bleeding in patients with cirrhosis.

Beta-blockers plus isosorbide mononitrate versus band ligation

Endoscopic variceal band ligation is highly effective in obliterating varices. A meta-analysis performed with 20 trials showed that band ligation is associated with a lower risk of rebleeding than sclerotherapy, fewer complications and higher survival rates[12]. As a result, band ligation has replaced endoscopic sclerotherapy.

Three trials have compared the efficacy of beta-blockers plus nitrate and band ligation[13–15]. In one trial the rebleeding rate was significantly lower in the pharmacological group; in a second trial the rebleeding rate was significantly lower in the band ligation group and in a third study there was no significant difference in the rebleeding rate between the two groups. None of these trials showed a significant difference in survival rate. These findings suggest that both treatments are effective in preventing rebleeding.

Beta-blockers plus band ligation versus band ligation

In a recent trial the combination of beta-blockers plus band ligation was compared to band ligation alone for the prevention of rebleeding[16]. This trial showed that the combination of pharmacological and endoscopic treatment is more effective in reducing the risk of rebleeding but the mortality rate was not significantly different between the two groups. These results suggest that the combination of these two treatments is better than one treatment alone, but further clinical trials are needed to confirm this hypothesis.

Beta-blockers plus isosorbide mononitrate plus band ligation versus beta-blockers plus isosorbide mononitrate

A preliminary report comparing different combinations has shown that nadolol plus nitrate plus band ligation is not different from nadolol plus nitrate for the rebleeding and mortality rates[17]. However, the variceal rebleeding rate was significantly lower in the pharmacological and endoscopic group than in the pharmacological group.

Beta-blockers plus band ligation plus sucralfate versus band ligation

One trial has shown that combination of nadolol, sucralfate and band ligation was better than band ligation alone in controlling the variceal rebleeding rate and variceal recurrence[18]. However, the risk of side-effects was higher in the former group. In addition, the mortality rate was not significantly different between the two groups.

ENDOSCOPIC TREATMENTS VERSUS TIPS

There are no trials comparing TIPS and pharmacological or endoscopic treatments in patients with refractory recurrent variceal bleeding. TIPS has only been compared to endoscopic treatments with or without pharmacological treatments to prevent 'non-refractory' recurrent variceal bleeding. Thirteen controlled studies were performed showing discrepant results. A meta-analysis showed that the rebleeding rate was significantly lower in the TIPS group than in the endoscopic group, but with no benefit on the mortality rate[19]. In addition, these studies showed that the risk of hepatic encephalopathy was significantly higher in the TIPS group than in the endoscopic group. These findings confirm that TIPS should be used only in patients with refractory rebleeding.

TIPS VERSUS DISTAL SPLENORENAL SHUNTS

One controlled trial showed that non-selective shunts and TIPS are effective in preventing recurrent refractory bleeding but are associated with significant peroperative and postoperative complications such as encephalopathy[20]. However re-intervention was significantly more frequent in the TIPS group.

CONCLUSIONS

This conclusion is similar to that reported during Baveno IV Consensus held in April 2005[21]: Prevention of rebleeding should start as soon as possible. In patients who have not received primary prophylaxis: beta-blockers, band ligation or both should be used. In patients who are on beta-blockers, band ligation should be added. Band ligation is the preferred treatment in patients with contraindications or intolerance to beta-blockers. In patients who do not respond to pharmacological and endoscopic treatment, TIPS or surgical shunt are effective for patients with Child A–B cirrhosis. Liver transplantation provides good long-term outcome in Child B–C cirrhosis.

References

1. Lebrec D. Pharmacological treatment of portal hypertension: present and future. J Hepatol. 2000;28:896–907.
2. Lebrec D, Nouel O, Corbic M et al. Propranolol: a medical treatment for portal hypertension. Lancet. 1980;i:121–4.
3. D'Amico G, Pagliaro L, Bosch J. The treatment of portal hypertension: a meta-analytic review. Hepatology. 1995;22:332–53.
4. Bernard B, Lebrec D, Mathurin P et al. Beta-adrenergic antagonists in the prevention of gastronintestinal rebleeding in patients with cirrhosis. A meta-analysis. Hepatology. 1997;25:63–70.
5. Poynard T, Lebrec D, Hillon P et al. Propranolol for prevention of recurrent gastrointestinal bleeding in patients with cirrhosis: a prospective study of factors associated with rebleeding. Hepatology. 1987;7:447–51.
6. Thalheimer U, Mela M, Patch D et al. Monitoring target reduction in hepatic venous pressure gradient during pharmacological therapy of portal hypertension close look at the evidence. Gut. 2004;53:43–8.
7. de Franchis R. Evolving consensus on portal hypertension: report of the IV consensus workshop on methodology of diagnosis and therapy in portal hypertension. J Hepatol. 2005;43:167–76.
8. Bernard B, Lebrec D, Mathurin P et al. Propranolol and sclerotherapy in the prevention of gastrointestinal rebleeding in patients with cirrhosis. J Hepatol. 1997;26:312–24.

9. Gournay J, Masliah C, Martin T et al. Isosorbide mononitrate and propranolol compared with propranolol alone for the prevention of variceal rebleeding. Hepatology. 2000;31:1239-45.
10. Patti R, D'Amico G, Pasta L et al. Isosorbide mononitrate with nadolol compared to nadolol alone for prevention of recurrent bleeding in cirrhosis. A double-blind placebo-controlled randomised trial. J Hepatol. 1999;30(Suppl. 1):81 (Abstract).
11. Zhang Qyuan R, Wang H. The randomized controlled trial of isosorbide mononitrate plus propranolol compared with propranolol alone for the prevention of variceal rebleeding. Zhonghua Yi Xue Za Zhi. 2002;8217:1157-9.
12. Goulis J, Burrough AK. Portal hypertensive bleeding. In: McDonald J, Burroughs AK, Feagen B, editors. Evidence-based Gastroenterology and Hepatology. London: BMJ Books, 2004.
13. Villanueva C, Minana J, Ortiz J et al. Endoscopic ligation compared with combined treatment with nadolol plus isosorbide mononitrate to prevent recurrent variceal bleeding. N Engl J Med. 2001;345:647-55.
14. Lo GH, Chen WC, Hsu PI et al. Banding ligation versus nadolol and isosorbide mononitrate for the prevention of esophageal variceal bleeding. Gastroenterology. 2002;123:728-34.
15. Patch D, Sabin CA, Goulis J et al. A randomized, controlled trial of medical therapy versus endoscopic ligation for the prevention of variceal rebleeding in patients with cirrhosis. Gastroenterology. 2002;123:1013-19.
16. de La Pena J, Sanchez-Hernandez E, Rivero M et al. Variceal ligation plus nadolol compared with ligation for prophylaxis of variceal rebleeding: a multi-center trial. Hepatology. 2005;41:572-8.
17. Study Group Spanish Cooperative Variceal Rebleeding. Multicenter RCT comparing drug therapy vs the combination of drug therapy + endoscopic band ligation in the prevention of rebleeding in patients with cirrhosis. Hepatology. 2006;44(Suppl. 1):202A (Abstract).
18. Lo GH, Lai KH, Cheng JS et al. Endoscopic variceal ligation plus nadolol and sucralfate compared with ligation alone for the prevention of variceal rebleeding: a prospective, randomised trial. Hepatology. 2000;32:461-5.
19. Papatheodoridis GV, Goulis J, Leandro G et al. Transjugular intrahepatic portosystemic shunt compared with endoscopic treatment for prevention of variceal rebleeding: a meta-analysis. Hepatology. 1999;30:612-22.
20. Henderson JM, Boyer TD, Kutner MH et al. Distal splenorenal shunt versus transjugular intrahepatic portal systematic shunt for variceal bleeding: a randomized trial. Gastroenterology. 2006;130:1643-51.
21. Lebrec D, Sauerbruch T, Bernard-Chabert B et al. Baveno IV consensus statements: Prevention of rebleeding. In: de Franchis R, editor. Proceedings of the Fourth Baveno International Consensus Workshop on Methodology of Diagnosis and Treatment. London: Blackwell, 2006:283-4.

23
From sodium retention to refractory ascites: the role of new drugs

F. WONG

INTRODUCTION

Abnormal renal sodium handling is an early and common complication of liver cirrhosis and eventually results in ascites formation. The development of ascites significantly increases the morbidity of these patients and adversely affects their prognosis, with a 50% 2-year survival at the time of development of ascites[1], worsening significantly to 20–50% at 1 year when the ascites becomes refractory to medical therapy[2].

SODIUM RETENTION IN CIRRHOSIS

Pre-ascitic cirrhosis

The pathophysiology leading to ascites formation is complex. Subtle sodium retention is evident early in cirrhosis[3]. Several mechanisms are operational at this stage to retain sodium (Figure 1). Sodium retention occurs mostly in the erect posture in pre-ascitic cirrhosis, associated with abnormalities in the renin–angiotensin–aldosterone system (RAAS). There is increased intra-renal angiotensin II production in the erect posture, leading to sodium retention via an increase in the sodium reabsorption in the proximal renal tubule[4]. The fact that angiotensin receptor antagonists are able to improve renal sodium excretion provides confirmatory evidence for the presence of this mechanism[5,6]. The assumption of the erect posture also results in an increase in serum aldosterone in pre-ascitic cirrhosis, although still within normal levels[7], associated with a reduction in glomerular filtration rate[8]; both changes also favour renal sodium retention. The latter may be related to a deranged tubuloglomerular feedback mechanism in the erect posture in pre-ascitic cirrhosis. This is a physiological response whereby the glomerular filtration rate increases when there is a reduction in the amount of sodium being delivered to the distal renal tubule. Failure to improve the glomerular filtration rate in the erect posture has been demonstrated in pre-ascitic

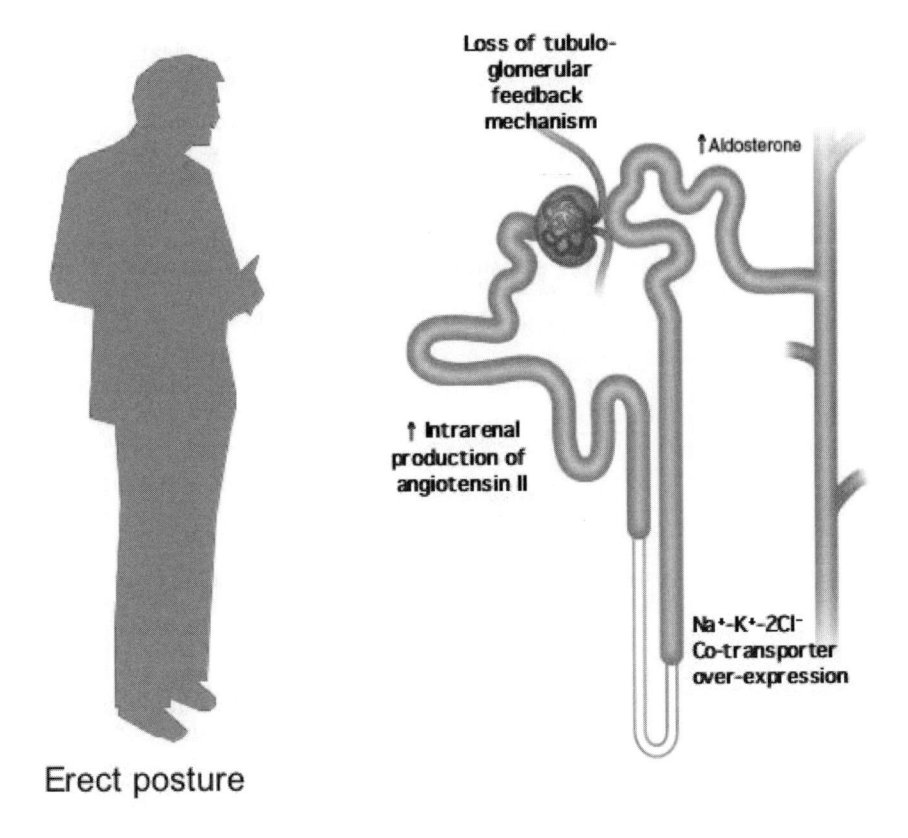

Figure 1 Summary of the proposed pathogenetic mechanisms that lead to subtle sodium retention in pre-ascitic cirrhosis

cirrhosis despite increased proximal renal sodium retention, and hence reduced distal delivery[9], and this may also contribute to the sodium retention observed with posture change in these patients.

More recently, the loop of Henle has also been shown to be involved in sodium retention in pre-ascitic cirrhosis. In animal models of pre-ascitic cirrhosis, there is hypertrophy of the thick ascending limb of the loop of Henle, associated with an increase in the expression of Na^+-K^+-$2Cl^-$ cotransporter, which is involved with sodium reabsorption at that site[10,11]. Calcium is an inhibitor of the Na^+-K^+-$2Cl^-$ cotransporter. Pre-ascitic cirrhotic patients, when given intravenous calcium, were able to increase their renal sodium excretion and urinary volume[12] significantly more compared to controls, confirming the involvement of the loop of Henle in renal sodium retention in these patients. Calcium also decreases norepinephrine release, and this may also contribute to the increased renal sodium excretion associated with calcium, as norepinephrine is known to stimulate renal sodium retention along the proximal renal tubule[13] and at the thick ascending limb of Henle's

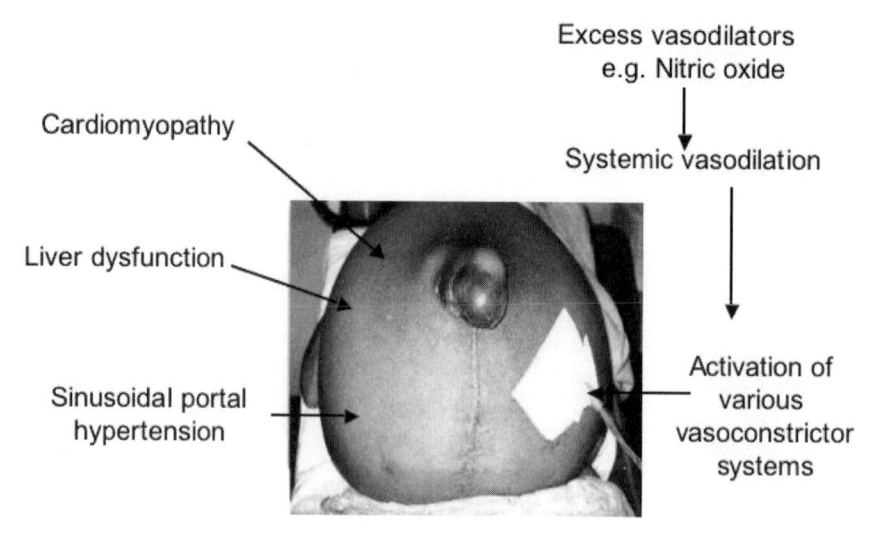

Figure 2 Summary of the proposed pathogenetic mechanisms that lead to avid sodium retention in ascitic cirrhosis

loop[14]. Thus, calcium could potentially be used in the management of the subtle sodium retention in pre-ascitic cirrhosis, although this is yet to be studied.

Ascitic cirrhosis

Sodium retention at the ascitic stage of cirrhosis is the result of the interplay of many pathophysiological changes (Figure 2). All the pathogenetic factors that are operational at the pre-ascitic stage of the disease are present at the ascitic stage of cirrhosis. In addition, ascitic patients have systemic arterial vasodilation and effective arterial underfilling, which worsens as the cirrhotic process progresses. There is activation of various compensatory neurohumoral vasoconstrictor mechanisms in an attempt to correct this effective arterial underfilling. These mechanisms also affect the renal circulation and renal tubular function to promote renal sodium and water retention[15]. Aside from the haemodynamic changes, there are many other factors that promote sodium and water retention in patients with cirrhosis and ascites. For example, a threshold of 50% reduction in liver function was identified below which sodium retention and ascites formation would occur[16], although for every patient who has a 50% reduction in hepatic function, the extent of sodium retention will vary[16]. The sinusoidal portal pressure in ascitic cirrhotic patients frequently continues to rise due to ongoing liver necrosis and fibrosis. An increase in sinusoidal portal pressure stimulates an intrahepatic baroreceptor, which in turn activates the afferent hepatic nerves, followed by activation of the efferent renal nerves with increased sympathetic nervous activity to the kidneys. Transection of either the hepatic nerves or the renal nerves abolishes this hepatorenal reflex[17]. Indeed, acute creation of sinusoidal portal hypertension in cirrhosis by blocking a functioning transjugular intrahepatic portosystemic shunt (TIPS) with an angioplasty balloon was associated with an acute reduction in renal blood flow, and release of the angioplasty balloon with reduction of sinusoidal portal hypertension returned the renal blood flow to baseline levels[18]. The fact that lumbar sympathetic blockade in patients with cirrhosis, ascites and hepatorenal syndrome was able to increase renal blood flow[19] would suggest that the renal sympathetic activity is indeed implicated in the efferent arm of this hepatorenal reflex. Absence of sinusoidal portal hypertension post-TIPS in cirrhotic patients with previous ascites was associated with an increased renal sodium excretion following a saline load, even better than that observed in pre-ascitic cirrhotic patients, thereby confirming the role of sinusoidal portal hypertension in mediating sodium retention in cirrhosis[20].

There are many other factors that promote renal sodium and water retention in patients with cirrhosis and ascites. The recently recognized entity known as cirrhotic cardiomyopathy can contribute to sodium retention in cirrhosis with ascites by reducing the 'effective' circulatory volume further, secondary to reduced contractile function (systolic incompetence), or increased myocardial stiffness (diastolic dysfunction) due to myocardial hypertrophy, or both. Perhaps the link between cirrhotic cardiomyopathy and sodium retention may be through a defect in α-adrenoreceptor function, possibly inherent to cirrhosis[21]. Various other vasoactive factors such as nitric oxide, endothelins and tumour necrosis factor alpha may contribute to renal sodium and water retention in patients with cirrhosis and ascites by affecting systemic and renal haemodynamics. Tumour necrosis factor alpha appears to act via stimulation of nitric oxide, a potent vasodilator which worsens the systemic arterial vasodilation of advanced cirrhosis[22]. Endothelins are potent vasoconstrictors, which may adversely affect renal perfusion and sodium handling leading to an exacerbation of ascites[23]. It is difficult to distinguish for any particular patient which pathogenetic factor predominates. Eventually, all of these lead to progressive renal vasoconstriction, enhanced proximal renal sodium reabsorption and reduced distal sodium delivery, and the patient evolves through the stages of responsive ascites, refractory ascites and finally hepatorenal syndrome.

THE STAGE OF REFRACTORY ASCITES

Refractory ascites is defined as a prolonged history of ascites unresponsive to 400 mg of spironolactone or 30 mg of amiloride plus up to 160 mg of furosemide daily for 2 weeks while on a sodium-restricted diet of 50 mmol or less per day. Patients who cannot tolerate diuretics because of side-effects are also regarded as diuretic-resistant[2] (Table 1). Patients are no longer responsive to diuretic treatment because there is insufficient sodium being delivered to the sites of diuretic action, namely the loop of Henle and distal convoluted tubule. This is due to avid sodium reabsorption at the proximal renal tubule, which in turn is due to reduced renal blood flow and decreased glomerular filtration,

Table 1 Definition of refractory ascites (adapted from ref. 2)

Failure to lose weight of $\geqslant 1.5$ kg/week while on:
400 mg spironolactone per day
or
30 mg amiloride per day
plus
160 mg furosemide per day for more than 2 weeks
and
dietary sodium restriction of $\leqslant 50$ mmol/day

---

secondary to renal vasoconstriction. Therefore, treatment for refractory ascites is aimed at either removing the ascites (repeat large volume paracentesis), which does not affect any of the underlying pathogenetic mechanisms, or correcting one or more of the many pathogenetic mechanisms of sodium retention. Non-pharmacological treatments of ascites include insertion of a TIPS, which reduces the sinusoidal portal pressure; or liver transplantation, which will correct the liver dysfunction and sinusoidal portal hypertension, as well as the abnormal haemodynamics associated with advanced cirrhosis. However, not all cirrhotic patients with ascites will be suitable for TIPS placement. Liver transplantation is a scarce resource that is available to a selected few; therefore, recent efforts have been made to evaluate other effective therapies for the management of refractory ascites, since repeat large-volume paracenteses are inconvenient and time-consuming both for the patient and the physician, as well as being associated with various side-effects[24].

THE USE OF ALBUMIN IN REFRACTORY ASCITES

Albumin is the most abundant plasma protein in healthy individuals, but in patients with refractory ascites, hypoalbuminaemia is common due to liver dysfunction. Albumin infusions have been used to prevent the development of circulatory dysfunction and hence renal failure associated with large-volume paracentesis in these patients for at least two decades[25]. The rationale for using albumin in this setting is to take advantage of its volume-expanding property, since patients with ascites have a reduction in their effective arterial blood volume[26,27]. However, recently, albumin has been found to have other properties that could potentially be beneficial to the cirrhotic patient with ascites. Albumin has been shown to have ligand-binding, anti-oxidant, anti-inflammatory and endothelial stabilizing properties[28], all of which help in improving the haemodynamics in cirrhotic patients with ascites; therefore albumin has also been used in settings other than those associated with large-volume paracentesis. For example, albumin has been used as an adjunct therapy in addition to diuretics in the management of ascites in cirrhosis. The chronic use of albumin, at the dose of 25 g/week for 1 year, followed by 25 g every 2 weeks, in addition to standard diuretics, has been shown to significantly improve the diuretic response in cirrhotic patients with ascites[29]. In addition, the possibility of ascites re-accumulation (Figure 3a), as well as hospital readmission for the treatment of ascites, were significantly less in those who received the combination of albumin plus diuretics when compared to those who received diuretic alone[29]. The same investigators have reported that, over a mean period of 84 months, patients who received chronic albumin infusion had a better cumulative survival[30] (Figure 3b). The survival of these patients was extended by 16 months. In another study in patients with refractory ascites, the use of albumin, at a dose of 50 g/week for 8 weeks, resulted in a significant decrease in water weight, hence their ascites, without changing their liver or renal function, or the Model of End-Stage Liver Disease (MELD) score[31]. Whether the use of albumin impacted the survival of these patients was not

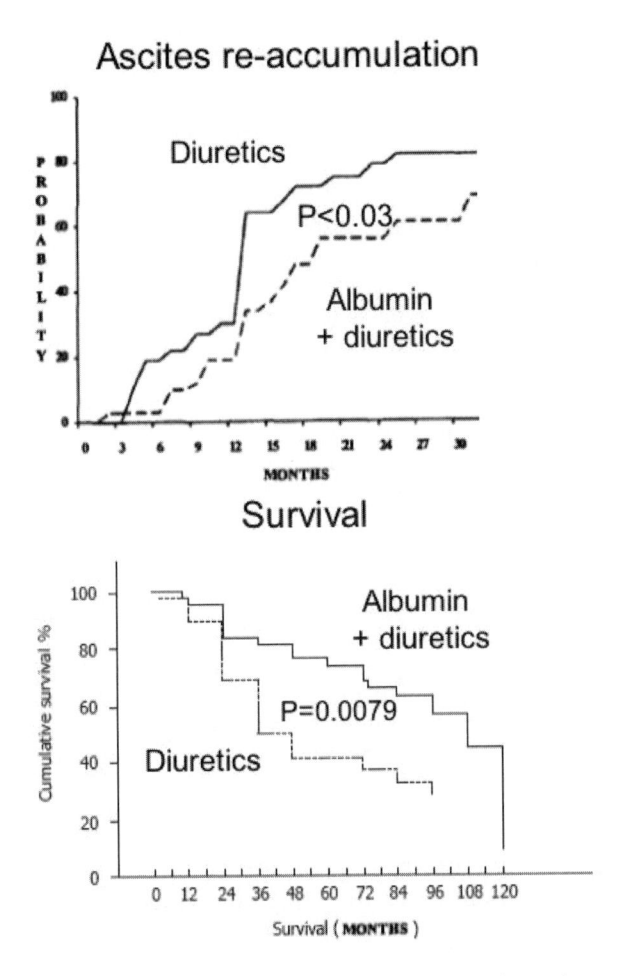

Figure 3 Probability of ascites re-accumulation and survival in patients who receive long-term albumin infusion in addition to diuretics versus those who received diuretics alone (reprinted from ref. 29 with permission of Elsevier and ref. 30 with permission of World J Gastroenterol., respectively)

assessed. The cost of albumin in certain countries can be enormous, and it is not universally available. There is the associated manpower cost in administering the albumin; therefore, before albumin is established as the standard adjunct therapy in addition to diuretics in the management of ascites, this 'new' indication for albumin use will have to await the results of definitive randomized controlled trials.

VASOACTIVE AGENTS

Since one of the pathogenetic mechanisms in the development of ascites in cirrhosis is a reduction of the effective arterial blood volume secondary to systemic arterial vasodilation, it stands to reason that agents such as systemic vasoconstrictors, by reducing the extent of arterial vasodilation, should be able to improve the effective arterial circulation, with possible beneficial effects on the renal circulation. In a study of 12 cirrhotic patients with bleeding oesophageal varices, with ascites ($n = 5$) or without ascites ($n = 7$), the use of a intravenous single dose of 2 mg of terlipressin, a potent systemic vasoconstrictor, resulted in significant improvement in systemic haemodynamics[32]. The systemic vascular resistance, and hence the mean arterial pressure, increased. The hyperdynamic circulation consequent upon the presence of systemic arterial vasodilation also improved. However, there were no measurements of renal haemodynamics. Renal sodium excretion improved in the non-ascitic, but not the ascitic patients. In a special subgroup of cirrhotic patients with refractory ascites and type 2 hepatorenal syndrome, the use of terlipressin at the dose of 1 mg 4-hourly for 7 days resulted in an improvement of renal haemodynamics without improvement of renal sodium excretion[33]. Whether the longer-term use of terlipressin in cirrhotic patients with ascites but without renal dysfunction will improve renal sodium excretion remains to be studied.

Midodrine is an orally active alpha-agonist, which has been widely used in the treatment of hypotensive disorders unrelated to cirrhosis. It was postulated that the same alpha-agonist effect could also be used to improve systemic arterial pressure in cirrhosis. In a study involving 17 patients with cirrhosis and ascites, a single oral dose of 15 mg of midodrine was able to increase the systemic vascular resistance, and the mean arterial blood pressure, together with an improvement in the hyperdynamic circulation in these patients[34]. Both the renal blood flow and the glomerular filtration rate increased, associated with a significant increase in urinary sodium excretion. Plasma renin activity and plasma vasopressin levels decreased significantly after the administration of midodrine, confirming better filling of the effective arterial circulation. All of these changes were maintained for up to 6 h after midodrine administration[34]. The same beneficial results were also observed in another cohort of cirrhotic patients with ascites after they were given 7 days of midodrine at a dose of 10 mg three times a day[35] (Figure 4). Moreover, there was a significant correlation between the increase in systemic vascular resistance and the increase in glomerular filtration rate, and the increase in renal sodium excretion. That is, the more the systemic circulation becomes vasoconstricted, the better the renal

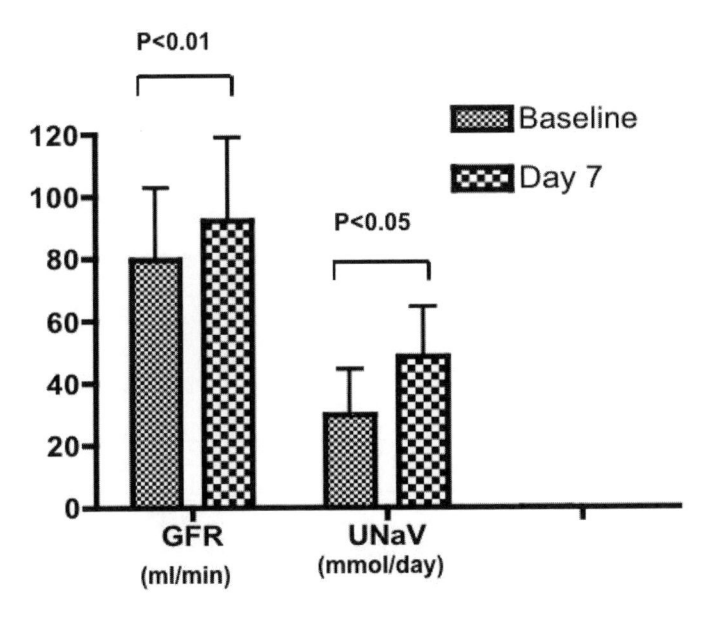

Figure 4 Renal effects of 7 days of midodrine at 7.5 mg t.i.d. in cirrhotic patients with ascites (data obtained from ref. 35)

haemodynamics and the greater the renal excretion of sodium. Suppression of activities of the various vasoconstrictor systems was also observed. It is interesting that the improvement in systemic haemodynamics and renal function in this study did not occur until 3 days after the patients had started the midodrine, whereas the study previously mentioned[34] noted a positive haemodynamic response 3 h after administration of midodrine. This may be related to the different dosing regiments used in these two studies. Currently, there are no data on the long-term effects of midodrine. It is also unclear whether the use of midodrine could have an additive effect to diuretics in effecting an increased renal sodium excretion.

AQUARETIC AGENTS

Patients with refractory ascites often cannot tolerate diuretics because of the development of electrolyte abnormalities. The prevalence of hyponatraemia in patients with ascites has been estimated to be almost 50%[36]. When this occurs, the management of ascites becomes problematic, as continued use of diuretics tends to reduce the effective arterial blood volume further and exaggerate the hyponatraemia. The recent advent of aquaretic agents, collectively known as 'vaptans', which act selectively at the renal collecting duct to block the action of vasopressin, has proven to be most useful in correcting hyponatraemia in

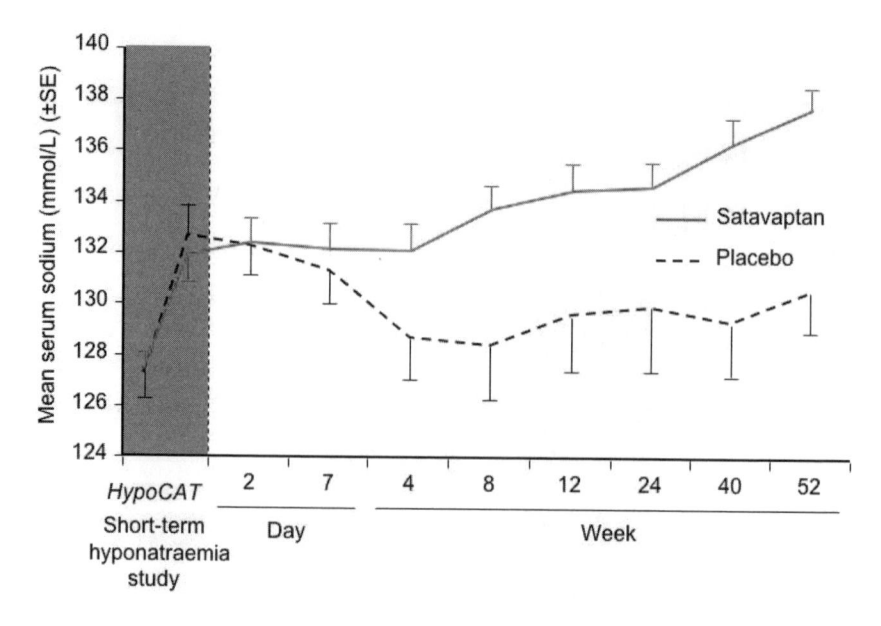

Figure 5 Long-term effects of satavaptan on serum sodium concentration in cirrhotic patients with ascites and hyponatraemia while on diuretic therapy (data obtained from ref. 39)

conditions of water excess including cirrhosis[37,38]. The long-term use of one of these agents, satavaptan of 5–25 mg over a 12-month period, in patients with hyponatraemia, not only corrected the hyponatraemia, it also allowed for the maintenance of normal serum sodium concentrations despite continued use of diuretics[39] (Figure 5). These vaptan agents are not yet available for commercial use; however, it is envisaged that these agents will convert some of the cirrhotic patients with diuretic-resistant ascites into diuretic-responsive ascites, as hyponatraemia will no longer be a barrier to continued use of diuretic therapy.

In cirrhotic patients with ascites and minimal hyponatraemia (serum sodium >130 mmol/L), the short-term and medium-term use of satavaptan has also been shown to be effective in reducing ascites. In a 2-week study involving 148 mostly normonatraemic cirrhotic patients with ascites, the use of various doses (5–25 mg) of satavaptan for 2 weeks was associated with a significant reduction in body weight of approximately 2 kg, together with a significant reduction in abdominal girth, compared to no change in either parameter in patients who were on placebo[40]. The use of the same doses of satavaptan for 12 weeks in cirrhotic patients with ascites who required frequent large-volume paracentesis in addition to standard doses of diuretics resulted in a reduction in the volume of ascites accumulated per week, together with a prolongation of the time to first paracentesis after starting the first dose of satavaptan, leading to a significant reduction in the cumulative number of paracenteses over the 12-week period ($p<0.05$ for all doses of satavaptan)[41] (Figure 6). These results

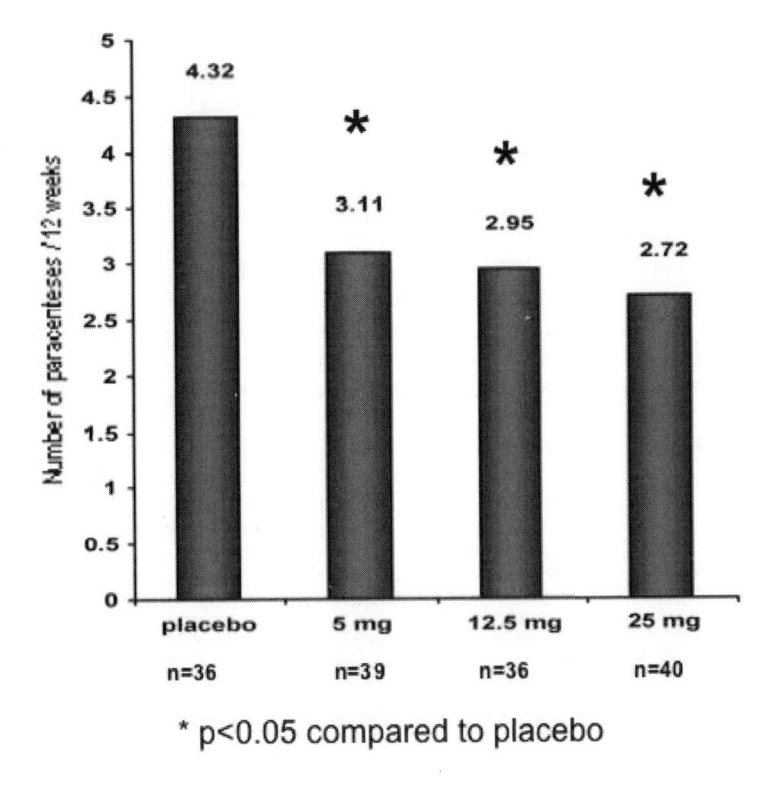

Figure 6 Mean number of paracenteses in cirrhotic patients with ascites while taking diuretics plus satavaptan versus diuretics plus placebo (data obtained from ref. 41)

suggest that the vaptans, apart from improving serum sodium concentrations in cirrhosis, may also be beneficial in the control of ascites in these patients. If confirmed in the currently ongoing phase III clinical trials, the vaptans could represent a novel pharmacological agent in the management of ascites in advanced cirrhosis.

SUMMARY

The understanding of the pathophysiology leading to the development of ascites in advanced cirrhosis in recent years has helped to improve the management of these patients. The advent of living-related liver transplantation means that more and more of these patients will need to be optimized to receive a liver transplant. Sodium restriction remains the mainstay of treatment for ascites, as reducing the sodium intake can reduce the rate of ascites accumulation, thus making it easier for a natriuretic effect with diuretics. Regular administration of albumin on a long-term basis can improve the natriuretic response of diuretics. In patients with diuretic-responsive ascites, albumin can also improve survival. The use of vasoconstrictor to improve system haemodynamics makes physiological sense, but it appears that not all vasoconstrictors are equally effective. Furthermore, there are no long-term data on the use of vasoconstrictors and further studies are needed before they can be established as an adjunct therapy for ascites. Finally, vasopressin receptor antagonists hold promise as the next class of drugs that can improve the management of cirrhotic ascites. These are aquaretic agents that can improve serum sodium concentrations in cirrhotic patients with ascites and hyponatraemia, thus permitting the continued use of diuretics. Aquaretic agents have also been shown to reduce ascites independent of their effects on serum sodium concentrations, and therefore may potentiate the effects of diuretics in achieving better control of ascites.

References

1. D'Amico G, Garcia-Tsao G, Pagliaro L. Natural history and prognostic indicators of survival in cirrhosis: a systemic review of 118 studies. J Hepatol. 2006;44:217–31.
2. Moore KP, Wong F, Gines P et al. The management of ascites – report on the consensus conference of the International Ascites Club. Hepatology. 2003;38:258–66.
3. Wong F, Liu P, Blendis LM. Sodium homeostasis with chronic sodium loading in pre-ascitic cirrhosis. Gut. 2001;49:847–51.
4. Wong F, Sniderman K, Blendis LM. The renal sympathetic and renin–angiotensin response to lower body negative pressure in well-compensated cirrhosis. Gastroenterology. 1998;115:397–405.
5. Wong F, Liu P, Blendis LM. The mechanism of improved sodium homeostasis of low-dose losartan in pre-ascitic cirrhosis. Hepatology. 2002;35:1449–58.
6. Schepke M, Wiest R, Flacke S et al. Irbesartan plus low-dose propranolol versus propranolol alone in cirrhosis: a placebo-controlled double-blind study. Am J Gastroenterol. 2008 (In press).
7. Bernardi M, Di Marco C, Trevisani F et al. Renal sodium retention during upright posture in preascitic cirrhosis. Gastroenterology. 1993;105:188–93.
8. Gentilini P, Romanelli RG, Laffi G et al. Cardiovascular and renal function in normotensive and hypertensive patients with compensated cirrhosis: effects of posture. J Hepatol. 1999;30:632–8.
9. Sansoe G, Biava AM, Silvano S et al. Renal tubular events following passage from the supine to the standing position in patients with compensated liver cirrhosis: loss of tubuloglomerular feedback. Gut. 2002;51:736–41.
10. Jonassen TE, Marcussen N, Haugan K et al. Functional and structural changes in the thick ascending limb of Henle's loop in rats with liver cirrhosis. Am J Physiol. 1997;273:R568–72.
11 Fernandez-Llama P, Ageloff S, Fernandez-Varo G et al. Sodium retention in cirrhotic rats is associated with increased renal abundance of sodium transporter proteins. Kidney Int. 2005;67:622–30.
12. Sansoe G, Wong F. Natriuretic and aquaretic effects of intravenous calcium in pre-ascitic cirrhosis: a pathophysiological study. Gut. 2007;56:1117–23.
13. Simón MA, Díez J, Prieto J. Abnormal sympathetic and renal response to sodium restriction in compensated cirrhosis. Gastroenterology. 1991;101:1354–60.
14. Bailly C. Transducing pathways involved in the control of NaCl reabsorption in the thick ascending limb of Henle's loop. Kidney Int. 1998;53(Suppl. 65):S29–35.
15. Schrier RW, Arroyo V, Bernardi M, Epstein M, Henriksen JH, Rodes J. Peripheral arterial vasodilation hypothesis: a proposal for the initiation of renal sodium and water retention in cirrhosis. Hepatology. 1988;8:1151–7.

16. Wensing G, Lotterer E, Link I, Hahn EG, Fleig WE. Urinary sodium balance in patients with cirrhosis: relationship to quantitative parameters of liver function. Hepatology. 1997;26:1149–55.
17. Kostreva DR, Castaner A, Kampine JP. Reflex effects of hepatic baroreceptors on renal and cardiac sympathetic nerve activity. Am J Physiol. 1980;238:R390–4.
18. Jalan R, Forrest EH, Redhead DN, Dillon JF, Hayes PC. Reduction in renal blood flow following acute increase in the portal pressure: evidence for the existence of a hepatorenal reflex in man? Gut. 1997;40:664–70.
19. Solis-Herruzo JA, Duran A, Favela V et al. Effects of lumbar sympathetic block on kidney function in cirrhotic patients with hepatorenal syndrome. J Hepatol. 1987;5:167–73.
20. Jalan R, Hayes PC. Sodium handling in patients with well-compensated cirrhosis is dependent on the severity of liver disease and portal pressure. Gut. 2000;46:527–33.
21. Ma Z, Miyamoto A, Lee SS. Role of altered beta-adrenoceptor signal transduction in the pathogenesis of cirrhotic cardiomyopathy in rats. Gastroenterology. 1996;110:1191–8.
22. Kilbourn RG, Gross SS, Jubran A et al. NG-methyl-L-arginine inhibits tumor necrosis factor-induced hypotension: implications for the involvement of nitric oxide. Proc Natl Acad Sci USA. 1990;87:3629–32.
23. Bernardi M, Gulberg V, Colantoni A, Trevisani F, Gasbarrini A, Gerbes AL. Plasma endothelin-1 and -3 in cirrhosis: relationship with systemic hemodynamics, renal function and neurohumoral systems. J Hepatol. 1996;24:161–8.
24. Thomsen TW, Shaffer RW, White B, Setnik GS. Videos in clinical medicine: paracentesis. N Engl J Med. 2006;355:e21.
25. Gines P, Arroyo V, Quintero E et al. Comparison of paracentesis and diuretics in the treatment of cirrhosis with tense ascites. Result of a randomized study. Gastroenterology. 1987;93:234–41.
26. Wong F, Legault L, Tobe S, Skorecki K, Logan AG, Blendis LM. Refractory ascites in cirrhosis: the roles of volume expansion and plasma atrial natriuretic factor elevation. Hepatology. 1993;18:519–28.
27. Wong F, Sniderman K, Liu P, Allidina Y, Sherman M, Blendis LM. The effects of transjugular intrahepatic portosystemic shunt on systemic and renal hemodynamics and sodium homeostasis in cirrhotic patients with refractory ascites. Ann Intern Med. 1995;122:816–22.
28. Wong F. The role of albumin in the management of chronic liver disease. Nat Clin Pract Gastroenterol Hepatol. 2007;4:43–51.
29. Gentilini P, Casini-Raggi G, Di Fiore G et al. Albumin improves the response to diuretic in patients with cirrhosis and ascites. J Hepatol. 1999;30:639–45.
30. Romanelli RG, La Villa G, Barletta G et al. Long-term albumin infusion improves survival in patients with cirrhosis and ascites: an unblinded randomized trial. World J Gastroenterol. 2006;12:1403–7.
31. Trotter J Pieramici E, Everson GT. Chronic albumin infusions to achieve diuresis in patients with ascites who are not candidates for transjugular intrahepatic portosystemic shunt (TIPS). Dig Dis Sci. 2005;50:1356–60.
32. Kalambokis G, Economou M, Paraskevi K et al. Effects of somatostatin, terlipressin and somatostatin plus terlipressin on portal and systemic hemodynamics and renal sodium excretion in patients with cirrhosis. J Gastroenterol Hepatol. 2005;20:1075–81.
33. Alessandria C, Venon WD, Marzano A, Barletti C, Fadda M, Rizetto M. Renal failure in cirrhotic patients: role of terlipressin in clinical approach to hepatorenal syndrome type 2. Eur J Gastroenterol Hepatol. 2002;14:1363–8.
34. Angeli P, Volpin R, Piovan D et al. Acute effects of the oral administration of midodrine, an alpha-adrenergic agonist, on renal hemodynamics and renal function in cirrhotic patients with ascites. Hepatology. 1998;28:937–43.
35. Kalambokis G, Fotopoulos A, Economou M, Pappas K, Tsianos EV. Effects of a 7-day treatment with midodrine in non-azotemic cirrhotic patients with and without ascites. J Hepatol. 2007;46:213–21.
36. Angeli P, Wong F, Watson H, Gines P and the participants to the CAPPS study. Hyponatremia in cirrhosis: results of the Cirrhotic Ascites Patient Population Survey (CAPPS). Hepatology. 2006;44:1535–42.
37. Wong F, Blei A, Blendis LM, Robertson G, Thuluvath PJ, and the North American VPA-985 Study Group. The effects of VPA-985, a vasopressin receptor antagonist, on water

metabolism in patients with hyponatremia: a multi-center randomized placebo controlled trial. Hepatology. 2003;37:182–91.
38. Gerbes AL, Gülberg V, Ginès P et al.; VPA Study Group. Therapy of hyponatremia in cirrhosis with a vasopressin receptor antagonist: a randomized double-blind multicenter trial. Gastroenterology. 2003;124:933–9.
39. Gines P, Wong F, Watson H, for ExpoCAT Study Investigators. Long-term improvement of serum sodium by the V2-receptor antagonist satavaptan in patients with cirrhosis and hyponatremia. J Hepatol. 2007;41(Suppl. 1):S41 (Abstract).
40. Gines P, Wong F, Watson HR, Ruiz del Arbol LR, Bilic A, Dobru D. Effects of a selective vasopressin V2 receptor antagonist, satavaptan (SR121463B), in patients with cirrhosis and ascites without hyponatremia. Hepatology. 2006;44(Suppl. 1):445A (Abstract).
41. Wong F, Gines P, Watson H, Kujundzic M, Angeli P, Horsmans Y. Effects of a selective vasopressin V2 receptor antagonist, satavaptan (SR121463B), on recurrence of ascites after large volume paracentesis. Hepatology. 2006;44(Suppl. 1):256A (Abstract).

24
Transjugular intrahepatic portosystemic shunt versus paracentesis: a critical review of randomized studies and meta-analyses

M. RÖSSLE and W. EURINGER

INTRODUCTION

For the treatment of patients with refractory ascites mainly two options exist: large-volume paracentesis and the transjugular intrahepatic portosystemic shunt (TIPS). Five randomized studies have been published[1-5] showing worsened, comparable or improved survival with TIPS. This is surprising since the design and population of the five studies is comparable and results are relatively consistent in terms of other outcome variables such as ascites and hepatic encephalopathy. Looking at the four meta-analyses including these five studies[6-9], results were also different. This is even more surprising since the calculations were done on an identical body of data. The aim of this study was to discover potential reasons for the varying results of the five randomized studies (RCT) and to identify the causes for the inconsistent results of the meta-analyses. Our evaluation is limited to survival/mortality since this is not only the most important but also the most objective outcome parameter.

RANDOMIZED STUDIES

The 2-year probability of survival of the five RCT is shown in Table 1. Two studies, the French and the Spanish one, found a very poor survival of TIPS patients of <30% while survival was 58%, 62% and 79% in the other three studies. Similarly, two studies found a very good survival of paracentesis patients with about 60%, while the remaining three studies had a survival of only about 30%. Comparing the study groups, one study found an improved survival with paracentesis, two studies found an improved survival with TIPS,

Table 1 2-year survival rates of randomized studies

		2-year survival (%)	
Study	n	TIPS	Paracentesis
France 1996[1]	25	29	60
Germany 2000[2]	60	58	32
Spain/USA 2002[3]	70	26	30
USA/Canada 2003[4]	109	62	62
Italy 2004[5]	66	79	29

Table 2 Variables assessing technical quality of the TIPS intervention; the secondary patency rate is the patency achieved by shunt revision

	Technical success (%)	Reduction in portosystemic pressure gradient mmHg	Reduction in portosystemic pressure gradient (%)	Secondary patency rate (%)
France 1996	77	6	30	46
Germany 2000	100	14	58	93
Spain/USA 2002	97	10.4	54	91
USA/Canada 2003	94	11.5	58	>90
Italy 2004	89	13.8	61	82

and two studies found similar survival rates between the groups. What are the reasons for the differences in survival?

Technique

One reason for variable results may be differences in technical skills to perform the TIPS intervention, which is one of the most ambitious radiological interventions. Table 2 shows three technical quality parameters of the TIPS procedure: the success rate of the TIPS intervention, the degree of reduction of the portosystemic pressure gradient, and the rate of secondary patency. As shown, the French study published in 1996 differs considerably with respect to technical success (77%), reduction in pressure gradient (6 mmHg), and rate of secondary TIPS patency (46%). As demonstrated by D'Amico et al.[9] the technical variables correspond to the odds ratios for mortality, suggesting that technical disability was the reason for the poor outcome of the TIPS patients in the French study. D'Amico and coauthors therefore concluded that the French study should be regarded as an outlier.

Selection

Selection is the ratio of patients included to patients screened. As shown in Table 3 about 40–60% of patients screened were included with the exception of the American study. This study included only 21% of the source population. A more detailed look shows that inclusion varies from centre to centre with the laziest centre including only 11% and the busiest centre including 40%. Overall, from the 525 patients screened only 109 patients were included. Surprisingly, 180 patients, who were obviously eligible, disappeared. Without doubt, loss of most of the eligible patients has to be regarded as a severe selection bias influencing the result of the study[10].

Selection bias may also be due to unbalanced inclusion or exclusion criteria. Thus, the use of different thresholds for the bilirubin and creatinine concentrations may be a source of bias. Both parameters are equally important as markers for liver or kidney function. They are also similar in a quantitative aspect. A value of 1 represents good organ function and a value of 6 indicates failure requiring organ replacement or haemodialysis. Since the TIPS may worsen liver function (but improves kidney function) and the paracentesis worsens kidney function (but has no effect on liver function) one should request similar concentrations of bilirubin and creatinine to provide equal chances for the treatment arms and to avoid a selection bias. Table 4 shows that all studies disfavoured the TIPS groups by including patients with much higher bilrubin than creatinine concentrations. The Spanish study even included patients with a bilirubin concentration as high as 10 mg/dl, which

Table 3 Selection of patients in the five randomized studies; centres, patients included, patients per centre included, and percentage of patients selected

	No. of study centres and no. of patients included		Patients included per centre	Percentage of patients included (selection) (%)
France 1996	1	25	25	50
Germany 2000	2	60	20, 40	40
Spain/USA 2002	4	70	n.d.	59
USA/Canada 2003	6	109	7, 11, 12, 21, 22, 36	21 (11–40)
Italy 2004	3	66	n.d.	48

n.d. = not determined

Table 4 Inclusion and exclusion threshold values for bilirubin and creatinine concentrations

	Bilirubin (mg/dl)	Creatinine (mg/dl)
France 1996	n.d.	n.d.
Germany 2000	<5	<3
Spain/USA 2002	<10	<3
USA/Canada 2003	<5	<1.5
Italy 2004	<6	<3

n.d. = not determined

seems to be a clear contraindication for a portosystemic shunt. On the other hand, very low creatinine concentrations are a fine condition for paracentesis, providing a clear advantage for this arm. Based on these considerations the American study should be regarded as severely biased by selecting patients with an almost normal renal function but with severe liver dysfunction.

Analysis

In all studies survival/mortality was analysed according to the method described by Kaplan and Meier. However, studies differ in providing transplant-free survival (Table 5). The more patients being transplanted the more important will it be to assess transplant-free survival. This is particularly important when the time to transplantation differs between the groups. In the two studies where the time to transplantation is given, the TIPS patients had a much longer time to transplantation than the paracentesis patients. Considering this, it is incomprehensible that the American study did not present transplant-free survival, which would be a more appropriate measure to compare survival of the two treatment arms.

META-ANALYSES

Four meta-analyses are published so far and are summarized in Table 6. The first study[6] presents survival as percentages. A sophisticated statistical evaluation has not been performed and also a calculation of heterogeneity is lacking. Overall, this study is of insufficient quality and should be disregarded.

The second study[7] gives relative risks which are not identical to the commonly used odds ratios and comparison is therefore limited. Considering survival, significant heterogeneity between the studies was found but authors made no effort to investigate and eliminate its source. The presence of heterogeneity, however, prohibits the use of the data, because studies involved differ so much that combined statistical evaluation is not meaningful.

Table 5 Numbers and percentages of liver transplantation, time to transplantation and survival analysis

	Patients receiving transplantation		Time to transplantation (months)		Analysis of transplant-free survival
	TIPS	Paracentesis	TIPS	Paracentesis	
France 1996	0	0			No
Germany 2000	1	2	n.d.	n.d.	Yes
Spain/USA 2002	7	7	n.d.	n.d.	Yes
USA/Canada 2003	16	17	19.6	12.4	No
Italy 2004	4	4	20 ± 4	13 ± 4	Yes

n.d. = not determined

Table 6 Odds ratios, confidence intervals and heterogeneities of meta-analyses. Results vary in spite of identical data source

Reference	24-month mortality	Confidence interval	Heterogeneity POR (p-value)
Deltenre et al., 2005[6]	50% vs 42.8%	−10–23.6	n.d.
Albillos et al., 2005[7]	0.93 (RR)	0.67–1.28	(0.09)
D'Amico et al., 2005[9]	0.90 (POR)	0.44–1.82	9.2 (0.056)
	0.74*	0.40–1.37*	5.27 (0.15)*
Saab 2004[8]	1.26 (POR)	0.65–2.56	7.75 (0.1)

*Excluding Lebrec.

n.d. = not determined

Table 7 Transplant-free 1 and 2-year survival probabilities and estimated 12-month mortality according to various MELD scores after TIPS or paracentesis treatment. Data are derived from the meta-analysis of individual patient data[11]

	TIPS (%)	Paracentesis (%)
1-year survival	65	55
2-year survival	50	36
12-month mortality		
MELD 10	28	42
MELD 15	44	68
MELD 19	62	84

A third study comes from the Cochrane Institute[8]. This study is hampered by picking up wrong figures from the Italian publication[5]. They erroneously picked up the number of patients in study (TIPS 9 and paracentesis 5) instead of the number of patients who died (TIPS 14, paracentesis 23). This is why their odds ratio for survival differs from the other studies. They also found heterogeneity but made no effort to provide a meaningful result without it.

The remaining study, by D'Amico[9], found that the French study is the source of heterogeneity of survival. After defining this study as an outlier, and after its elimination, heterogeneity disappeared and actuarial rates of survival became different, favouring TIPS (POR 0.74).

META-ANALYSIS OF INDIVIDUAL PATIENT DATA

The study by D'Amico was the first to create reliable data for survival by eliminating heterogeneity. However, the inappropriate survival analysis in the American study[4] could not be corrected. This was overcome by Salerno et al.[11], who analysed individual patient data. The findings with respect to survival/mortality are reproduced in Table 7. By excluding the French study and analysing transplant-free survival the TIPS patients lived significantly longer than the patients receiving paracentesis. The TIPS also improves the estimated transplant-free survival in patients with higher Model for End-stage Liver Disease (MELD) scores, suggesting that even advanced patients benefit from this treatment.

CONCLUSIONS

RCT comparing TIPS and paracentesis are biased by technical disability, selection, and inappropriate survival analysis. Three of the four meta-analyses published are not meaningful because they delivered data originating from studies with significant heterogeneity. The meta-analysis which obtained homogeneity by excluding the outlier[9] found improved survival in the TIPS arm (POR 0.74). Furthermore, in the meta-analysis using individual patient data, the TIPS resulted in a significant improvement in transplant-free survival. Based on these findings, TIPS may now be regarded as the first-line treatment for refractory and recidivant ascites.

References

1. Lebrec D, Giuily N, Hadengue A et al. Transjugular intrahepatic portosystemic shunt: comparison with paracentesis in patients with cirrhosis and refractory ascites: a randomized trial. J Hepatol. 1996;25:135–44.
2. Rössle M, Ochs A, Gulberg V et al. A comparison of paracentesis and transjugular intrahepatic portosystemic shunting in patients with ascites. N Engl J Med. 2000;342:1701–7.
3. Ginès P, Uriz J, Calahorra B et al. Transjugular intrahepatic portosystemic shunting versus paracentesis plus albumin for refractory ascites in cirrhosis. Gastroenterology. 2002;123:1839–47.
4. Sanyal AJ, Genning C, Reddy KR et al. The North American Study for the treatment of refractory ascites. Gastroenterology. 2003;124:634–41.
5. Salerno F, Merli M, Riggio O et al., and GIST. Randomized controlled study of TIPS versus paracentesis plus albumin in cirrhosis with severe ascites. Hepatology. 2004;40:629–35.
6. Deltenre P, Mathurin P, Dharancy S et al. Transjugular intrahepatic portosystemic shunt in refractory ascites: a meta-analysis. Liver Int. 2005;25:349–56.
7. Albillos A, Banares R, Gonzalez M, Catalina MV, Molinero LM. A meta-analysis of transjugular intrahepatic portosystemic shunt versus paracentesis for refractory ascites. J Hepatol. 2005;43:990–6.
8. Saab S, Nieto JM, Ly D, Runyon BA. TIPS versus paracentesis for cirrhotic patients with refractory ascites. Cochrane Database Syst Rev 2004;3:CD004889.
9. D'Amico G, Luca A, Morabito A, Miraglia R, D'Amico M. Uncovered transjugular intrahepatic portosystemic shunt for refractory ascites: a meta-analysis. Gastroenterology. 2005;129:1282–93.
10. Rössle M. Discussion of the North American study for the treatment of refractory ascites. Gastroenterology. 2004;126:1214–15.
11. Salerno F, Camma C, Enea A, Rössle M, Wong F. Transjugular intrahepatic portosystemic shunt for refractory ascites: a meta-analysis of individual patient data. Gastroenterology. 2007;133:825–34.

25
Spontaneous bacterial peritonitis – a disease of the gut? Therapeutic implications

J. FERNÁNDEZ, A. CÁRDENAS and P. GINES

INTRODUCTION

Spontaneous bacterial peritonitis (SBP) is one of the most frequent complications in cirrhosis. It is defined as the infection of a previously sterile ascitic fluid without an apparent intra-abdominal source of infection[1]. Although the pathogenesis of this severe complication of cirrhosis is very complex, intestinal bacterial overgrowth and translocation of enteric bacteria from the intestinal lumen to the systemic circulation constitute two of the main mechanisms involved. The prevalence of SBP in cirrhotic patients with ascites admitted to the hospital ranges between 10% and 30%[2]. Diagnosis is established by paracentesis when the polymorphonuclear cell count in ascitic fluid is >250 cells/mm^3. During the past 25 years, the outcome of cirrhotic patients with SBP has dramatically improved with significant improvement in cure rates (90%) and hospital survival rates (70–90%)[1-3]. The aim of this chapter is to review the current knowledge on the pathophysiology and current treatment options in preventing and managing patients with SBP.

PATHOGENESIS

Colonization of the ascitic fluid from an episode of bacteraemia is the most accepted hypothesis that explains the pathogenesis of SBP[2,4]. Since most organisms causing SBP are Gram-negative bacteria of enteric origin[2,4], it is believed that passage of enteric organisms from the intestinal lumen to the systemic circulation plays a key role in the development of SBP. Bacterial translocation, or the process by which viable enteric bacteria normally present in the gastrointestinal lumen cross the enteric mucosa, colonize the mesenteric lymph nodes and reach the blood stream through the intestinal lymphatic circulation, plays a major role in the pathogenesis of SBP. Patients with advanced liver disease have an impaired reticuloendothelial system (RES) which facilitates the free passage of microorganisms from the intestinal lumen, skin, urinary and respiratory tracts to the systemic circulation[2]. Once bacteria reach the ascitic fluid the development of SBP depends on the antimicrobial capacity within the peritoneal fluid. Thus patients with cirrhosis and a decreased defensive capacity of ascitic fluid are prone to develop the infection.

Bacterial translocation

Bacterial translocation in cirrhosis may develop due to several factors; the most important are the presence of intestinal bacterial overgrowth with Gram-negative bacilli, an increase in gut permeability and decreased local and systemic immunity. Previous studies in carbon tetrachloride-induced cirrhotic rats with ascites have demonstrated an increased passage of bacteria from the intestinal lumen to extraintestinal sites, including regional lymph nodes and the systemic circulation[5-11]. The simultaneous presence of intestinal bacterial overgrowth and alterations in the permeability of the intestinal barrier is probably required for bacterial translocation to occur and spread to mesenteric lymph nodes[6,7] (Figure 1). The alteration in gut permeability could be partially due to portal hypertension that causes marked oedema and inflammation in the submucosa of the caecum, as has been demonstrated in cirrhotic rats with ascites[10]. Circumstances decreasing mucosal blood flow

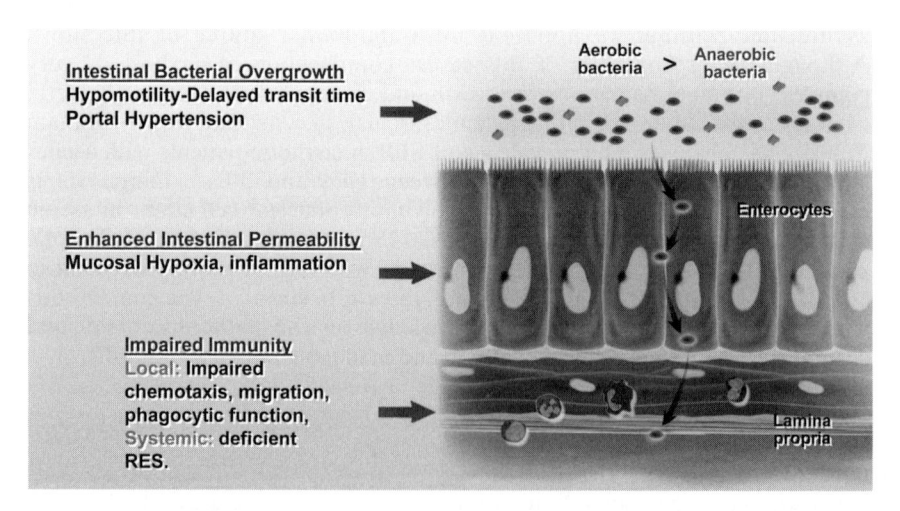

Figure 1 The three mechanisms involved in bacterial translocation include bacterial overgrowth, enhanced intestinal permeability and impared immunity. Although anaerobic bacteria outnumber aerobic bacteria in the intestinal lumen, it is aerobic Gram-negative bacteria that translocate across an intact intestinal epithelium. Bacterial overgrowth (aerobic bacteria) occurs in cirrhosis and seems to be due to delayed small bowel motility. In cirrhosis there are structural and functional alterations in the intestinal mucosa that may increase permeability to bacteria. Finally, for bacterial translocation to lead to a systemic/local inflammatory response or infection, a failure of local and systemic immune defences should also be present. Reprinted with permission from Garcia-Tsao and Wiest. Best Pract Res Clin Gastroenterol. 2004;18:353

such as haemorrhagic shock or sepsis, two frequent events in cirrhotic patients, also increase gut permeability[11]. An increase in aerobic Gram-negative bacilli in the intestinal flora of cirrhotic patients has also been demonstrated in the jejunal flora of cirrhotic patients[6]. Bacterial overgrowth is probably due to intestinal hypomotility caused by the sympathetic overactivity characteristic in advanced cirrhosis[7]. This change in the intestinal flora facilitates the passage of aerobic Gram-negative bacteria across the intestine and further spread into the blood stream (Figure 1). Finally, bacterial translocation seems to be related to the presence of ascites and to the degree of hepatic insufficiency, since it is significantly increased in Child C patients[12].

Depression of activity of the reticuloendothelial system

Although the RES is widely distributed throughout the body, approximately 90% of this defensive system is in the liver, where Kupffer cells and endothelial sinusoidal cells are its major components[13]. Cirrhotic patients may have a depressed RES function. Intrahepatic shunting and a reduction in the phagocytic capacity of monocytes, the Kupffer cell precursors, contribute to the impairment of the phagocytic activity of the RES observed in cirrhosis[13-15]. Moreover, serum opsonic activity is also markedly reduced in most cirrhotic patients, probably as a consequence of a decreased serum concentration of complement and fibronectin. Survival and the risk of bacteraemia and SBP in cirrhosis are directly related to the degree of RES dysfunction[16,17].

Decreased opsonic activity of ascitic fluid

The non-specific antimicrobial capacity of ascitic fluid in cirrhosis varies greatly from patient to patient and this variability may be involved in the pathogenesis of SBP. There is an inverse significant correlation between the opsonic activity of ascitic fluid and the risk of developing SBP[18]. The opsonic activity of ascitic fluid is directly correlated with the total protein level in ascites and with the concentration of defensive substances, such as immunoglobulins, leucocytes, complement, and fibronectin[18-24]. The concentration of total protein in ascitic fluid correlates directly with the risk of developing SBP. The probabilities of developing SBP during hospital stay and during the first year of follow-up, 15% and 20% respectively, are significantly greater in patients with low protein concentration in ascitic fluid (<10 g/L)[19,21,22]. This variation in the antimicrobial properties of ascites could be related to: (a) the serum levels of the defensive proteins involved in antibacterial mechanisms of ascitic fluid; (b) the degree of portal hypertension and hepatic insufficiency; and (c) the volume of water diluting ascitic fluid solutes. This last possibility is supported by the finding that diuretics increase the total protein concentration and the antibacterial capacity of ascites, and by the common observation in clinical practice that SBP occurs predominantly in cirrhotic patients with large-volume ascites.

Iatrogenic factors

Some procedures disrupt the natural defensive barriers and therefore predispose to infection in cirrhosis. Endoscopic sclerotherapy for bleeding oesophageal varices, particularly emergency sclerotherapy, is associated with bacteraemia (incidence ranging from 5% to 30%); however, this is transient and prophylactic antibiotics are not recommended[25]. Other invasive procedures commonly performed in patients with cirrhosis – such as diagnostic or therapeutic paracentesis, variceal band ligation, percutaneous ethanol injection or transcatheter arterial embolization – also have a very low risk of clinically relevant infections, and prophylactic antibiotics are not recommended. At present, antibiotic prophylaxis with first- or second-generation cephalosporins is advised only prior to transjugular intrahepatic portosystemic shunt insertion or surgical intervention[3].

DIAGNOSIS

Clinical characteristics

The clinical presentation of SBP depends on the stage at which the infection is diagnosed. Some patients present signs or symptoms clearly suggestive of peritoneal infection, but others, especially in the initial stages of the infection, are asymptomatic. Abdominal pain and fever are the most frequent symptoms. Diarrhoea, vomiting, ileus, hepatic encephalopathy, gastrointestinal bleeding, and renal impairment are other possible clinical signs or symptoms of the infection[1,2]. Early diagnosis of SBP relies on the performance of diagnostic paracentesis at hospital admission in all cirrhotic patients with ascites, and in hospitalized patients with ascites with deterioration of the clinical status[1].

Laboratory and microbiological data

The diagnosis of SBP is based on clinical suspicion and on ascitic fluid analysis by paracentesis. An ascitic fluid polymorphonuclear (PMN) count >250 cells/mm^3 is considered diagnostic of SBP and constitutes an indication to empirically initiate antibiotic treatment[1,2]. The measurement of lactic dehydrogenase concentration, glucose levels and total protein concentration in ascitic fluid may be helpful in establishing a differential diagnosis when secondary peritonitis is being considered. Secondary peritonitis should be suspected when at least two of the following features are present in ascitic fluid: glucose levels <50 mg/dl, protein concentration >10 g/L, lactic dehydrogenase concentration > normal serum levels. Gram's stain of a smear of sediment obtained after centrifugation of ascitic fluid is frequently negative in SBP, as the concentration of bacteria is usually low (one organism per millilitre or less). Nevertheless, it may be helpful in identifying patients with gut perforation in whom multiple types of bacteria can be seen[1]. Table 1 shows the most common organisms responsible for SBP.

Table 1 Bacteria responsible for spontaneous bacterial peritonitis (percentages)

Culture positive SBP	40–65
Gram-negative bacilli	31–50
E. coli	25–37
Klebsiella spp.	2–6
Enterobacter spp.	1–2
Others	3–7
Gram-positive cocci	8–17
Streptococcus pneumoniae	1–10
Other streptococci	6
Staphylococcus aureus	1
Culture-negative SBP	35–60

Table 2 Antibiotic therapy and spontaneous bacterial peritonitis outcome

Antibiotic	Resolution rate (%)	Hospital survival (%)
Cefotaxime (i.v.)		
2 g/12 h	79	79
2 g/8 h for 5 days	93	67
2 g/8 h for 10 days	91	58
Ceftriaxone (i.v.)	91	70
Cefonicid (i.v.)	94	63
Amoxicillin- clavulanic acid (i.v.)	85	63
Aztreonam (i.v.)	71	57
Ofloxacin (oral)	84	81

i.v. = intravenous.

TREATMENT

Antibiotic regimen

Antibiotic therapy must be started immediately after the diagnosis of SBP is established. Third-generation cephalosporins are considered the empirical antibiotic of choice in the treatment of SBP[1,2,26–31]. However, other antibiotics such as amoxicillin-clavulanic acid are also effective[32,33]. Quinolones should not be employed in the treatment of SBP in patients on long-term norfloxacin prophylaxis since in these patients there is an increased risk of developing infections caused by quinolone-resistant bacteria[3]. Table 2 shows the outcome of SBP depending on the antibiotic therapy employed.

Intravenous albumin infusion

Intravenous albumin (1.5 g/kg of body weight at the time of diagnosis, followed by 1 g/kg of body weight on day 3) reduces the incidence of renal impairment (33% vs 10%) and improves hospital survival (29% vs 10%) in

SBP[34]. Patients with abnormal renal or hepatic function at diagnosis of the infection (BUN >30 mg/dl and/or creatinine >1.0 mg/dl and/or bilirubin >4 mg/dl) clearly benefit from administration of albumin. The usefulness of albumin administration in patients with normal baseline renal and hepatic function is doubtful, since the incidence of renal impairment in this subgroup is low in both treatment groups (7% and 0%). A recent study suggests that albumin cannot be substituted by artificial plasma expanders in SBP[35].

Since renal dysfunction results from an aggravation in vasodilation and a decrease in effective arterial blood volume, the use of diuretics and large-volume paracentesis should probably be avoided during SBP, but information on this issue is not available[36].

Liver transplantation

SBP carries a very poor prognosis. The 1-year and 2-year probability of survival after an episode of SBP is 30–50% and 25–30%, respectively[2]. Therefore, patients recovering from an episode of SBP should be considered as potential candidates for liver transplantation.

PROPHYLAXIS

Antibiotic prophylaxis in cirrhosis should be restricted to selected patients at a high risk for the developmnent of SBP. Current indications of antibiotic prophylaxis are shown in Table 3.

Gastrointestinal bleeding

Cirrhotic patients with upper gastrointestinal haemorrhage are predisposed to develop SBP and other severe bacterial infections during or immediately after the bleeding episode. Approximately 20% are already infected at admission and 50% develop infections during the first days of hospitalization in the absence of antibiotic prophylaxis[1].

Because most bacteria causing infections are of enteric origin, the initial investigations addressed the effectiveness of oral intestinal decontamination in these patients. Two randomized, controlled studies demonstrated that selective intestinal decontamination with norfloxacin or a combination of oral non-absorbable antibiotics is effective in preventing SBP and other infections in cirrhotic patients with gastrointestinal haemorrhage[37,38]. The role of systemic antibiotics in this setting has also been investigated in four controlled studies. Ofloxacin, ofloxacin plus amoxicillin-clavulanic acid (before each endoscopy), ciprofloxacin plus amoxicillin-clavulanic acid, and oral ciprofloxacin were the antibiotics evaluated in these studies[39–42]. The incidence of bacterial infections was significantly lower in the treated groups (10–20%) than in the corresponding control groups (45–66%). A meta-analysis including all but one of these studies showed a significant improvement in survival in the group of patients receiving antibiotic prophylaxis[43]. Based on all these data current guidelines strongly recommend antibiotic prophylaxis in all cirrhotic patients

Table 3 Current indications of SBP prophylaxis in cirrhosis

Indication	Type	Duration of prophylaxis
Cirrhotic patients recovering from a previous episode of SBP	Norfloxacin 400 mg/day	Indefinitely
Cirrhotic patients with upper gastrointestinal bleeding Preserved liver function Severe liver failure*	Norfloxacin 400 mg/12 h Ceftriaxone 1 g/day	Seven days Seven days
Cirrhotic patients with low ascitic fluid protein levels (≤ 15 g/L) and severe liver failure*, renal failure** and hyponatraemia***	Norfloxacin 400 mg/day	Indefinitely

* Child–Pugh score ≥ 9 points with malnutrition and serum bilirubin ≥ 3 mg/dl.

** Serum creatinine ≥ 1.2 mg/dl, BUN ≥ 25 mg/dl.

*** Serum sodium ≤ 130 mEq/L).

with gastrointestinal haemorrhage independently of the presence or absence of ascites[1]. Oral norfloxacin (400 mg/12 h) during 7 days is the first-line antibiotic prophylaxis recommended in these patients due to its simpler administration and lower cost.

A recent study indicates that intravenous ceftriaxone is more effective than oral norfloxacin in the prophylaxis of bacterial infections in patients with cirrhosis, gastrointestinal haemorrhage and severe liver failure[44]. The study compared ceftriaxone (1 g/day for 7 days) and norfloxacin (400 mg/12 h for 7 days) in the prophylaxis of bacterial infection in 111 patients with advanced cirrhosis (at least two of the following: ascites, severe malnutrition, encephalopathy or bilirubin >3 mg/dl) and gastrointestinal bleeding. The probability of developing possible infections, proved infections, spontaneous bacteraemia or SBP was significantly higher in patients receiving norfloxacin (33% vs 11%, $p = 0.003$; 26% vs 11%, $p = 0.03$ and 12% vs 2%, $p = 0.03$, respectively). The type of antibiotic used, transfusion requirements at inclusion and failure to control bleeding were independent predictors of infection. The results of this study suggest that intravenous ceftriaxone should be used instead of oral norfloxacin in the prophylaxis of bacterial infections in patients with advanced liver disease and acute gastrointestinal haemorrhage[44].

Low protein ascites in advanced cirrhosis

Patients with low protein content in ascitic fluid and without a past history of SBP may be a second group of cirrhotic patients who may benefit from selective intestinal decontamination. The 1-year and 3-year probabilities of developing the first episode of SBP in patients with ascitic fluid protein content lower than 10 g/L are 20% and 24%, respectively[21]. However, this risk factor alone (low protein ascites) does not identify patients at a very high risk for the development of the first episode of SBP. Severe liver failure and low platelet count appear to be associated with an increased risk of SBP in these patients[22,23]. However, the specific subsets of patients who clearly benefit from this therapy have not been well defined[45–48].

Recently, a double-blind randomized placebo-controlled study evaluated the efficacy of primary prophylaxis with norfloxacin in cirrhotic patients at high risk of developing SBP and hepatorenal syndrome. Patients with low protein ascites (<15 g/L) and advanced liver failure (Child–Pugh score ≥9 points with serum bilirubin ≥3 mg/dl) or impaired renal function (serum creatinine ≥1.2 mg/dl, BUN ≥25 mg/dl or serum sodium ≤130 mEq/L) were randomized to receive norfloxacin (35 patients) or placebo (33 patients)[49]. Norfloxacin administration reduced the 1-year probability of developing SBP (7% vs 61%, $p<0.001$) and hepatorenal syndrome (28% vs 41%, $p = 0.02$) and improved the 3-month (94% vs 62%, $p = 0.003$) and the 1-year (60% vs 48%, $p = 0.05$) probability of survival compared to placebo (Figure 2). Long-term norfloxacin administration is, therefore, clearly indicated in these patients, particularly if they are awaiting liver transplantation, because it may increase the applicability of this procedure.

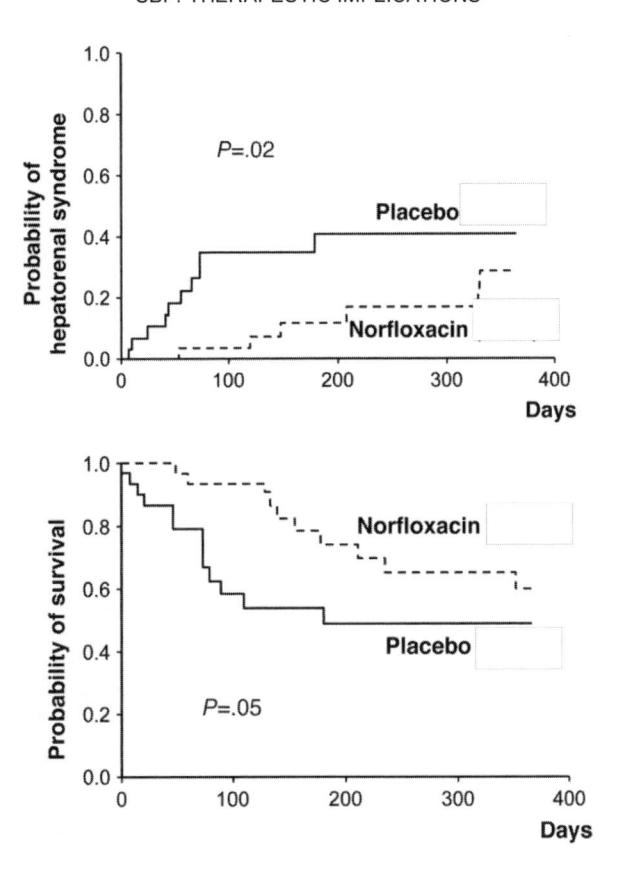

Figure 2 The effect of selective intestinal decontamination (norfloxacin 400 mg/day) on the probability of developing hepatorenal syndrome and survival in patients with advanced cirrhosis and low protein level in ascitic fluid (<15 g/L). With permission from ref. 49

Secondary prophylaxis

Patients recovering from a previous episode of SBP are at a very high risk of SBP recurrence in the absence of antibiotic prophylaxis. In a double-blind placebo-controlled trial including 80 cirrhotic patients who had recovered from an episode of SBP, norfloxacin administration was superior to placebo in the prevention of SBP. The overall probability of SBP recurrence at 1 year of follow-up was 20% in the norfloxacin group and 68% in the placebo group, and the probabilities of SBP caused by aerobic Gram-negative bacilli at 1 year of follow-up were 3% and 60%, respectively[50]. Long-term selective intestinal decontamination, therefore, markedly decreases the rate of SBP recurrence in patients with SBP.

The problem of quinolone-resistant bacteria

A review of the published data indicates that we have moved from an initial stage in which norfloxacin prophylaxis was considered effective and not associated with the development of quinolone-resistant bacteria, to the current stage in which quinolone-resistant bacteria may cause severe infections in patients with cirrhosis. Initial studies suggested that the risk of developing SBP or other infections caused by quinolone-resistant strains of Gram-negative bacilli was low, since the majority of SBP recurrences in patients on norfloxacin prophylaxis were caused by Gram-positive cocci, mainly streptococci[50–52]. Thereafter, a high incidence of quinolone-resistant strains of *Escherichia coli* in stools of cirrhotic patients undergoing long-term quinolone prophylaxis was reported in several studies[53,54]. In 1997 the first study on long-term norfloxacin prophylaxis in SBP revealed a relevant emergence of infections, mainly mild urinary infections, caused by Gram-negative bacilli resistant to quinolones[55]. However, development of SBP due to quinolone-resistant *E. coli* in decontaminated patients was scarcely reported[56]. In 2002 a study in patients with cirrhosis showed a clear relationship between long-term prophylaxis with norfloxacin and the development of SBP caused by quinolone-resistant bacteria[3]. In patients on long-term norfloxacin prophylaxis, 50% of culture-positive SBP were caused by quinolone-resistant Gram-negative bacilli, compared to only 16% in patients not receiving this prophylaxis. Thus, quinolone-resistant SBP emerged for the first time as a real problem in clinical hepatology. This study also showed a high rate of SBP caused by trimethoprim-sulphamethoxazole-resistant Gram-negative bacteria in patients on long-term treatment with norfloxacin (44%), suggesting that this antibiotic is not an alternative to norfloxacin. These results also suggest that the effectiveness of norfloxacin in the prevention of SBP in cirrhosis may decrease in the near future. In that sense further studies are needed to evaluate alternative prophylactic measures such as other antibiotic regimes and non-antibiotic procedures in SBP prophylaxis. Until then the administration of prophylactic antibiotics should be restricted to those patients at the greatest risk of SBP.

References

1. Rimola A, Garcia-Tsao G, Navasa M et al. Diagnosis, treatment and prophylaxis of spontaneous bacterial peritonitis: a consensus document. J Hepatol. 2000;32:142–53.
2. Navasa M, Rodés J. Bacterial infections in cirrhosis. Liver Int. 2004;24:277–80.
3. Fernández J, Navasa M, Gomez J et al. Bacterial infections in cirrosis: epidemiological changes with invasive procedures and norfloxacin prophylaxis. Hepatology. 2002;35:140–8.
4. Runyon BA, Hoefs JC. Culture-negative neutrocytic ascites: a variant of spontaneous bacterial peritonitis. Hepatology. 1984;4:1209–11.
5. Runyon BA, Squier S, Borzio M. Translocation of gut bacteria in rats with cirrhosis to mesenteric lymph nodes partially explains the pathogenesis of spontaneous bacterial peritonitis. J Hepatol. 1994;21:792–6.
6. Casafont Morencos F, de las Heras Castaño G, Martín Ramos L et al. Small bowel bacterial overgrowth in patients with alcoholic cirrhosis. Dig Dis Sci. 1995;40:1252–6.
7. Perez-Paramo MP, Muñoz J, Albillos A et al. Effect of propranolol on the factors promoting bacterial translocation in cirrhotic rats with ascites. Hepatology. 2000;31:43–8.

8. Sorell WT, Quigley EMM, Jin G et al. Bacterial translocation in the portal-hypertensive rat: studies in basal conditions and on exposure to haemorrhagic shock. Gastroenterology. 1993;104:1722–6.
9. Llovet JM, Bartoli R, Planas R et al. Bacterial translocation in cirrhotic rats. Its role in the development of spontaneous bacterial peritonitis. Gut. 1994;35:1648–52.
10. Garcia-Tsao G, Lee FY, Barden GE et al. Bacterial translocation to mesenteric lymph nodes is increased in cirrhotic rats with ascites. Gastroenterology. 1995;108:1835–41.
11. Llovet JM, Bartoli R, Planas R et al. Selective intestinal decontamination with norfloxacin reduces bacterial translocation in ascitic cirrhotic rats exposed to haemorrhagic shock. Hepatology. 1996;23:781–7.
12. Cirera I, Bauer TM, Navasa M et al. Bacterial translocation of enteric organisms in patients with cirrhosis. J Hepatol. 2001;34:32–7.
13. Jones EA, Summerfield JA. Kupffer cells. In: Arias IM, Jakoby WB, Popper H, Schacter D, Shafritz DA, editors. The Liver: Biology and Pathobiology, 2nd edn. New York: Raven Press, 1988:683–704.
14. Guarner C, Runyon BA. Macrophage function in cirrhosis and the risk of bacterial infection. Hepatology. 1995;22:367–9.
15. Gomez F, Ruiz P, Schreiber AD. Impaired function of macrophage Fc gamma receptors and bacterial infection in alcoholic cirrhosis. N Engl J Med. 1994:331:1122–8.
16. Rimola A, Soto R, Bory F et al. Reticuloendothelial system phagocytic activity in cirrhosis and its relation to bacterial infections and prognosis. Hepatology. 1984;4:53–8.
17. Bolognesi M, Merkel C, Bianco S et al. Clinical significance of the evaluation of hepatic reticuloendothelial removal capacity in patients with cirrhosis. Hepatology. 1994;19:628–34.
18. Runyon BA. Patients with deficient ascitic fluid opsonic activity are predisposed to spontaneous bacterial peritonitis. Hepatology. 1988;8:632–5.
19. Runyon BA. Low-protein-concentration ascitic fluid is predisposed to spontaneous bacterial peritonitis. Gastroenterology. 1986;91:1343–6.
20. Tito Ll, Rimola A, Gines P et al. Recurrence of spontaneous bacterial peritonitis in cirrhosis: frequency and predictive factors. Hepatology. 1988;8:27–31.
21. Llach J, Rimola A, Navasa M et al. Incidence and predictive factors of first episode of spontaneous bacterial peritonitis in cirrhosis with ascites: relevance of ascitic fluid protein concentration. Hepatology. 1992;16:724–7.
22. Andreu M, Solá R, Sitges-Serra A et al. Risk factors for spontaneous bacterial peritonitis. Gastroenterology. 1993;104:1133–8.
23. Guarner C, Sola R, Soriano G et al. Risk of a first community-acquired spontaneous bacterial peritonitis in cirrhotics with low ascitic protein levels. Gastroenterology 1999; 117: 414-419.
24. Garcia-Gonzalez M, Boixeda D, Herrero D et al. Effect of granulocyte-macrophage colony-stimulating factor on leukocyte function in cirrhosis. Gastroenterology. 1993;105:527–31.
25. Rolando N, Gimson A, Philpott-Howard J et al. Infectious sequel after endoscopic sclerotherapy of oesophageal varices: role of antibiotic prophylaxis. J Hepatol. 1993;18:290–4.
26. Felisart J, Rimola A, Arroyo V et al. Cefotaxime is more effective than is ampicillin–tobramycin in cirrhotics with severe infections. Hepatology. 1985;5:457–62.
27. Runyon BA, McHutchison JG, Antillon MR et al. Short-course versus long-course antibiotic treatment of spontaneous bacterial peritonitis. A randomized controlled study of 100 patients. Gastroenterology. 1991;100:1737–42.
28. Rimola A, Salmeron JM, Clemente G et al. Two different dosages of cefotaxime in the treatment of spontaneous bacterial peritonitis in cirrhosis: results of a prospective, randomized, multicenter study. Hepatology. 1995;21:674–9.
29. Mercader J, Gómez J, Ruiz J et al. Use of ceftriaxone in the treatment of bacterial infections in cirrhotic patients. Chemotherap. 1989;35(Suppl. 2):23–6.
30. Gómez-Jimenez J, Ribera E, Gasser I et al. Randomized trial comparing ceftriaxone with cefonicid for treatment of spontaneous bacterial peritonitis in cirrhotic patients. Antimicrob Agents Chemother. 1993;37:1587–92.
31. Ariza J, Xiol X, Esteve M et al. Aztreonam vs. cefotaxime in the treatment of Gram-negative spontaneous peritonitis in cirrhotic patients. Hepatology. 1991;14:91–8.

32. Grange JD, Amiot X, Grange V et al. Amoxicillin-clavulanic acid therapy of spontaneous bacterial peritonitis: a prospective study of twenty-seven cases in cirrhotic patients. Hepatology. 1990;11:360–4.
33. Ricart E, Soriano G, Novella MT et al. Amoxicillin-clavulanic acid versus cefotaxime in the therapy of bacterial infections in cirrhotic patients. J Hepatol. 2000;32:596–602.
34. Sort P, Navasa M, Arroyo V et al. Effect of intravenous albumin on renal impairment and mortality in patients with cirrhosis and spontaneous bacterial peritonitis. N Engl J Med. 1999;5:403–9.
35. Fernández J, Monteagudo J, Bargalló X et al. A randomized unblinded pilot study comparing albumin versus hydroxyethyl starch in spontaneous bacterial peritonitis. Hepatology. 2005;42:627–34.
36. Ruiz del Arbol L, Urman J, Fernández J et al. Cardiovascular, renal and hepatic hemodynamic derangement in cirrhotic patients with spontaneous bacterial peritonitis. Hepatology. 2003;38;1210–18.
37. Rimola A, Bory F, Terés J et al. Oral non-absorbable antibiotics prevent infection in cirrhosis with gastrointestinal haemorrhage. Hepatology. 1985;5:463–7.
38. Soriano G, Guarner C, Tomás A et al. Norfloxacin prevents bacterial infection in cirrhotics with gastrointestinal haemorrhage. Gastroenterology. 1992;103:1267–72.
39. Blaise M, Pateron D, Trinchet J-C et al. Systemic antibiotic therapy prevents bacterial infection in cirrhotic patients with gastrointestinal haemorrhage. Hepatology. 1994;20:34–8.
40. Pauwels A, Mostefa-Kara N, Debenes B et al. Systemic antibiotic prophylaxis after gastrointestinal haemorrhage in cirrhotic patients with a high risk of infection. Hepatology. 1996;24:802–6.
41. Hsieh W-J, Lin H-C, Hwang S-J et al. The effect of ciprofloxacin in the prevention of bacterial infections in patients with cirrhosis after upper gastrointestinal bleeding. Am J Gastroenterol. 1998;93:962–6.
42. Hou MC, Lin HC, Liu TT et al. Antibiotic prophylaxis after endoscopic therapy prevents rebleeding in acute variceal hemorrhage: a randomized trial. Hepatology. 2004;39:746–53.
43. Bernard B, Grange JD, Khac EN et al. Antibiotic prophylaxis for the prevention of bacterial infections in cirrhotic patients with gastrointestinal bleeding: a meta-analysis. Hepatology. 1999; 29:1655–61.
44. Fernandez J, Ruiz del Arbol L, Gomez C et al. Norfloxacin vs ceftriaxone in the prophylaxis of infections in patients with advanced cirrhosis and hemorrhage. Gastroenterology. 2006;131:1049–56.
45. Soriano G, Guarner C, Teixidó M et al. Selective intestinal decontamination prevents spontaneous bacterial peritonitis. Gastroenterology. 1991;100:477–81.
46. Grange J-D, Roulot D, Pelletier G et al. Norfloxacin primary prophylaxis of bacterial infections in cirrhotic patients with ascites: a double-blind randomised trial. J Hepatol. 1998;29:430–6.
47. Rolanchon A, Cordier L, Bacq Y et al. Ciprofloxacin and long-term prevention of spontaneous bacterial peritonitis: results of a prospective controlled trial. Hepatology. 1995;22:1171–4.
48. Singh N, Gayowski T, Yu VL et al. Trimethoprim-sulfamethoxazole for the prevention of spontaneous bacterial peritonitis in cirrhosis: a randomized trial. Ann Intern Med. 1995;122:595–8.
49. Fernandez J, Navasa N, Planas R et al. Primary prophylaxis of spontaneous bacterial peritonitis delays hepatorenal syndrome and improves survival in cirrhosis. Gastroenterology. 2007;133:818–24.
50. Ginès P, Rimola A, Planas R et al. Norfloxacin prevents spontaneous bacterial peritonitis recurrence in cirrhosis: results of a double-blind, placebo-controlled trial. Hepatology. 1990;12:716–24.
51. Llovet JM, Rodríguez-Iglesias P, Moitinho E et al. Spontaneous bacterial peritonitis in patients with cirrhosis undergoing selective intestinal decontamination. J Hepatol. 1997;26:88–95.
52. Campillo B, Dupeyron C, Richardet J-P et al. Epidemiology of severe hospital-acquired infections in patients with liver cirrhosis: effect of long-term administration of norfloxacin. Clin Infect Dis. 1998;26:1066–70.

53. Dupeyron C, Mangeney N, Sedrati L et al. Rapid emergence of quinolone resistance in cirrhotic patients treated with norfloxacin to prevent spontaneous bacterial peritonitis. Antimicrob Agents Chemother. 1994;38:340–4.
54. Aparicio JR, Such J, Pascual S et al. Development of quinolone-resistant strains of *Escherichia coli* in stools of patients with cirrhosis undergoing norfloxacin prophylaxis: clinical consequences. J Hepatol. 1999;31:277–83.
55. Novella M, Solà R, Soriano G et al. Continuous versus inpatient prophylaxis of the first episode of spontaneous bacterial peritonitis with norfloxacin. Hepatology. 1997;25:532–36.
56. Ortiz J, Vila MC, Soriano G et al. Infections caused by *Escherichia coli* resistant to norfloxacin in hospitalized cirrhotic patients. Hepatology. 1999;29:1064–69.

26
Hepatorenal syndrome – a defined entity with a standard treatment?

A. L. GERBES

INTRODUCTION

Definition and diagnostic criteria for hepatorenal syndrome (HRS) established in 1994[1] were based on the following three concepts:

1. Renal failure in HRS is functional and caused by marked intrarenal arteriolar vasoconstriction.
2. HRS occurs in the setting of a systemic circulatory dysfunction caused by extrarenal vasodilation.
3. Plasma volume expansion does not improve renal failure.

Four new concepts have emerged since then:

4. Extrarenal arterial vasodilation mainly occurs in the splanchnic bed, whereas other major vascular beds, such as the brain and the liver, may be vasoconstricted. This may contribute to some of the frequent extrarenal complications, i.e. progressive hepatic failure and encephalopathy.
5. Cardiac output in patients with HRS may be low, normal, or high, but all the same it is insufficient because of reduced peripheral vascular resistance. This may aggravate the systemic circulatory dysfunction of HRS.
6. The most frequent trigger of type 1 HRS is bacterial infection, mainly spontaneous bacterial peritonitis (SBP).
7. HRS is not always a terminal event as it can be improved by medical treatment, and the improvement is associated with improved survival.

Background for the new concepts

The first of these concepts was discovered during investigations carried out using Doppler ultrasonography or plethysmography both before and after 1994. These studies were performed in patients with varying severity of cirrhosis, and reveal arterial vasodilation in the splanchnic circulation as well as arterial vasoconstriction in other areas such as brain, kidneys, and liver[2-9], whereas cutaneous and muscular blood flow is low, normal, or even increased[9-12]. The dilation of the splanchnic vessels is mainly caused by local release of potent vasodilators such as nitric oxide (NO)[13]. These vasodilators also make the splanchnic circulation resistant to the vasoconstrictive effect of angiotensin II, noradrenalin, vasopressin, and endothelin[14-20]. Consequently, the homeostasis of arterial pressure in cirrhosis depends on the effect exerted by the endogenous vasoconstrictor systems in extrasplanchnic organs. As arterial vasodilation increases with progression of cirrhosis, the role of vasoconstrictors in maintaining haemodynamic stability becomes critical. This explains why cirrhotic patients with HRS are predisposed to develop renal, hepatic, and cerebral vasoconstriction.

Regarding the second new concept, insufficient cardiac output contributing to renal hypoperfusion in patients with HRS was first suggested by Tristani and Cohn[21], but two more recent studies have provided further evidence[22,23]. The first study showed that the cardiac output of cirrhotic patients with SBP who developed progressive renal failure was relatively low, in spite of infection resolution, compared to the cardiac output measured before renal failure and to that of patients with SBP who did not develop renal failure[22]. The second study compared non-azotaemic cirrhotic patients who developed HRS with similar patients who did not, and showed that low cardiac output and high plasma renin activity (PRA) were independent predictors of HRS[23]. Moreover, in patients developing HRS, the progression of circulatory dysfunction leading to arterial hypotension and renal failure occurred in the setting of continued decrease in cardiac output and increase in PRA. These findings support the hypothesis that hyperdynamic circulation is essential to maintain central blood volume and renal perfusion in cirrhosis. Therefore, when cardiac output decreases, effective hypovolaemia occurs leading to renal hypoperfusion and HRS. Why cardiac output becomes relatively insufficient in patients developing HRS is unknown. The role of so-called 'cirrhotic cardiomyopathy' is a reliable hypothesis that needs to be validated.

HRS can be triggered by precipitating events. The most important are infections, bleeding, and large-volume paracentesis without albumin administration[24-27]. The role of SBP has recently been emphasized. Changes in circulatory function, endogenous vasoactive systems, and renal function in patients developing renal failure triggered by SBP are identical to those observed in patients with HRS unrelated to infection, suggesting that the pathogenesis of progressive renal failure in cirrhotic patients with infection is the same as HRS.

The most important concept of HRS, however, arises out of studies exploring new therapeutic strategies[28]. Since type 1 HRS is often associated with a rapid deterioration of liver function with increased levels of bilirubin and prothrombin time, it has traditionally been viewed as a manifestation of terminal hepatic failure, but type 1 HRS was known as 'terminal functional renal failure'. The corollary of this was that patients with type 1 HRS died because of irreversible liver failure and that liver transplantation (LT) was the only effective treatment. Therefore, the demonstration that type 1 HRS can be improved by vasoconstrictors or by transjugular intrahepatic portosystemic shunt (TIPS)[29-34], and that reversal of type 1 HRS is associated with improved survival, represents a major change in the notion of the syndrome.

In conclusion, the main pathogenetic mechanism in type 1 HRS is a potentially reversible deterioration of systemic circulatory function, mostly due to splanchnic vasodilation and renal vasoconstriction, and often triggered by a precipitating event (Figure 1). In addition to renal failure, the syndrome may be associated with other organ dysfunctions, such as decreased cardiac output, hepatic failure, and encephalopathy.

Altogether, portal hypertension, peripheral vasodilation and markedly decreased centrally effective blood volume are the triggers for hepatorenal syndrome. Thus, any novel concepts for treatment will have to counteract these changes.

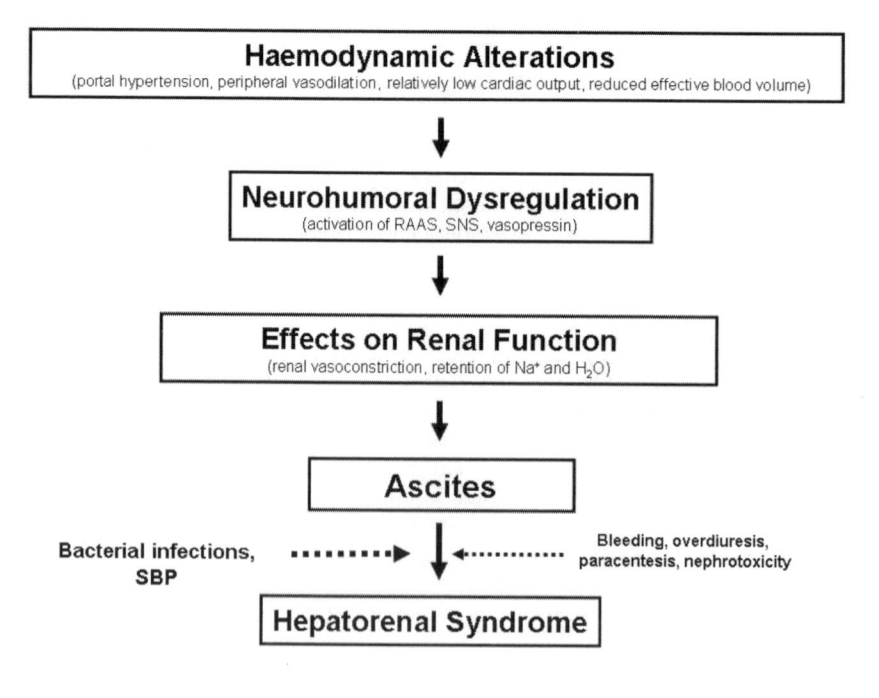

Figure 1 Pathogenetic mechanisms of hepatorenal syndrome

NEW DEFINITION OF HRS

HRS is a potentially reversible syndrome that mainly occurs in patients with cirrhosis, ascites, and liver failure, and less frequently in patients with acute liver failure or acute alcoholic hepatitis. It is characterized by impaired renal function, marked alterations in cardiovascular function and overactivity in the endogenous vasoactive systems. Intrarenal vasoconstriction causes low glomerular filtration rate (GFR), whereas in systemic circulation vascular resistance decreases due to splanchnic and peripheral arterial vasodilation. There are two types of HRS. Type 2 HRS is characterized by moderate renal failure (serum creatinine from 133 to 226 µmol/L or 1.5–2.5 mg/dl), with a steady or slowly progressive course. It appears spontaneously, but can also follow a precipitating event. Type 2 HRS is typically associated with refractory ascites. Survival of patients with type 2 HRS is shorter than that of non-azotaemic cirrhotic patients with ascites, but better than that of patients with type 1 HRS.

Type 1 HRS is characterized by rapid progressive renal failure defined by doubling of the initial serum creatinine concentration to a level greater than 226 µmol/L (2.5 mg/dl) in less than 2 weeks. It may appear spontaneously, but often develops after a precipitating event, particularly SBP. Type 1 HRS usually occurs within the setting of an acute deterioration of circulatory function characterized by arterial hypotension and activation of endogenous vasoconstrictor systems, and may be associated with impaired cardiac and liver functions as well as encephalopathy. The natural prognosis of type 1 HRS is very poor.

The main differences with the definition reported in 1996[1] are:

1. the potential reversibility of HRS without LT;
2. the dominant role of the splanchnic bed in arterial vasodilation;
3. the frequent role of SBP as an event precipitating type 1 HRS;
4. the concept that, in addition to renal failure, the function of other organs is frequently impaired.

Revised diagnostic criteria of HRS

As there are no specific hallmarks of HRS, the diagnosis is based on the exclusion of other types of renal failure. The criteria necessary to diagnose HRS are listed in Table 1. The main differences between these criteria[35] and those previously established[1] are:

1. Creatinine clearance has been excluded because it is more complicated than simple serum creatinine for routine purposes, and it does not increase the accuracy of renal function estimation in cirrhotic patients.

2. Renal failure in the setting of ongoing bacterial infection, but in the absence of septic shock, is now considered HRS. This means treatment of HRS can be started without waiting for complete recovery from the infection.

Table 1 New diagnostic criteria of hepatorenal syndrome

1. Cirrhosis with ascites.
2. Serum creatinine >133 μmol/L (1.5 mg/dl).
3. No improvement of serum creatinine (decrease to a level of 133 μmol/L or less) after at least 2 days with diuretic withdrawal and volume expansion with albumin. The recommended dose of albumin is 1 g/kg of body weight per day up to a maximum of 100 g/day.
4. Absence of shock.
5. No current or recent treatment with nephrotoxic drugs.
6. Absence of parenchymal kidney disease as indicated by proteinuria >500 mg/day, microhaematuria (>50 red blood cells per high-power field), and/or abnormal renal ultrasonography.

3. Plasma volume expansion should be performed with albumin rather than saline. It is generally agreed that albumin causes a greater and more sustained expansion than saline.
4. Minor diagnostic criteria have been removed as they are not essential.

TREATMENT OF HRS

New treatments of HRS are designed to expand central blood volume by simultaneously increasing total plasma volume and reducing intense peripheral vasodilation. This strategy is not entirely new, as in 1967 Tristani and Cohn[21] showed that dextran infusion improved cardiac output and renal perfusion in oliguric cirrhotic patients, and 18 years later Shapiro et al.[32] showed that the urine water and sodium excretion in cirrhotic patients with ascites was improved by the administration of norepinephrine combined with head-out water immersion, a manoeuvre aimed at expanding central blood volume. However, clinically relevant results have only been obtained more recently with the use of albumin and various vasoconstrictors.

The mechanism by which vasoconstrictors and albumin improve GFR in patients with HRS has yet to be completely clarified. Nevertheless, it is known that a 2-day administration of terlipressin to patients with HRS induces a vasopressor effect associated with a significant decrease in PRA and increase in GFR[33], indirectly indicating correction of circulatory dysfunction. It is conceivable that vasopressin analogues cause vasoconstriction of the splanchnic bed, allowing redistribution of the total blood volume from this bed to some of the extrasplanchnic organs including the kidneys. In addition, the inhibition of the sympathetic nervous and renin–angiotensin systems shifts the autoregulatory curve to the left, making renal blood flow and GFR more responsive to changes in blood pressure. Albumin is traditionally considered to improve circulatory function in cirrhosis by expanding central blood volume and increasing cardiac output[38]. Moreover, recent studies have shown that the administration of albumin to cirrhotic patients with SBP causes arterial vasoconstriction and blood pressure increase[37], probably attributable to the ability of albumin to bind vasodilators[36]. It is therefore conceivable that an improvement of renal function in patients with HRS treated with vasoconstrictors and albumin is due to the additive effects that the two compounds have on cardiac function and peripheral arterial circulation.

Vasoconstrictors and albumin

Lenz et al.[34] showed that GFR may be moderately improved by ornipressin infusion in patients with HRS, but the drug was given for only 4 h therefore precluding assessment of its long-term effects. Two more studies demonstrated that a long-term (1–2 weeks) infusion of ornipressin, combined with albumin or dopamine, normalized serum creatinine concentrations in many patients with type 1 HRS[29,38]. Interestingly, recurrence of renal failure rarely occurred after treatment withdrawal and, in the few cases where it did recur, a second course of therapy was successful. However, there was a drawback with ornipressin: the frequent occurrence of ischaemic complications[29,38].

Widespread use of vasoconstrictors in patients with HRS has therefore become reality only after the use of safer compounds such as terlipressin[39–41], a vasopressin analogue with longer activity, and the α_2-agonist midodrine combined with octreotide[42,43]. Table 2 summarizes the data available on the use of terlipressin in type 1 HRS. This includes three randomized controlled trials (RCT), and many pilot or retrospective studies. These studies show that: (a) although GFR rarely reaches normal levels, a short period of treatment with terlipressin can improve renal function in up to 65% of patients with type 1 HRS; (b) the effectiveness of terlipressin is probably enhanced by albumin[41]; (c) HRS recurs after treatment withdrawal in approximately 20% of patients, but retreatment is often effective; (d) in most cases dilutional hyponatraemia associated with HRS improves with terlipressin treatment[40,41]; (e) severe side-effects of the treatment are rare (5–10%). With regard to survival, patients who experienced a complete reversal of type 1 HRS by terlipressin seem to have an improved short-term survival. Therefore, the long-term survival of patients with type 1 HRS treated with terlipressin merits further investigation.

The initial dose of terlipressin in many studies ranged from 0.5 to 1 mg every 4–6 h. This regimen was maintained until reversal of HRS, which usually occurred within the second week of treatment. In other studies the initial dose in cases without an early response was increased up to 2 mg every 4–6 h. Continuous terlipressin infusion is an interesting novel approach which may yield good response rates at very few severe adverse events[45].

The daily dose of albumin was generally 20–40 g, preceded in some studies by a load of 1 g/kg of body weight.

Experience of using midodrine in patients with type 1 HRS is more limited. To date there are only two pilot studies[42,43]. In both of these midodrine was combined with octreotide to enhance the effect of splanchnic vasoconstriction, but doses and routes of administration were quite different. Angeli et al.[42] used 7.5–12.5 mg t.i.d. of oral or intravenous midodrine plus 100–200 µg t.i.d. of subcutaneous octreotide, whereas Wong et al.[43] used 2.5 mg t.i.d. of oral midodrine plus an intravenous infusion of octreotide (25 µg/h after a bolus of 25 µg). The dose of midodrine was adjusted to increase mean arterial pressure to 90 mmHg. Albumin was also given in these studies. The results are similar to

Table 2 Characteristics and results of studies reporting the effect of terlipressin in patients with cirrhosis and type 1 HRS

Author, year (ref)	Type of study*	Success rate of treatment**	Dose (mg/day)	Duration (days)	Survival at 4 weeks**	Adverse events
Moreau, 2002[39]	R	53/99	3.2±1.2	11±12	37/99	23/99
Uriz, 2000[40]	PU	4/6	3–6	5–15	4/6	1/6
Mulkay, 2001[48]	PU	12/12	1–6	8–14	3/12	4/12
Angeli, 2006[42]	PU	12/19	2–12	≤15	13/19	n.d.
Ortega, 2002[41]	PU	T+A: 8/9	2	4–14	8/9	1/16
		T–A: 1/7			1/7	
Hadengue, 1998[33]	RCT	6/9	2	2	n.d.	0/9
Solanki, 2003[44]	RCT	T: 5/12	2	14	n.d.	5/12
		P: 0/12				
Sanyal, 2006[52]	RCT	T+A: 19/56	4–8	14	27/56***	
		A: 7/56			27/56***	
Total		120/229	2–12	2–27	93/208	34/154

*R = retrospective; PU = prospective uncontrolled; RCT = randomized controlled trial.

** Successful treatment means partial or complete response in renal function improvement. T+A = terlipressin + albumin; T–A = terlipressin without albumin; T = terlipressin; P = placebo; A = albumin.

*** Survival was reported at 60 days.

n.d. = not determined.

those obtained using terlipressin, although response was slower. Since octreotide alone had no impact on GFR in patients with HRS[46], it is likely that midodrine plays the main role in improving GFR.

A pilot study explored the effect of norepinephrine infusion (0.5–3 mg/h) combined with albumin and furosemide in type 1 HRS[47]. The doses were titrated to increase mean arterial pressure by 10 mmHg. Reversal of HRS was achieved in 10 out of 12 cases and was associated with improvement in urinary sodium excretion and decrease in PRA. Norepinephrine is cheaper and more widely available than terlipressin, but it can induce arrhythmias more often. Therefore, the role of norepinephrine in patients with type 1 HRS should still be established on the basis of future comparisons with terlipressin or midodrine/octreotide.

Only a few patients with type 2 HRS have been specifically treated using terlipressin and albumin. In most cases normalization of serum creatinine was observed, but in contrast to type 1 HRS, renal failure invariably recurred after treatment withdrawal.

Transjugular intrahepatic portosystemic stent–shunt (TIPS)

Only a few studies have assessed the role of TIPS in HRS – 91 patients in total. Most were prospective but uncontrolled studies[30,31,43,49,50]. Three were performed in patients with type 1 HRS, one in patients with type 1 HRS and patients with type 2 HRS, and the last specifically investigated type 2 HRS. The following can be observed:

1. Significant suppression of the endogenous vasoactive systems, particularly the renin–angiotensin system[31], and a decrease of creatinine levels were recorded after TIPS in most patients with type 1 HRS. The rate of the creatinine decrease was slower than is usually obtained using terlipressin plus albumin.

2. Recurrence of HRS was rare, provided that there was no shunt malfunction.

3. Hepatic encephalopathy was a frequent complication of TIPS but was adequately managed by medical treatment.

4. TIPS almost always induced a reduction of ascites volume.

5. Resolution of type 1 HRS by TIPS can improve survival.

6. Sequential treatment with vasoconstrictors and albumin followed by TIPS could be used as an alternative approach to increasing the probability of long-term success[43].

7. Although TIPS may improve renal function and refractory ascites in patients with type 2 HRS, its effect on survival is still undefined.

However, since almost all studies excluded patients with a history of severe encephalopathy, or serum bilirubin levels over 85 μmol/L (5 mg/dl), or Child–Pugh score over 12, the applicability of TIPS may be rather limited in patients with HRS who frequently show jaundice, encephalopathy, and high Child–Pugh scores[50].

There has been little investigation into the mechanism through which TIPS exerts beneficial effects in patients with HRS. Nevertheless, as TIPS functions as a side-to-side portacaval shunt, it is expected to relieve portal hypertension, which plays a pivotal role in the pathogenesis of splanchnic arterial vasodilation[51]. Moreover, TIPS insertion is associated with an increase in cardiac output and an expansion in central blood volume[53,54]. The simultaneous effects on the splanchnic and systemic circulation may represent the mechanism by which TIPS improves renal perfusion, GFR, urine sodium and water excretion, and hyponatraemia.

Take-home messages[55,56]

1. HRS type 1 is rapidly progressive with poor prognosis.

2. Infections, particularly SBP, have a high risk for HRS; therefore prophylaxis with albumin is recommended for patients with SBP.

3. Patients with HRS waiting for liver transplantation should be offered TIPS (at bilirubin <3–5 mg/dl) or vasoconstrictors (terlipressin) plus albumin.

4. These novel therapeutic strategies seem to improve short-term survival.

References

1. Arroyo V, Gines P, Gerbes A et al. Definition and diagnostic criteria of refractory ascites and hepatorenal syndrome in cirrhosis. Hepatology. 1996;23:164–76.
2. Fernandez-Seara J, Prieto J, Quiroga J et al. Systemic and regional hemodynamics in patients with liver cirrhosis and ascites with and without functional renal failure. Gastroenterology. 1989;97:1304–312.
3. Maroto A, Gines P, Arroyo V et al. Brachial and femoral artery blood flow in cirrhosis: relationship to kidney dysfunction. Hepatology. 1993;17:788–93.
4. Rivolta R, Maggi A, Cazzaniga M et al. Reduction of renal cortical blood flow assessed by Doppler in cirrhotic patients with refractory ascites. Hepatology. 1998;28:1235–40
5. Guevara M, Bru C, Gines P et al. Increased cerebrovascular resistance in cirrhotic patients with ascites. Hepatology. 1998;28:39–44.
6. Sacerdoti D, Bolognesi M, Merkel C, Angeli P, Gatta A. Renal vasoconstriction in cirrhosis evaluated by duplex Doppler ultrasonography. Hepatology. 1993;17:219–24.
7. Sugano S, Yamamoto K, Atobe T et al. Postprandial middle cerebral arterial vasoconstriction in cirrhotic patients. A placebo, controlled evaluation. J Hepatol. 2001;34:373–7.
8. Dillon JF, Plevris JN, Wong FC et al. Middle cerebral artery blood flow velocity in patients with cirrhosis. Eur J Gastroenterol Hepatol. 1995;7:1087–91.
9. Moller S, Henriksen J. The systemic circulation in cirrhosis. In: Gines P, Arroyo V, Rodes J, Schrier RW, editors. Ascites and Renal Dysfunction in Liver Disease, 2nd edn. Oxford: Blackwell, 2005:139–55.
10. Luca A, Garcia-Pagan JC, Feu F et al. Noninvasive measurement of femoral blood flow and portal pressure response to propranolol in patients with cirrhosis. Hepatology. 1995;21:83–8.
11. Piscaglia F, Zironi G, Gaiani S et al. Relationship between splanchnic, peripheral and cardiac hemodynamics in cirrhosis of different degrees of severity. Eur J Gastroenterol Hepatol. 1997;9:799–804.
12. Wong F, Logan A, Blendis L. Hyperinsulinemia in preascitic cirrhosis: effects on systemic and renal hemodynamics, sodium homeostasis, forearm blood flow and sympathetic nervous activity. Hepatology. 1996;23:414–22.

13. Mitamura K, Kawauchi A, Sasaki K et al. Measurement of renal artery blood flow velocity by Doppler ultrasonography in chronic liver disease. Hepatol Res. 1999;15:201–14.
14. Domenicali M, Ros J, Fernandez-Varo G et al. Increased anandamide induced relaxation in mesenteric arteries of cirrhotic rats: role of cannabinoid and vanilloid receptors. Gut. 2005;54:522–7.
15. Castro A, Jimenez W, Claria J et al. Impaired response to angiotensin II in experimental cirrhosis: role of nitric oxide. Hepatology. 1993;18:367–72.
16. Heller J, Schepke M, Gehnen N et al. Altered adrenergic responsiveness of endothelium-denuded hepatic arteries and portal veins in patients with cirrhosis. Gastroenterology. 1999;116:387–93.
17. Hartleb M, Moreau R, Cailmail S, Gaudin C, Lebrec D. Vascular hyporesponsiveness to endothelin 1 in rats with cirrhosis. Gastroenterology. 1994;107:1085–93.
18. Michielsen PP, Boeckxstaens GE, Sys SU, Herman AG, Pelckmans PA. The role of increased nitric oxide in the vascular hyporeactivity to noradrenaline in long-term portal vein ligated rats. J Hepatol. 1995;23:341–7.
19. Islam M, Williams B, Madhavan K, Hayes P, Hadoke P. Selective alteration of agonist-mediated contraction in hepatic arteries isolated from patients with cirrhosis. Gastroenterology. 2000;118:765–71.
20. Helmy A, Newby DE, Jalan R et al. Nitric oxide mediates the reduced vasoconstrictor response to angiotensina II in patients with preascitic cirrhosis. J Hepatol. 2003;38:44–50.
21. Tristani FE, Cohn JN. Systemic and renal hemodynamics in oliguric hepatic failure: effect of volume expansion. J Clin Invest. 1967;46:1894–6.
22. Ruiz del Arbol L., Urman J, Fernandez J et al. Systemic, renal, and hepatic hemodynamic derangement in cirrhotic patients with spontaneous bacterial peritonitis. Hepatology. 2003;38:1210–18.
23. Ruiz del Arbol L, Monescillo A et al. Circulatory function and hepatorenal syndrome in cirrhosis. Hepatology. 2005;42:439–47.
24. Follo A, Llovet JM, Navasa M et al. Renal impairment after spontaneous bacterial peritonitis in cirrhosis: incidence, clinical course, predictive factors and prognosis. Hepatology. 1994;20:1495–501.
25. Terra C, Guevara M, Torre A et al. Renal failure in patients with cirrhosis and sepsis unrelated to spontaneous bacterial peritonitis: value of MELD score. Gastroenterology. 2005;129:1944–53.
26. Cardenas A, Gines P, Uriz J et al. Renal failure after upper gastrointestinal bleeding in cirrhosis: incidence, clinical course, predictive factors, and short-term prognosis. Hepatology. 2001;34:671–6.
27. Salerno F, Badalamenti S. Drug-induced renal failure in cirrhosis. In: Gines P, Arroyo V, Rodes J, Schrier RW, editors. Ascites and Renal Dysfunction in Liver Disease, 2nd edn. Oxford: Blackwell, 2005:372–82.
28. Moreau R, Lebrec D. The use of vasoconstrictors in patients with cirrhosis: type 1 HRS and beyond. Hepatology. 2006;43:385–94.
29. Guevara M, Ginès P, Fernandez-Esparrach G et al. Reversibility of hepatorenal syndrome by prolonged administration of ornipressin and plasma volume expansion. Hepatology. 1998;27:35–41.
30. Brensing KA, Textor J, Perz J et al. Long term outcome after transjugular intrahepatic portosystemic stent-shunt in non-transplant cirrhotics with hepatorenal syndrome: a phase II study. Gut. 2000;47:288–95.
31. Guevara M, Gines P, Bandi JC et al. Transjugular intrahepatic portosystemic shunt in hepatorenal syndrome: effects on renal function and vasoactive systems. Hepatology. 1998;28:416–22.
32. Shapiro MD, Nichols KM et al. Interrelationship between cardiac output and vascular resistance as determinant of effective arterial blood volume in cirrhotic patients. Kidney Int. 1985;28:206–11.
33. Hadengue A, Gadano A, Moreau R et al. Beneficial effects of the two-day administration of terlipressin in patients with cirrhosis and hepatorenal syndrome. J Hepatol. 1998;29:565–70.
34. Lenz K, Hortnagl H, Druml W et al. Ornipressin in the treatment of functional renal failure in decompensated cirrhosis: effects on renal hemodynamics and atrial natriuretic factor. Gastroenterology. 1991;101:1060–7.

35. Salerno F, Gerbes AL, Gines P, Wong F, Arroyo V. Definition, diagnosis, prevention and treatment of hepatorenal syndrome in cirrhosis. A consensus workshop of the international ascites club. Gut. 2007;56:1310–18.
36. Bevers LM, van Faassen EE, Vuong TD et al. Low albumin levels increased endothelial NO production and decrease vascular NO sensitivity. Nephrol Dial Transplant. 2006;21:3443–9.
37. Sort P, Navasa M, Arroyo V et al. Effect of intravenous albumin on renal impairment and mortality in patients with cirrhosis and spontaneous bacterial peritonitis. N Engl J Med. 1999;5:403–9.
38. Gülberg V, Bilzer M, Gerbes AL. Long-term therapy and retreatment of hepatorenal syndrome type 1 with ornipressin and dopamine. Hepatology. 1999;30:870–5.
39. Moreau R, Durand F, Poynard T et al. Terlipressin in patients with cirrhosis and type 1 hepatorenal syndrome: a retrospective multicenter study. Gastroenterology. 2002;122:923–30.
40. Uriz J, Ginès P, Cardenas A et al. Terlipressin plus albumin infusion: an effective and safe therapy of hepatorenal syndrome. J Hepatol. 2000;33:43–8.
41. Ortega R, Ginès P, Uriz J et al. Terlipressin therapy with and without albumin for patients with hepatorenal syndrome: results of a prospective nonrandomized study. Hepatology. 2002;36:941–8.
42. Angeli P, Volpin R, Gerunda G et al. Reversal of type 1 hepatorenal syndrome with the administration of midodrine and octreotide. Hepatology. 1999;29:1690–7.
43. Wong F, Pantea L, Sniderman K. Midodrine, octreotide, albumin, and TIPS in selected patients with cirrhosis and type 1 hepatorenal syndrome. Hepatology. 2004;40:55–64.
44. Solanki P, Chawla A, Garg R et al. Beneficial effects of terlipressin in hepatorenal syndrome: a prospective, randomized placebo-controlled clinical trial. J Gastroenterol Hepatol. 2003;18:152–6.
45. Gülberg V, Huber E, Gerbes AL. Terlipressin infusion improves renal function in patients with hepatorenal syndrome. Hepatology. 2007;46;(Suppl. 1) 865A.
46. Pomier-Layrargues G, Paquin SC, Hassoun Z et al. Octreotide in hepatorenal syndrome: a randomized, double-blind, placebo-controlled, crossover study. Hepatology. 2003;38:238–43.
47. Duvoux C, Zanditenas D, Hezode C et al. Effects of noradrenalin and albumin in patients with type 1 hepatorenal syndrome: a pilot study. Hepatology. 2002;36:374–80.
48. Mulkay JP, Louis H, Donckier V et al. Long-term terlipressin administration improves renal function in cirrhotic patients with type 1 hepatorenal syndrome: a pilot study. Acta Gastroenterol Belg. 2001;64:15–19.
49. Testino G, Ferro C, Sumberaz A et al. Type-2 hepatorenal syndrome and refractory ascites: role of transjugular intrahepatic portosystemic stent–shunt in eighteen patients with advanced cirrhosis awaiting orthotopic liver transplantation. Hepatogastroenterology. 2003; 50:1753–5.
50. Gerbes AL, Gulberg V. Benefit of TIPS for patients with refractory ascites: serum bilirubin may make the difference. Hepatology. 2005;41:217.
51. Jalan R, Forrest EH, Redhead DN, Dillon JF, Hayes PC. Reduction in renal blood flow following acute increase in the portal pressure: evidence for the existence of a hepatorenal reflex in man? Gut. 1997;40:664–70.
52. Sanyal A, Boyer T, Garcia-Tsao G et al. A prospective randomized double blind, placebo-controlled trial of terlipressin for type 1 hepatorenal syndrome (HRS). Hepatology. 2006;44 (Suppl.1):694A.
53. Salerno F, Cazzaniga M, Pagnozzi G et al. Humoral and cardiac effects of TIPS in cirrhotic patients with different 'effective' blood volume. Hepatology. 2003;38:1370–7.
54. Schwartz JM, Beymer C, Althaus SJ et al. Cardiopulmonary consequences of transjugular intrahepatic portosystemic shunts: role of increased pulmonary artery pressure. J Clin Gastroenterol. 2004;38:590–4.
55. Gerbes AL. The patient with refractory ascites. Best Pract Res Clin Gastroenterol. 2007;21:551–60.
56. Gerbes AL, Gulberg V. Progress in treatment of massive ascites and hepatorenal syndrome. World J Gastroenterol. 2006;12:516–19.

27
From infections to hepatic encephalopathy

D. HÄUSSINGER

INTRODUCTION

Hepatic encephalopathy (HE) defines a frequent neuropsychiatric manifestation of chronic and acute liver disease with disturbances of psychomotoric, intellectual, cognitive, emotional/affective, behavioural and fine motor functions of varying severity (for review see ref. 1). The syndrome is frequent and, depending on the population under study, 20–80% of cirrhotics may suffer from subclinical or manifest HE.

It is a long-standing clinical experience that cirrhotic patients are prone to episodes of HE in response to sepsis or infections. Several mechanisms may underlie this observation. First, infections are associated with a protein catabolic state, which increases the ammonia load to the liver and impairs ammonia detoxication in muscle. Second, lipopolysaccharide (LPS) injection, which is frequently used as a sepsis model in the rat, induces an inactivating tyrosine nitration of hepatic glutamine synthetase with impairment of hepatic ammonia detoxication. Third, inflammatory cytokines, such as tumour necrosis factor (TNF)-α can act directly on the brain and trigger pathophysiological events leading to HE.

LPS IMPAIRS HEPATIC AMMONIA DETOXICATION

The liver acinus exhibits a sophisticated structural and functional organization of ammonia-detoxifying pathways (for reviews see refs 2–4). Following the blood stream, the pathways of urea and glutamine synthesis are anatomically switched behind each other. Thus, the ammonia-rich portal blood first gets into contact with periportal hepatocytes, which contain urea cycle enzymes. Here, however, ammonia is detoxified with low affinity only, and considerable amounts of ammonia reach the perivenous hepatocytes, which are the only compartment containing glutamine synthetase. These cells eliminate ammonia with high affinity and have been termed perivenous scavenger cells. Destruction of these glutamine synthetase-containing perivenous hepatocytes causes hyperammonaemia. Interestingly, LPS injection into rats causes a rapid tyrosine nitration of hepatic glutamine synthetase, which inactivates the enzyme[5,6]. This is associated with a diminished hepatic ammonia removal and an increase of ammonia in the hepatic vein. Thus, LPS induces hyperammonaemia due to a scavenger cell defect and may by that means contribute to the development of HE in sepsis.

PATHOGENESIS OF HE: ROLE OF INFLAMMATORY CYTOKINES

There is consensus that ammonia is a key toxin in HE, which may sensitize the brain to the different precipitating factors[4-8]. HE in liver cirrhosis is seen as a clinical manifestation of a low-grade cerebral oedema, which exacerbates in response to ammonia and other precipitating factors[7,8]. Here, the pathogenetic action of ammonia and HE-precipitating factors integrates at the level of astrocyte swelling. This low-grade cerebral oedema triggers an oxidative and nitrosative stress response. Although human studies concerning the involvement of oxidative stress in HE are rare up to now, there is substantial evidence from animal and cell culture studies for an important role of oxidative/nitrosative stress in the pathogenesis of HE. In cultured astrocytes and in rat brain *in vivo*, ammonia, inflammatory cytokines, benzodiazepines and hyponatraemia induce the rapid formation of reactive oxygen species and nitric oxide (NO) through *N*-methyl-D-aspartate (NMDA)-receptor and Ca^{2+}-dependent mechanisms[9-12]. There is a close relationship between astrocyte swelling and oxidative stress. On the one hand, astrocyte swelling induces oxidative stress through NMDA receptor- and Ca^{2+}-dependent mechanisms and, on the other hand, NMDA receptor activation and oxidative stress trigger astrocyte swelling (for review see ref. 13). This points to an auto-amplificatory signalling loop between astrocyte swelling and oxidative stress. Activation of NADPH oxidase isoforms[12] and opening of the mitochondrial permeability transition pore[14] are the most likely sources for reactive oxygen species.

Although it would be an oversimplification to ascribe all pathogenetic effects of ammonia and HE-relevant toxins to astrocyte swelling and oxidative/nitrosative stress, current evidence suggests a major contribution of these events to HE pathophysiology. For example, nitrosative stress induces Zn^{2+} mobilization with an increased protein kinase C-dependent translocation of transcription factors such as SP1/3 to the nucleus and enhanced SP1/3 DNA binding in cultured astrocytes. These transcription factors participate in regulation of the expression of the peripheral benzodiazepine receptor (PBR). This protein is up-regulated in HE[15,16] and is also involved in the synthesis of neurosteroids, such as allopregnanolone and allotetrahydrodeoxy-corticosterone[15-18]. The positive $GABA_A$-receptor modulatory activity of these neurosteroids may contribute to the increased GABAergic tone found in patients with HE[18]. Another consequence of the ROS/RNS formation is protein tyrosine nitration (PTN), which is induced *in vivo* and *in vitro* in response to ammonia[10], benzodiazepines[11] or inflammatory cytokines[19], but also after experimental astrocyte swelling, indicating that astrocyte swelling is sufficient to induce PTN. These effectors act synergistically with respect to PTN induction, indicating that the known synergism between hyperammonaemia and inflammation in precipitating HE symptoms[20-23] is also reflected at the level of PTN.

PTN is a selective process and affects enzyme activities and signal transduction elements, and is most pronounced in perivascular astrocytes with potential impact on blood–brain barrier permeability. A novel finding is that the oxidative stress response, which is induced by ammonia, TNF-α, benzodiazepines or hyponatraemia, is associated with an increased oxidation of RNA[24]. RNA oxidation involves ribosomal and some mRNA species and oxidized RNA is also found in so-called RNA granules in neuronal dendrites. Such RNA granules participate in local postsynaptic protein synthesis, which is required for synaptic plasticity and the formation of long-term memory[25,26]. Oxidized RNA species exhibit altered translation efficacy and can result in the formation of defective proteins[27]. Thus, these findings could provide a link between ammonia, inflammatory cytokines and oxidative stress on the one hand and cognitive dysfunction on the other. In line with this, TNF-α affects synaptic plasticity by inhibiting long-term potentiation and can facilitate glutamate exitotoxicity in part by inhibiting glial glutamate transporters[28]. Indeed, oxidation of glutamate transporter GLAST mRNA occurs in response to ammonia-induced oxidative stress[24].

The *in vitro* synergism between ammonia and inflammatory cytokines with regard to oxidative/nitrosative stress is also reflected in *in vivo* studies. Induced hyperammonaemia results in a significant deterioration of neuropsychological test scores in cirrhotic patients during an inflammatory state, but not after its resolution[23]. Another study on cirrhotic patients showed that the presence of minimal hepatic encephalopathy was related to the presence of markers of inflammation, and again induction of hyperammonaemia in these patients caused a deterioration of neuropsychological test results[29]. Injection of LPS into bile duct-ligated rats induces precoma and exacerbates cerebral oedema[30]; this was also found when bile duct-ligated rats, which display signs of inflammation, received a hyperammonaemic diet[22]. These studies underline the synergistic effects of ammonia and inflammation in precipitating HE. The mechanisms by which peripheral inflammatory cytokines act on the brain are mechanistically poorly understood. Vagal afferences and a modulation of cerebral blood flow by cytokine interactions with the brain endothelium may play a role[31]. However, LPS injection increases brain TNF-α to levels of about one-third of those found in the plasma[30]; suggestive for an intracerebral TNF-α formation or TNF entry into the brain during systemic inflammation.

PATHOGENETIC MODEL

It remains to be established whether the functional sequelae of astrocyte swelling, oxidative/nitrosative stress and other actions of neurotoxins, which were mainly studied in *in vitro* or experimental animals, also apply for the cirrhotic human. In our current pathogenetic model for HE (Figure 1) ammonia triggers astrocytic glutamine accumulation, resulting in a compensatory depletion of osmolytes, such as taurine and myoinositol.

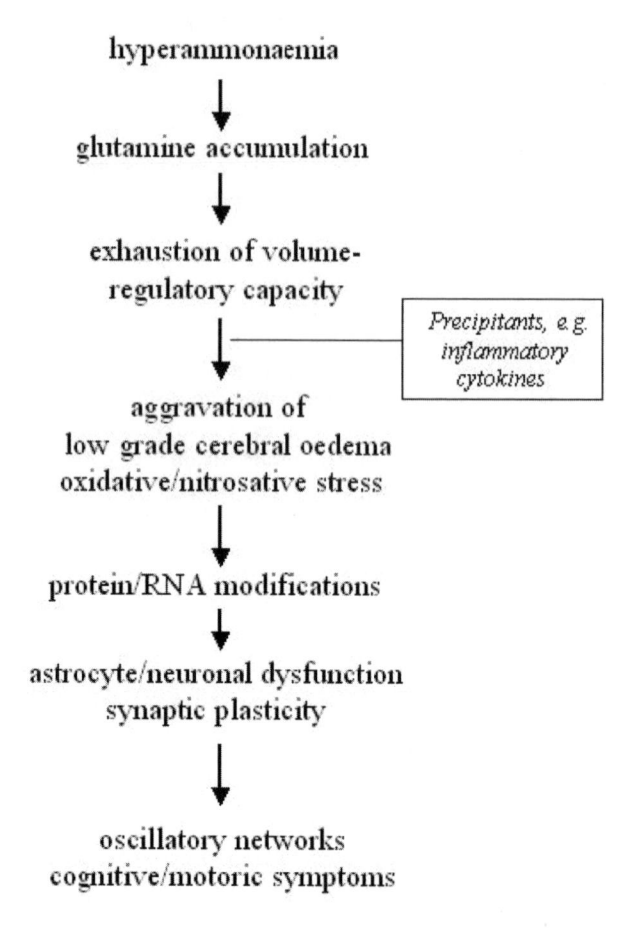

hyperammonaemia
↓
glutamine accumulation
↓
exhaustion of volume-
regulatory capacity
↓ ——— Precipitants, e.g. inflammatory cytokines
aggravation of
low grade cerebral oedema
oxidative/nitrosative stress
↓
protein/RNA modifications
↓
astrocyte/neuronal dysfunction
synaptic plasticity
↓
oscillatory networks
cognitive/motoric symptoms

Figure 1 Ammonia and inflammatory cytokines in the pathogenesis of hepatic encephalopathy

Exhaustion of the volume-regulatory capacity of astrocytes predisposes the brain to the induction of swelling by HE-precipitating factors, such as inflammatory cytokines, which synergistically promote a low-grade cerebral oedema. This mild, clinically silent hydration increase is sufficient to trigger multiple alterations of astrocyte function and gene expression in part through oxidative/nitrosative stress-dependent modifications of proteins and RNA. A mutual amplification of astroglial swelling and oxidative/nitrosative stress creates an autoamplificatory signalling loop and the action of various HE-precipitating factors, including inflammatory cytokines, integrates at least in part at this level. Oxidative/nitrosative stress induces protein modifications and RNA oxidation in the brain with impact on synaptic plasticity. As a result disturbances of oscillatory cerebral networks occur, which finally account for the symptoms of HE.

References

1. Häussinger D, Blei AT. Hepatic encephalopathy. In: Rodes J et al., editors. The Textbook of Hepatology. Oxford: Blackwell, 2007:728–60.
2. Häussinger D, Sies H, Gerok W. Functional hepatocyte heterogeneity in ammonia metabolism: the intercellular glutamine cycle. J Hepatol. 1984;1:3–14.
3. Häussinger D, Schliess F. Glutamine metabolism and signaling in the liver. Front Biosci. 2007;12:371–91.
4. Häussinger D. Ammonia, urea production and pH regulation. In: Rodes J et al., editors. The Textbook of Hepatology. Oxford: Blackwell, 2007:181–90.
5. Görg B, Wettstein M, Metzger S, Schliess F, Häussinger D. Lipopolysaccharide-induced tyrosine nitration and inactivation of hepatic glutamine synthetase in the rat. Hepatology. 2005;41:1065–73.
6. Görg B, Qvartskhava N, Voss P, Grune T, Schliess F. Reversible inhibition of mammalian glutamine synthetase by tyrosine nitration. FEBS Lett. 2007;581:84–90.
7. Häussinger D, Laubenberger J, vom Dahl S et al. Proton magnetic resonance spectroscopy studies on human brain myo-inositol in hypo-osmolarity and hepatic encephalopathy. Gastroenterology. 1994;107:1475–80.
8. Häussinger D. Low grade cerebral edema and the pathogenesis of hepatic encephalopathy in cirrhosis. Hepatology. 2006;43:1187–90.
9. Murthy CR, Rama Rao KV, Bai G, Norenberg MD. Ammonia-induced production of free radicals in primary cultures of rat astrocytes. J Neurosci Res. 2001; 66:282–8.
10. Schliess F, Görg B, Fischer R et al. Ammonia induces MK-801-sensitive nitration and phosphorylation of protein tyrosine residues in rat astrocytes. FASEB J. 2002;16:739–41.
11. Görg B, Foster N, Reinehr R et al. Benzodiazepine-induced protein tyrosine nitration in rat astrocytes. Hepatology. 2003;37:334–42.
12. Reinehr R, Görg B, Becker S et al. Hypoosmotic swelling and ammonia increase oxidative stress by NADPH oxidase in cultured astrocytes and vital brain slices. Glia. 2007;55:758–71.
13. Schliess F, Görg B, Reinehr RM, Bidmon HJ, Häussinger D. Osmotic and oxidative stress in hepatic encephalopathy. In: Häussinger D, Kircheis G, Schliess F, editors. Hepatic Encephalopathy and Nitrogen Metabolism. Dordrecht: Springer, 2006:20–42.
14. Rama Rao KV, Jayakumar AR, Norenberg MD. Induction of mitochondrial permeability transition in cultured astrocytes by glutamine. Neurochem Int. 2003;43:517–23.
15. Lavoie J, Layrargues GP, Butterworth RF. Increased densities of peripheral-type benzodiazepine receptors in brain autopsy samples from cirrhotic patients with hepatic encephalopathy. Hepatology. 1990;11:874–8.
16. Ahboucha S, Pomier-Layrargues G, Butterworth RF. Increased brain concentrations of endogenous (non-benzodiazepine) GABA-A receptor ligands in human hepatic encephalopathy. Metab Brain Dis. 2004;19:241–51.
17. Bender AS, Norenberg MD. Effect of benzodiazepines and neurosteroids on ammonia-induced swelling in cultured astrcytes. J Neurosci Res. 1998;54:673–80.
18. Butterworth RF. The astrocytic ('peripheral-type') benzodiazepine receptor: role in the pathogenesis of portal-systemic encephalopathy. Neurochem Int. 2000;36:411–16.
19. Görg B, Bidmon HJ, Keitel V et al. Inflammatory cytokines induce protein tyrosine nitration in rat astrocytes. Arch Biochem Biophys. 2006;449:104–14.
20. Shawcross D, Jalan R. The pathophysiologic basis of hepatic encephalopathy: central role for ammonia and inflammation. Cell Mol Life Sci. 2005;62:2295–304.
21. Blei AT. Infection, inflammation and hepatic encephalopathy: synergism redefined. J Hepatol. 2004;40:327–30.
22. Jover R, Rodrigo R, Felipo V et al. Brain edema and inflammatory activation in bile duct ligated rats with diet-induced hyperammonemia: a model of hepatic encephalopathy in cirrhosis. Hepatology. 2006;43:1257–66.
23. Shawcross DL, Davies NA, Williams R, Jalan R. Systemic inflammatory response exacerbates the neuropsychological effects of induced hyperammonemia in cirrhosis. J Hepatol. 2004;40:247–54.
24. Görg B, Qvartskhava N, Keitel V et al. Ammonia increases RNA oxidation in cultured astrocytes and brain *in vivo*. Hepatology (In press).

25. Kandel ER. The molecular biology of memory storage: a dialogue between genes and synapses. Science. 2001;294:1030–8.
26. Sutton MA, Schumann EM. Dendritic protein synthesis, synaptic plasticity, and memory. Cell. 2006;127:49–58.
27. Tanaka M, Chock PB, Stadtman ER. Oxidized messenger RNA induces translation errors. Proc Natl Acad Sci USA. 2007;104:66–71.
28. Pickering M, Cumiskey D, O'Connor JJ. Actions of TNF-alpha on glutamatergic synaptic transmission in the central nervous system. Exp Physiol. 2005;90:663–70.
29. Shawcross DL, Wright G, Olde Damink SWM, Jalan R. Role of ammonia and inflammation in minimal hepatic encephalopathy. Metab Brain Dis. 2007;22:125–38.
30. Wright G, Davies NA, Shawcross DL et al. Endotoxin produces coma and brain swelling in bile duct ligated rats. Hepatology. 2007;4:1517–26.
31. O'Beirne JP, Chouhan M, Hughes RD. The role of infection and inflammation in the pathogenesis of hepatic encephalopathy and cerebral edema in acute liver failure. Nature Clin Pract Gastroenterol Hepatol. 2006;3:118–19.

28
Liver and lung – treatment of hepatopulmonary diseases

P. SCHENK

INTRODUCTION

Pulmonary changes in patients with liver diseases are well known but infrequently recognized[1]. In recent years there has been increasing recognition of the importance of pulmonary vascular complications of liver diseases. These vascular complications, namely portopulmonary hypertension (PPHTN) and hepatopulmonary syndrome (HPS), usually present with dyspnoea and are not easily distinguished from other common reasons for dyspnoea in patients with advanced liver disease (such as anaemia, ascites, hepatic hydrothorax, muscle wasting, chronic obstructive pulmonary disease). PPHTN and HPS have a different prevalence, pathomechanism, clinical consequence and therapy.

PORTOPULMONARY HYPERTENSION

PPHTN is defined as pulmonary arterial hypertension (PAH) associated with portal hypertension in the presence or absence of liver disease. Diagnostic criteria for PAH according to the ERS Task Force consensus[2] are a mean pulmonary artery pressure (PAPmean) >25 mmHg at rest, a pulmonary capillary wedge pressure (PCP) <15 mmHg and a pulmonary vascular resistance (PVR) >240 dyn.s.cm^{-5}. This is to discriminate the moderate increases in PAP related to the commonly increased cardiac output (hyperdynamic circulatory state) and PCP (increased blood volume) that accompany liver disease.

A severity staging has been suggested which correlates with the increased mortality after orthotopic liver transplantation (OLT)[2,3]; see Table 1.

Prevalence in cirrhosis is 2–8.5% in catheter-based studies[4–9]. Echocardiography should be used as screening tool, right heart catheterization is recommended whenever PAPsyst is >50 mmHg. Acute vasodilator testing is useless, as calcium channel blockers are not indicated in PPHTN.

Table 1 Staging of severity of portopulmonary hypertension

Mild (early)	PAPmean	>25–34 mmHg
Moderate	PAPmean	⩾35–44 mmHg
Severe	PAPmean	⩾45 mmHg

PAPmean, mean pulmonary artery pressure.

Prognosis is worse compared to patients with idiopathic pulmonary artery hypertension, even when adjusted for laboratory values, haemodynamics and treatment[10]. Mean and median survivals of 15 and 6 months, respectively, were reported in the pre-OLT era[11].

TREATMENT

Oral anticoagulants should not be prescribed in PPHTN because of increased risk of gastrointestinal bleeding. Beta-blockers which are often administered for variceal bleeding prophylaxis can contribute to the clinical deterioration of PPHTN. In a prospective study, oral beta-blockers were discontinued in 10 patients with PPHTN[12]. Nine of 10 patients increased their 6-min walking distance with a mean increase in the whole group of 79±78 m, NYHA functional class improved in six patients (from class III to II). Cardiac output increased significantly by 28% with no change in mean pulmonary artery pressure, resulting in a 19% decrease in pulmonary vascular resistance. Increases in cardiac output were related to a 25% increase in heart rate, whereas stroke volume was unchanged.

Transjugular intrahepatic portosystemic shunt (TIPS) should be avoided because it may acutely enhance preload and thus increase PAP and PVR[13,14].

Vasodilator therapy

Calcium channel blockers are not recommended in patients with portal hypertension because they may increase hepatic venous pressure gradient.

Prostacyclin is a powerful systemic and pulmonary vasodilator, inhibitor of smooth muscle cell proliferation and platelet aggregation. It can be administered only by continuous intravenous infusion via a central venous catheter (e.g. Hickman catheter) or a Port-A-Cath, because of a short half-life (3–5 min). Fifty-two patients with continuous prostacyclin therapy have been reported so far (see Table 2) with favourable changes in PAPmean, PVR (reduction in the range from 22% to 71%), cardiac output, 6-min walk test and NYHA functional class. Common side-effects include jaw pain, headache, diarrhoea, flush, leg pain, nausea and vomiting. Serious and even fatal complications may occur due to the delivery system: catheter-related infection and sepsis, thrombosis, life-threatening interruption of the infusion (causing severe increase of pulmonary hypertension) due to pump failure. Progressive

Table 2 Long-term effects of intravenous prostacyclin in portopulmonary hypertension

No. of patients	Treatment time	PAPmean ↓ (%)	PVR ↓ (%)	Author
4	6–14 months	29–46	22–71	Kuo et al., Transplant, 1997
7	13 months	33	68	McLaughlin et al., Ann Intern Med., 1999
7	3–30 months	17	47	Krowka et al., Hepatology, 1999
1	4 months	24	54	Plotkin et al., Transplant, 1998
1	3 weeks	24	67	Ramsay et al., Anesthesiology, 1999
1	18 months	–4	52	Rafanan et al., Chest, 2000
1	5 months	24	40	Kähler et al., Wien Klin Wochenschr., 2000
1	29 months	31	43	Tan et al., Liver Transplant., 2001
1	4 days	29	15	Kett et al., Liver Transplant., 2001
1	7 weeks	6	57	Uchiyama et al., Liver Transplant., 2006
8	6.5 months	23	53	Sussman et al., Am J Transplant., 2006
19	15 months	25	55	Fix et al., Liver Transplant., 2007

PAPmean, mean pulmonary artery pressure; PVR, pulmonary vascular resistance.

splenomegaly with worsening thrombocytopenia and leucopenia occurred in four patients[15] and fatal gastrointestinal bleeding has been reported in a patient under continuous prostacyclin therapy[16].

The prostacyclin analogue treprostinil has been administered as long-term subcutaneous infusion in patients with PPHTN which resulted in an improved 6-min walk test, as published solely in abstract form[17].

Another prostacyclin analogue, iloprost, is effective for PAH when inhaled and therefore does not need an intravenous or subcutaneous access. In PPHTN, 16 patients treated with inhaled iloprost have been reported[18–21]. In the largest series ($n = 13$) published by Hoeper et al.[21], inhaled iloprost (six times daily at a dose of 5 µg) did not improve haemodynamic parameters after 6–18 months of treatment. Eight of the 13 patients died within 3 years (right heart failure: six, variceal bleeding: one, after liver and lung transplant: one) and in 9/13 patients a change of the treatment was necessary (five to intravenous prostacyclin and four to per os bosentan).

The dual receptor antagonist bosentan may cause a transient increase in hepatic enzyme levels (observed in 14% of patients)[22–24]. In a case series of 11 patients per os bosentan (started at 62.5 mg b.i.d. with increase to 125 mg b.i.d. after 4–8 weeks) significantly reduced PVR and improved exercise capacity[25]. The medication was well tolerated by all patients, and there was no evidence of drug-related liver injury. In a retrospective analysis of the same group, the efficacy and safety of inhaled iloprost ($n = 13$) and per os bosentan ($n = 18$) was assessed. In the iloprost group the survival rates at 1, 2 and 3 years were 77%, 62% and 46%, respectively. In the bosentan group the respective survival rates were 94%, 89% and 89% ($p = 0.029$ by log-rank analysis)[21]. Event-free survival rates, i.e. survival without transplantation, right heart failure or clinical worsening requiring the introduction of a new treatment for pulmonary hypertension, was also significantly better in the bosentan group. Bosentan had significantly better effects than inhaled iloprost on exercise capacity, as determined by the 6-min walk test, as well as on haemodynamics. Both treatments proved to be safe, especially with regard to liver function. In a multivariate Cox proportional hazard analysis relating survival time to selected variables only medication (iloprost vs bosentan) was significantly associated with survival ($p = 0.045$). According to the manufacturer's information bosentan is considered as a contraindication in Child B and C cirrhosis. However, in a case report low-dose bosentan (initially twice 31.25 mg/day and then twice 62.5 mg/day) was obviously effective and safe in a PPHTN patient with Child C cirrhosis and renal insufficiency[26].

Sildenafil, an oral phosphodiesterase-5 inhibitor, is registered for PH therapy[27] and is effective even in severe stages of PH[28]. It has the advantage of no detrimental effects on liver function, and is thus of interest in patients with severe liver disease. Seventeen patients have been reported to date[29–32]. In the largest series published recently by Reichenberger and co-workers[29], sildenafil at a dosage of 3×50 mg/day significantly improved PAPmean, PVR and cardiac index at 3 months and 6-min walk test at 3 and 12 months in 14 PPHTN patients in NYHA functional class III and IV. Mean pro-brain natriuretic peptide levels decreased significantly after 3 and 12 months. Patients with combination therapy (sildenafil + inhaled prostanoids) showed a trend to a higher improvement of 6-min walk test at 3 and 12 months compared to patients with sildenafil monotherapy. In addition, patients with Child A cirrhosis had a significantly higher increase of 6-min walk test at 3 months compared to patients with more advanced liver disease (Child B).

In contrast to HPS, PPHTN is not uniformly reversible after OLT. Moderate to severe PH (PAPmean >35 mmHg and PVR >250 dyn.s.cm^{-5}) is associated with increased risk of perioperative morbidity and mortality ($>50\%$)[33] and is therefore considered as a contraindication for OLT. There is no increase in mortality if PAPmean is $\leqslant 35$ mmHg[4,33]. The reason why OLT is dangerous for PPHTN patients is the sudden increase of right ventricular preload during reperfusion of the transplanted liver. During reperfusion PAPmean and right ventricular end-diastolic volume index increased by 40% and 39%, respectively in a group of patients with cirrhosis and mild PPHTN[34]. In patients with moderate to severe PH this may cause right ventricular failure; therefore all OLT candidates should be screened by echocardiography, and patients with PPHTN should be monitored by regular echocardiography examinations. Patients with moderate to severe PPHTN can be successfully treated with vasodilators to lower their PAP in the acceptable range for OLT (PAPmean <35 mmHg). Their postoperative survival is similar to that of transplanted patients without PPHTN, and in some patients vasodilator therapy can be stopped after a few months[35,36].

A practical recommendation for screening and therapy is provided in Figure 1.

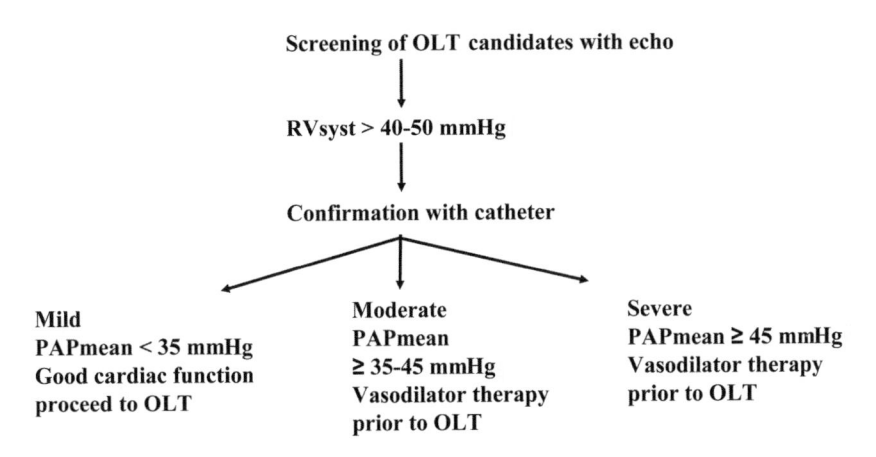

```
Screening of OLT candidates with echo
                │
    RVsyst > 40-50 mmHg
                │
    Confirmation with catheter
                │
    ┌───────────┼───────────┐
    ▼           ▼           ▼
Mild         Moderate      Severe
PAPmean < 35 mmHg   PAPmean      PAPmean ≥ 45 mmHg
Good cardiac function  ≥ 35-45 mmHg   Vasodilator therapy
proceed to OLT   Vasodilator therapy  prior to OLT
              prior to OLT
```

Figure 1 Algorithm for screening and therapeutic decisions in patients with portopulmonary hypertension, modified from Rodriguez-Roisin et al.[2]. OLT: orthotopic liver transplantation; RVsyst: right ventricular systolic pressure, PAPmean: mean pulmonary artery pressure

HEPATOPULMONARY SYNDROME

Definition

HPS is defined by the trias of liver disease, intrapulmonary vasodilation, and impaired arterial oxygenation[2,37,38]. The previous fourth point, the absence of intrinsic cardiopulmonary disease[39,40], has been removed because HPS may coexist with a primary cardiac or pulmonary disease[41]. According to the consensus of the ERS Task Force impaired arterial oxygenation is defined as $AaDO_2 > 15$ mmHg and $AaDO_2 > 20$ mmHg for patients older than 64 years[2].

Pathophysiology

The hallmark of pulmonary vascular changes in HPS are dilated vessels at the precapillary, capillary, and postcapillary level which enable mixed venous blood to pass into the pulmonary veins. In animal models, accumulation of macrophages in the pulmonary microcirculation and an increased number of pulmonary capillaries have been shown, suggesting a vasculogenic response[42,43].

Several mechanisms have been proposed to explain hypoxaemia in HPS: ventilation-perfusion (V'/Q') mismatch (impaired hypoxic pulmonary vasoconstriction, which is present in about 30% of patients with advanced liver disease, contributes mainly to V'/Q' mismatch), alveolo-capillary diffusion impairment to oxygen, and increased intrapulmonary shunt. The relative contributions of the three determinants appear to vary. Because the capillaries are dilated and have an expanded diameter (ranging from 15 to 500 µm), O_2 molecules from adjacent alveoli cannot diffuse to the centre in the dilated vessel to oxygenate haemoglobin in erythrocytes at the centre stream of venous blood. Supplemental O_2 provides enough driving pressure to partially overcome this relative diffusion defect.

Both acute and chronic liver diseases are associated with intrapulmonary vasodilation and arterial deoxygenation. The most frequent hepatic diagnoses are all different aetiologies of liver cirrhosis. Portal hypertension has been considered to be the most important determinant for development of HPS[44]. However, liver cirrhosis *per se* is not a prerequisite for the development of HPS, as patients with acute[45] and chronic non-cirrhotic hepatitis[46,47] with HPS have been reported, demonstrating that portal hypertension may not be present in all cases. HPS has also been described in patients after surgical portosystemic shunting[48], in the course of graft rejection after OLT[49], in extrahepatic portal venous obstruction[50] and hepatic venous obstruction without cirrhosis[51], and patients with hypoxic hepatitis[52].

Increased pulmonary production of nitric oxide (NO) is considered to play a central role in the pathogenesis of intrapulmonary vasodilation in cirrhotic patients with HPS[53–57]. Inhibition of NO synthase[58] by N^G-nitro-L-arginine methyl ester (L-NAME) prevented the development of hypoxaemia in rats with HPS, thereby supporting the pathogenetic role of NO[59]. Methylene blue, an oxidizing agent that blocks the stimulation of soluble guanylate cyclase by NO, improved hypoxaemia (by reduction of intrapulmonary shunt) and hyperdynamic circulation in patients with cirrhosis and moderate to severe HPS (see Figure 3)[60]. Further animal studies have shown that increased hepatic production and release of low levels of endothelin-1 (ET-1) is one mechanism for triggering an increased expression of eNOS with consecutive pulmonary vasodilation[61,62]. On the other hand, increased expression of iNOS is stimulated by elevated levels of cytokines (such as TNF-α, IL-6)[63] and endotoxin[63], caused by bacterial translocation (intestine barrier failure, occurring in up to 70% in cirrhotic rats). Suppression of the macrophages-iNOS by pentoxifyllin[64] reduced the NO production; prevention of bacterial translocation by antibiotic prophylaxis improved HPS severity in the rat model[65]. In recent years the findings of increased haem oxygenase 1 expression and carbon monoxide production in animal[66,67] and human studies[68] support their role for development of intrapulmonary vasodilation and HPS.

SYMPTOMS AND CLINICAL PRESENTATION

Cutaneous spider naevi are found in a significantly higher rate in HPS patients[69] and are considered as a cutaneous marker for intrapulmonary vasodilation. More specific pulmonary signs are dyspnoea (at exertion and later on at rest), platypnoea, orthodeoxia, cyanosis, and digital clubbing. Characteristic but not pathognomic symptoms are platypnoea, that is increased dyspnoea in upright position and less dyspnoea in supine position[70], and the associated finding of orthodeoxia (decrease of PaO_2 ⩾5% or >4 mmHg from the supine to upright position)[71–73].

PREVALENCE AND PROGNOSIS OF HPS IN PATIENTS WITH CIRRHOSIS

Patients with cirrhosis and HPS have a worse prognosis compared to patients without HPS (Figure 2)[74]. This is independent from severity of liver disease. Even after exclusion of patients who underwent OLT, HPS was associated with a worse prognosis. In HPS the severity of hypoxaemia correlates with prognosis (Figure 3). The presence of HPS has been shown to be a strong independent predictor of survival. Candidates for OLT should be screened for HPS and hypoxaemic patients with HPS should receive additional Model of End-Stage Liver Disease (MELD) points to be prioritized on the transplant waiting list.

THERAPEUTIC MANAGEMENT

Orthotopic liver transplantation

Since 1990 several case reports have shown complete resolution of HPS after OLT [75-80], PaO_2 returned to the normal range. Complete resolution of HPS has been observed in >80% of patients; however, it may take from 2 weeks up to 14 months to reach normal arterial oxygenation[76-81]. HPS is currently recognized as an indication for OLT in many centres[39,82-85], especially in the paediatric population[48,86,87]. Patients with severe HPS (PaO_2 <50 mmHg) have a higher postoperative mortality (30%)[88]; a recent study showed that a PaO_2 ⩽50 mmHg alone or in combination with a shunt fraction ⩾20% (perfusion lung scan) were the strongest predictors of postoperative mortality[89].

Long-term O₂ therapy

HPS patients with severe hypoxaemia (PaO_2 <60 mmHg) at rest should receive continuous long-term low-flow O_2 therapy[2]. Interestingly, as postulated in our publication[74], long-term O_2 therapy improved liver function in two patients with cirrhosis and HPS[58].

Embolization

Coil embolization of focal pulmonary arteriovenous communications has been reported to improve arterial oxygenation in a single case report[90].

Pharmacological treatment

A number of small uncontrolled clinical trials have been performed; however, none of the studies demonstrated consistent improvement in arterial oxygenation[2].

111 patients with cirrhosis, 27 with HPS

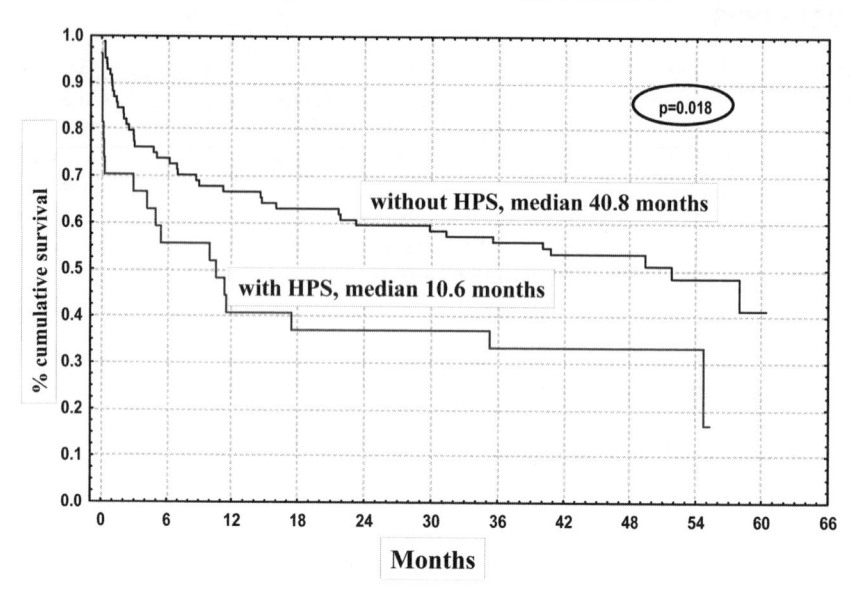

Figure 2 Cumulative survival of patients with cirrhosis with and without HPS

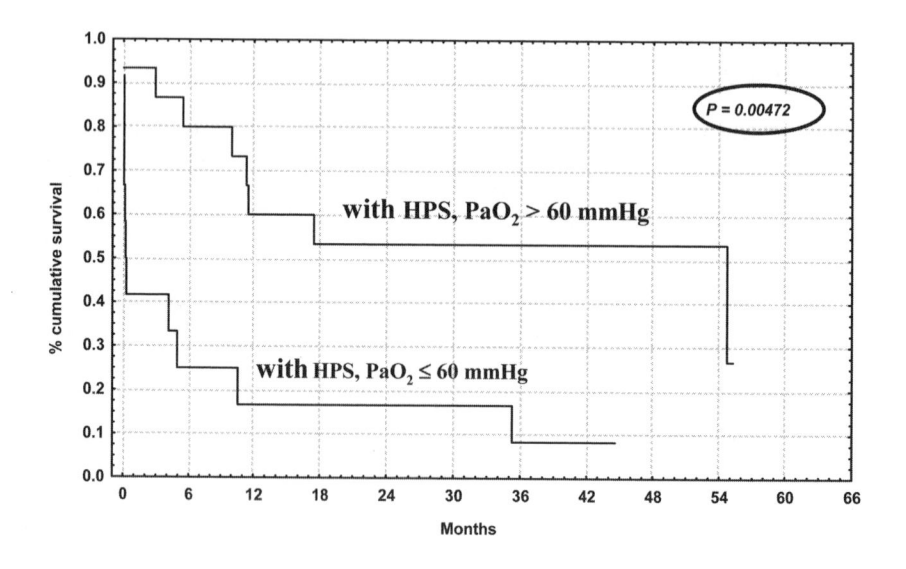

Figure 3 Prognosis of HPS according to the severity of hypoxaemia

References

1. Sherlock S. Disorders of the Liver and the Biliary System, 8th edn. Oxford: Blackwell, 1989:82–6.
2. Rodriguez-Roisin R et al. Pulmonary-hepatic vascular disorders (PHD). Eur Respir J. 2004;24:861–80.
3. Chemla D et al. Haemodynamic evaluation of pulmonary hypertension. Eur Respir J. 2002;20:1314–31.
4. Castro M et al. Frequency and clinical implications of increased pulmonary artery pressures in liver transplant patients. Mayo Clin Proc. 1996;71:543–51.
5. Hadengue A et al. Pulmonary hypertension complicating portal hypertension: prevalence and relation to splanchnic hemodynamics. Gastroenterology. 1991;100:520–8.
6. Ramsay MA et al. Severe pulmonary hypertension in liver transplant candidates. Liver Transplant Surg. 1997;3:494–500.
7. Sen S et al. Primary pulmonary hypertension in cirrhosis of liver. Indian J Gastroenterol. 1999;18:158–60.
8. Taura P et al. Moderate primary pulmonary hypertension in patients undergoing liver transplantation. Anesth Analg. 1996;83:675–80.
9. Yang YY et al. Portopulmonary hypertension: distinctive hemodynamic and clinical manifestations. J Gastroenterol. 2001;36:181–6.
10. Kawut SM et al. Hemodynamics and survival of patients with portopulmonary hypertension. Liver Transplant. 2005;1:1107–11.
11. Robalino BD, Moodie DS. Association between primary pulmonary hypertension and portal hypertension: analysis of its pathophysiology and clinical, laboratory and hemodynamic manifestations. J Am Coll Cardiol. 1991;17:492–8.
12. Provencher S et al. Deleterious effects of beta-blockers on exercise capacity and hemodynamics in patients with portopulmonary hypertension. Gastroenterology. 2006;130:120–6.
13. Azoulay D et al. Transjugular intrahepatic portosystemic shunt worsens the hyperdynamic circulatory state of the cirrhotic patient: preliminary report of a prospective study. Hepatology. 1994;19:129–32.
14. Van der Linden P et al. Pulmonary hypertension after transjugular intrahepatic portosystemic shunt: effects on right ventricular function. Hepatology. 1996;23:982–7.
15. Findlay JY et al. Progressive splenomegaly after epoprostenol therapy in portopulmonary hypertension. Liver Transplant Surg. 1999;5:362–5.
16. McLaughlin VV et al. Compassionate use of continuous prostacyclin in the management of secondary pulmonary hypertension: a case series. Ann Intern Med. 1999;130:740–3.
17. Benza RL et al. Safety and efficacy of treprostinil in cirrhosis-related pulmonary artery hypertension. Hepatology. 2003;38:A530.
18. Schroeder RA et al. Use of aerosolized inhaled epoprostenol in the treatment of portopulmonary hypertension. Transplantation. 2000;70:548–50.
19. Halank M et al. Use of aerosolized inhaled iloprost in the treatment of portopulmonary hypertension. J Gastroenterol. 2004;39:1222–3.
20. Molnar C et al. Successful switch from inhalative iloprost to oral bosentan in portopulmonary hypertension associated with liver cirrhosis. Wien Klin Wochenschr. 2004;116:627–30.
21. Hoeper MM et al. Experience with inhaled iloprost and bosentan in portopulmonary hypertension. Eur Respir J. 2007;30:1096–102.
22. van Giersbergen PL et al. Influence of mild liver impairment on the pharmacokinetics and metabolism of bosentan, a dual endothelin receptor antagonist. J Clin Pharmacol. 2003;43:15–22.
23. Channick RN et al. Effects of the dual endothelin-receptor antagonist bosentan in patients with pulmonary hypertension: a randomised placebo-controlled study. Lancet. 2001;358:1119–23.
24. Sitbon O et al. Effects of the dual endothelin receptor antagonist bosentan in patients with pulmonary arterial hypertension: a 1-year follow-up study. Chest. 2003;124:247–54.
25. Hoeper MM et al. Bosentan therapy for portopulmonary hypertension. Eur Respir J. 2005;25:502–8.

26. Barth F et al. Efficiency and safety of bosentan in Child C cirrhosis with portopulmonary hypertension and renal insufficiency. Eur J Gastroenterol Hepatol. 2006;18:1117–19.
27. Galie N et al. Sildenafil citrate therapy for pulmonary arterial hypertension. N Engl J Med. 2005;353:2148–57.
28. Singh TP et al. A randomized, placebo-controlled, double-blind, crossover study to evaluate the efficacy of oral sildenafil therapy in severe pulmonary artery hypertension. Am Heart J. 2006;151: 851 e1-5.
29. Reichenberger F et al. Sildenafil treatment for portopulmonary hypertension. Eur Respir J. 2006;28:563–7.
30. Chua R, Keogh A, Miyashita M. Novel use of sildenafil in the treatment of portopulmonary hypertension. J Heart Lung Transplant. 2005;24:498–500.
31. Makisalo H et al. Sildenafil for portopulmonary hypertension in a patient undergoing liver transplantation. Liver Transplant. 2004;10:945–50.
32. Rubio JLC. Successful treatment of severe portopulmonary hypertension in a patient with Child C cirrhosis by sildenafil. Liver Transplant. 2006;12:690–1.
33. Krowka MJ et al. Pulmonary hemodynamics and perioperative cardiopulmonary-related mortality in patients with portopulmonary hypertension undergoing liver transplantation. Liver Transplant. 2000;6:443–50.
34. Acosta F et al. Portopulmonary hypertension and liver transplantation: hemodynamic consequences at reperfusion. Transplant Proc. 2005;37:3865–6.
35. Sussman N et al. Successful liver transplantation following medical management of portopulmonary hypertension: a single-center series. Am J Transplant. 2006;6:2177–82.
36. Ashfaq M et al. The impact of treatment of portopulmonary hypertension on survival following liver transplantation. Am J Transplant. 2007;7:1258–64.
37. Lange PA, Stoller JK. The hepatopulmonary syndrome. Ann Intern Med. 1995;122:521–9.
38. Rodriguez-Roisin R, Agusti AG, Roca J. The hepatopulmonary syndrome: new name, old complexities. Thorax. 1992;47:897–902.
39. Krowka MJ, Cortese DA. Hepatopulmonary syndrome: an evolving perspective in the era of liver transplantation. Hepatology. 1990;11:138–42.
40. Rodriguez-Roisin R, Roca J. Hepatopulmonary syndrome: the paradigm of liver-induced hypoxaemia. Baillieres Clin Gastroenterol. 1997;11:387–406.
41. Martinez G et al. Hepatopulmonary syndrome associated with cardiorespiratory disease. J Hepatol. 1999;30:882–9.
42. Chang SW, Ohara N. Chronic biliary obstruction induces pulmonary intravascular phagocytosis and endotoxin sensitivity in rats. J Clin Invest. 1994;94:2009–19.
43. Schraufnagel DE et al. Lung capillary changes in hepatic cirrhosis in rats. Am J Physiol. 1997;272:L139–47.
44. Caruso G, Catalano D. Esophageal varices and hepato-pulmonary syndrome in liver cirrhosis. J Hepatol. 1991;12:262–3.
45. Regev A et al. Transient hepatopulmonary syndrome in a patient with acute hepatitis A. J Viral Hepatatis. 2001;8:83–6.
46. Silverman A et al. Syndrome of cyanosis, digital clubbing, and hepatic disease in siblings. J Pediatr. 1968;72:70–80.
47. Teuber G et al. Pulmonary dysfunction in non-cirrhotic patients with chronic viral hepatitis. Eur J Intern Med. 2002;13:311–18.
48. Laberge JM et al. Reversal of cirrhosis-related pulmonary shunting in two children by orthotopic liver transplantation. Transplantation. 1992;53:1135–8.
49. Crary GS et al. Radiological cases of the month. Pulmonary arteriovenous shunting in a child with cirrhosis of the liver. Am J Dis Child. 1989;143:749–51.
50. Gupta D et al. Prevalence of hepatopulmonary syndrome in cirrhosis and extrahepatic portal venous obstruction. Am J Gastroenterol. 2001;96:3395–9.
51. De BK et al. Hepatopulmonary syndrome in inferior vena cava obstruction responding to cavoplasty. Gastroenterology. 2000;118:192–6.
52. Fuhrmann V et al. Hepatopulmonary syndrome in patients with hypoxic hepatitis. Gastroenterology. 2006;131:69–75.
53. Cremona G et al. Elevated exhaled nitric oxide in patients with hepatopulmonary syndrome. Eur Respir J. 1995;8:1883–5.
54. Rolla G et al. Exhaled nitric oxide and oxygenation abnormalities in hepatic cirrhosis. Hepatology. 1997;26:842–7.

55. Rolla G et al. Exhaled nitric oxide and impaired oxygenation in cirrhotic patients before and after liver transplantation. Ann Intern Med. 1998;129:375–8.
56. Rolla G, Bucca C, Brussino L. Methylene blue in the hepatopulmonary syndrome. N Engl J Med. 1994;331:1098.
57. Vallance P, Moncada S. Hyperdynamic circulation in cirrhosis: a role for nitric oxide? Lancet. 1991;337:776–8.
58. Fukushima KY et al. Two cases of hepatopulmonary syndrome with improved liver function following long-term oxygen therapy. J Gastroenterol. 2007;42:176–80.
59. Zhang XJ et al. Intrapulmonary vascular dilatation and nitric oxide in hypoxemic rats with chronic bile duct ligation. J Hepatol. 2003;39:724–30.
60. Schenk P, Lehr S, Müller C. Methylene blue improves the hepatopulmonary syndrome (Letter). Ann Intern Med. 2001;133:738–40.
61. Luo B, Abrams GA, Fallon MB. Endothelin-1 in the rat bile duct ligation model of hepatopulmonary syndrome: correlation with pulmonary dysfunction. J Hepatol. 1998;29:571–8.
62. Zhang M et al. Endothelin-1 stimulation of endothelial nitric oxide synthase in the pathogenesis of hepatopulmonary syndrome. Am J Physiol. 1999;277:G944–52.
63. Genesca J et al. Nitric oxide may contribute to nocturnal hemodynamic changes in cirrhotic patients. Am J Gastroenterol. 2000;95:1539–44.
64. Beshay E, Croze F, Prud'homme GJ. The phosphodiesterase inhibitors pentoxifylline and rolipram suppress macrophage activation and nitric oxide production *in vitro* and *in vivo*. Clin Immunol. 2001;98:272–9.
65. Rabiller A et al. Prevention of gram-negative translocation reduces the severity of hepatopulmonary syndrome. Am J Respir Crit Care Med. 2002;166:514–17.
66. Carter EP et al. Regulation of heme oxygenase-1 by nitric oxide during hepatopulmonary syndrome. Am J Physiol Lung Cell Mol Physiol. 2002;283:L346–53.
67. Zhang J et al. Analysis of pulmonary heme oxygenase-1 and nitric oxide synthase alterations in experimental hepatopulmonary syndrome. Gastroenterology. 2003;125:1441–51.
68. Arguedas MR et al. Carboxyhemoglobin levels in cirrhotic patients with and without hepatopulmonary syndrome. Gastroenterology. 2005;128:328–33.
69. Schenk P et al. Hepatopulmonary syndrome: prevalence and predictive value of various cut offs for arterial oxygenation and their clinical consequences. Gut. 2002;51:853–9.
70. Robin ED et al. Platypnea related to orthodeoxia caused by true vascular lung shunts. N Engl J Med. 1976;294:941–3.
71. Edell ES et al. Severe hypoxemia and liver disease. Am Rev Respir Dis. 1989;140:1631–5.
72. Gomez FP et al. Gas exchange mechanism of orthodeoxia in hepatopulmonary syndrome. Hepatology. 2004;40:660–6.
73. Krowka MJ, Cortese DA. Hepatopulmonary syndrome. Current concepts in diagnostic and therapeutic considerations. Chest. 1994;105:1528–37.
74. Schenk P et al. Prognostic significance of the hepatopulmonary syndrome in patients with cirrhosis. Gastroenterology. 2003;125:1042–52.
75. Stoller JK et al. Prevalence and reversibility of the hepatopulmonary syndrome after liver transplantation. The Cleveland Clinic experience. West J Med. 1995;163:133–8.
76. Barry S et al. Comparison of shunt fractions pre- and post-liver transplantation. Transplant Proc. 1993;25:1787–8.
77. Durand P et al. Reversal of hypoxemia by inhaled nitric oxide in children with severe hepatopulmonary syndrome, type 1, during and after liver transplantation. Transplantation. 1998;65:437–9.
78. Lange PA, Stoller JK. The hepatopulmonary syndrome. Effect of liver transplantation. Clin Chest Med. 1996;17:115–23.
79. Schwarzenberg SJ et al. Resolution of severe intrapulmonary shunting after liver transplantation. Chest. 1993;103:1271–3.
80. Stoller JK et al. Reduction of intrapulmonary shunt and resolution of digital clubbing associated with primary biliary cirrhosis after liver transplantation. Hepatology. 1990;11:54–8.
81. Philit F et al. Late resolution of hepatopulmonary syndrome after liver transplantation. Respiration. 1997;64:173–5.

82. Battaglia SE et al. Resolution of gas exchange abnormalities and intrapulmonary shunting following liver transplantation. Hepatology. 1997;25:1228–32.
83. Collisson EA et al. Retrospective analysis of the results of liver transplantation for adults with severe hepatopulmonary syndrome. Liver Transplant. 2002;8:925–31.
84. Krowk MJ. Hepatopulmonary syndrome: recent literature (1997 to 1999) and implications for liver transplantation. Liver Transplant. 2000;6:S31–5.
85. Rodriguez-Roisin R, Krowka MJ. Is severe arterial hypoxaemia due to hepatic disease an indication for liver transplantation? A new therapeutic approach. Eur Respir J. 1994;7:839–42.
86. Hobeika J et al. Orthotopic liver transplantation in children with chronic liver disease and severe hypoxemia. Transplantation. 1994;57:224–8.
87. Van Obbergh L et al. Liver transplantation and pulmonary gas exchanges in hypoxemic children. Am Rev Respir Dis. 1993;148:1408–10.
88. Krowka MJ et al. Hepatopulmonary syndrome with progressive hypoxemia as an indication for liver transplantation: case reports and literature review. Mayo Clin Proc. 1997;72:44–53.
89. Arguedas MR et al. Prospective evaluation of outcomes and predictors of mortality in patients with hepatopulmonary syndrome undergoing liver transplantation. Hepatology. 2003;37:192–7.
90. Poterucha JJ et al. Failure of hepatopulmonary syndrome to resolve after liver transplantation and successful treatment with embolotherapy. Hepatology. 1995;21:96–100.

29
Allocation in adult liver transplantation: is the Model for Endstage Liver Disease the solution?

D. M. HEUMAN

HISTORY OF MELD-BASED ORGAN ALLOCATION

In 1998, following years of study, the US Department of Health and Human Services issued its so-called Final Rule[1], mandating changes in organ allocation policy to eliminate waiting time as a criterion, reduce regional differences in organ availability, and establish more objective criteria for listing and transplantation. The intent of the rule was to make access to transplantation more equitable throughout the USA by eliminating discrepancies related to individual and regional variations in economic resources and in quality of health-care available. It was also intended to minimize the risk of abuses resulting from competition between transplant programmes, by providing a clear, uniform and unambiguous set of rules for organ allocation.

At that time, organ allocation for liver transplantation in the USA followed a four-tier system of priority, in order of descending urgency. Level 1 included patients with fulminant hepatic failure, early post-transplant complications (primary non-function, hepatic artery thrombosis) or acutely decompensated Wilson's disease. Level 2A included patients with acutely decompensated cirrhosis requiring intensive care. Level 2B included Child–Turcotte–Pugh (CTP) class C cirrhotics. Level 3 included CTP class B cirrhotics. Within each level, priority was determined by time spent on the waiting list. The system depended on clinical judgement in moving patients to status 2A, and in assigning points for ascites and encephalopathy when determining CTP scores. Experience had shown that these subjective components were frequently subject to manipulation in a competitive transplant environment.

To meet the requirements of the Final Rule, a new tool was needed for objectively assessing severity of liver disease. A candidate appeared in 2000, when Malinchoc and co-workers at the Mayo Clinic published a model for predicting 90-day survival in cirrhotic patients undergoing transjugular intrahepatic portosystemic shunting[2]. Components of the model included serum creatinine and bilirubin, plasma international normalized ratio (INR), and aetiology of liver disease (survival was significantly better in patients with cholestatic or alcoholic disease).

For the purposes of transplantation this model had a number of attractive features. It was based on an accepted sound statistical method, it required only easily obtainable laboratory data, it estimated disease severity on a continuous scale, and it had no subjective components. Some less attractive features included the possibility of negative scores (logarithms of numbers less than 1), difficulty in interpreting creatinine values in patients on dialysis, and an element of subjectivity in assigning aetiology. The latter problems were overcome arbitrarily by eliminating the aetiology component of the score, setting minimum values of 1 for each of the laboratory components, setting a maximum value of 4 to serum creatinine, and setting creatinine value to 4 in any patient requiring dialysis. While these changes were without *a priori* statistical justification, they were found to have only a minimal effect on the predictive power[3].

The resulting formula was renamed the Model for Endstage Liver Disease, or MELD. In a number of validation studies in different cirrhotic populations, MELD was found to be a good predictor of early mortality[3,4]. Some claims that MELD was superior to the more traditional CTP score were inflated by biases in patient selection[5], but MELD is at least as accurate as the CTP score for predicting short-term survival, and has the advantage of being based entirely on objective, easily determined, verifiable laboratory parameters.

MELD was adopted in the USA as the basis for most adult liver transplant organ allocation on 27 February 2002. For paediatric liver transplantation a somewhat different model, termed PELD, was implemented, following a similar process. Status 1 (not MELD/PELD-based) was retained for patients with fulminant hepatic failure, primary non-function, early hepatic artery thrombosis, and acute decompensated Wilson's disease, and these accounted for about 3% of liver transplants in 2005. Routine exceptions to MELD were permitted for patients with early-stage hepatocellular carcinoma (HCC), hepatopulmonary syndrome, and certain other rare conditions. Other individualized MELD exceptions could be requested and granted, subject to individual application and approval by regional review boards. In 2005 these exceptions accounted for 22% of all transplants (13% for HCC, 9% for other indications). In January 2005, allocation was further modified to discourage transplantation of low MELD patients, by requiring local organ procurement organizations to share organs regionally before allocating them to local patients with MELD scores under 15 (Share 15).

CONSEQUENCES OF MELD-BASED ORGAN ALLOCATION

The following analyses are based on publicly available data of the US Organ Procurement and Transplant Network and the Scientific Registry of Transplant Recipients, as updated through the end of 2006[6]; data are accessible on the internet at <www.unos.org> and <www.ustransplant.org>.

ALLOCATION IN ADULT LIVER TRANSPLANTATION

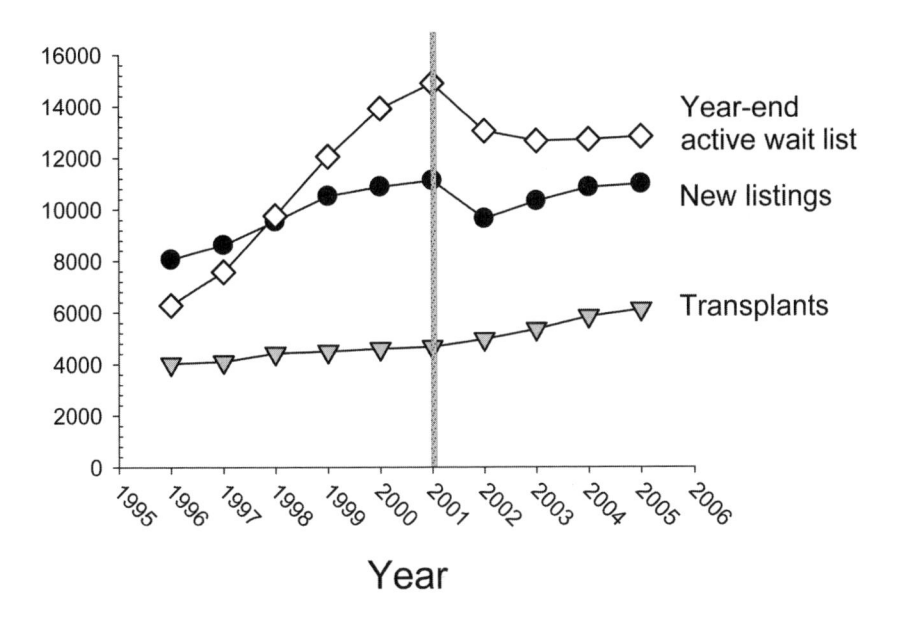

Figure 1 Effect of MELD-based organ allocation on the US liver transplant list. MELD-based 'sickest first' organ allocation was implemented on 27 February 2007. The year 2001 (vertical line) was therefore the last full year under the old system of organ allocation. The number of patients on the transplant list fell in 2002 and thereafter has remained constant. New transplant listings dropped during the year following implementation, but subsequently have returned to pre-MELD levels. A steady increase in total transplants has also been noted over this time period and helps to explain the lack of growth of the waiting list

Following implementation of the new system of MELD-based organ allocation there was an immediate decrease in new listings and a decline in the US liver transplant active waiting list (Figure 1). This reversed a trend of continuous growth over the preceding decade. For newly listed patients the waiting time to transplantation for sicker patients, which had been rising steadily, now dropped dramatically (Figure 2). For patients listed in 2000 and 2001 the median waiting time exceeded 5 years; by 2005 the median wait for newly listed patients was less than 1 year. This reflects the fact that listing of cirrhotic patients can now be put off until a more advanced stage of liver disease without loss of priority. While MELD was probably a major factor causing these changes, the shorter waiting list and shorter time to transplant were also partly explained by an increase in total adult liver transplants performed, from 4591 in 2001 to 6074 in 2006, due almost entirely to expanded use of extended criteria donor livers, especially those obtained following cardiac death.

The number of waiting-list deaths changed in parallel with the size of the waiting list (Figure 3). An initial drop in total waiting-list deaths was greeted with enthusiasm. However, when waiting-list mortality rate is expressed as a

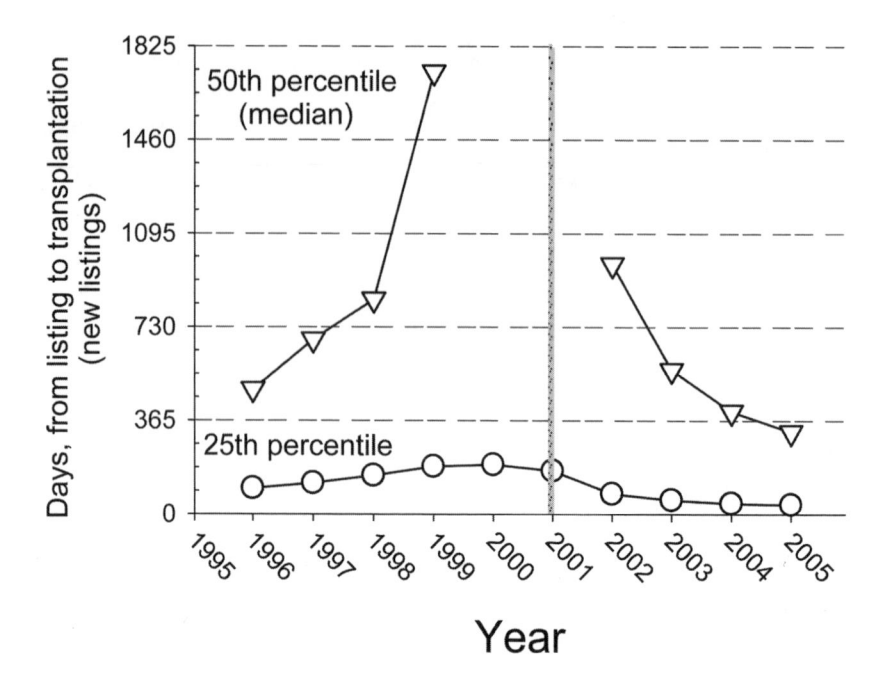

Figure 2 Effect of MELD-based 'sickest first' organ allocation on waiting time, by year of listing. Median waiting time for new listings, which had increased steadily prior to 2001, subsequently declined dramatically from >5 years to <1 year. Waiting time for the upper quartile of patients also decreased

function of total patient-years at risk, the benefits are less clear. Prior to adoption of MELD this mortality rate had shown progressive improvement. After 2002 little further improvement in adult US waiting-list mortality was noted, despite a substantial increase in number of adult liver transplants performed.

The trends in pretransplant mortality are complex and subject to varying interpretations. The advent of MELD produced an undercounting artifact, as physicians deferred listing potentially transplantable cirrhotics with low MELD scores, since deaths among these 'pre-list' cirrhotics are not tracked by the transplant system. This undercounting could largely explain the initial decrease in total waiting-list deaths after implementation of MELD. The decline in waiting-list mortality rate in the 1990s, prior to MELD, may reflect the disproportionate accumulation of relatively low-risk patients with uncomplicated cirrhosis who were being listed prematurely in order to accrue waiting time. If patients on the transplant list are now sicker, the stable mortality rate may in fact represent a significant achievement[7]. However, the distribution of MELD scores among newly listed patients, and on the waiting list as a whole, has been essentially constant at least since 2002. Pretransplant

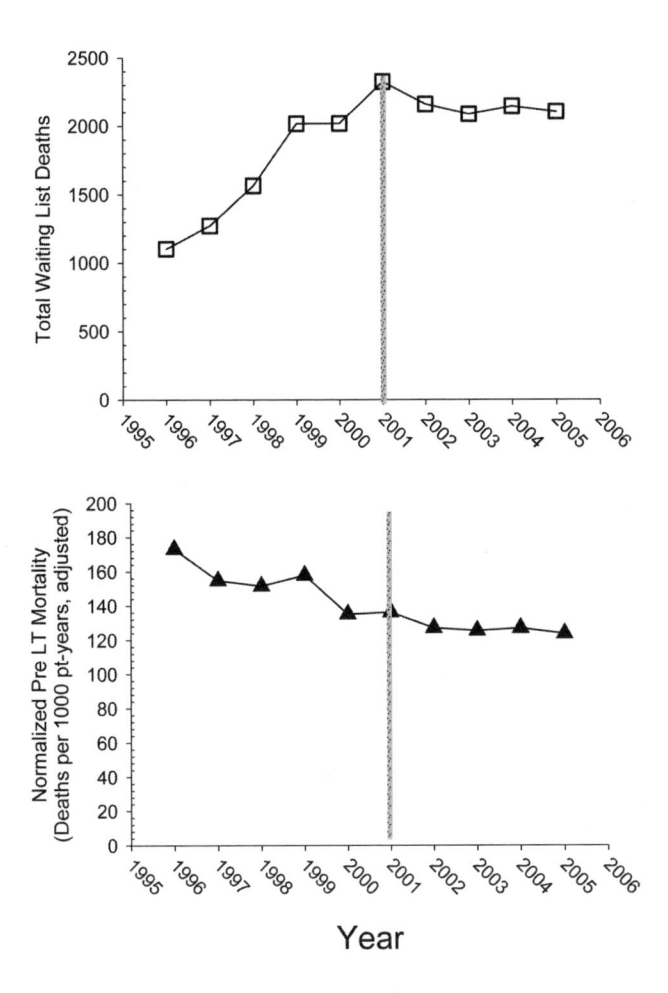

Figure 3 Effect of MELD-based organ allocation on pre-transplant mortality. The number of waiting-list deaths (upper graph) increased with growth in the waiting list through 2001, but declined and levelled off after implementation of MELD-based organ allocation. But when normalized for the number of patient-years at risk (lower figure), the pretransplant waiting-list mortality rate, which had decreased significantly in the previous 5 years, has shown little further improvement in the MELD era

deaths remain common among patients with high MELD. In a snapshot of patients listed actively for transplantation on 1 January 2005, 90-day pretransplant mortality exceeded 30% in patients with MELD >30 and 10% in patients with MELD of 21–30. The effects of Share 15 are not fully evaluable at this time, but preliminary figures showing a 7% decline in total waiting-list deaths in 2006 suggest that we may at last be seeing some real benefit.

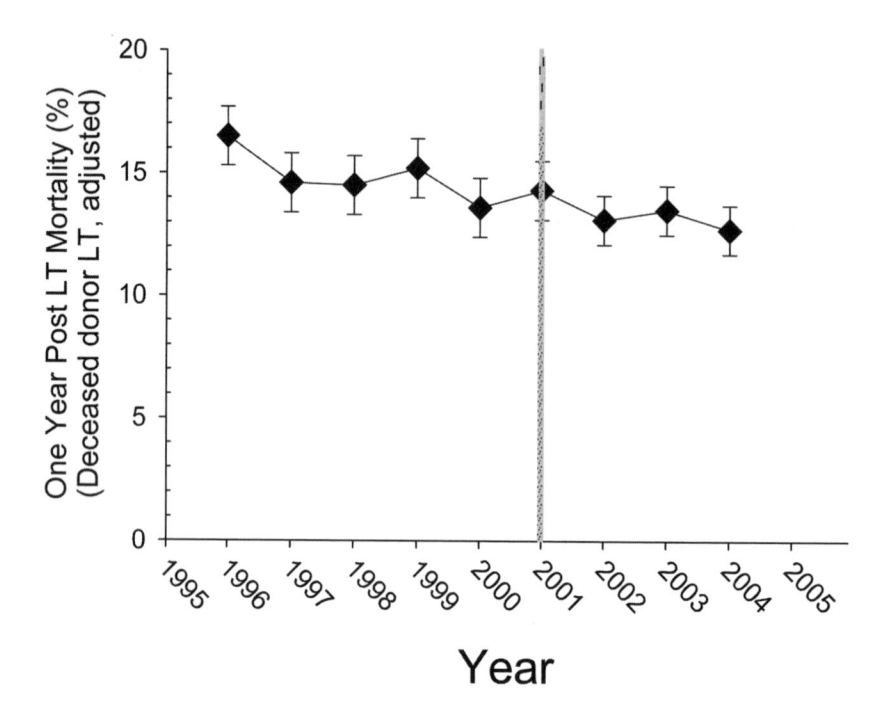

Figure 4 Effect of MELD-based organ allocation on post-liver transplant outcome. Slow improvement in post-transplant mortality (1 year) preceded implementation. Since 2001 mortality has been stable or slightly improved, despite the fact that patients transplanted at MELD scores > 30 have significantly worse outcomes

The impact of MELD-based organ allocation on post-transplant outcomes is also hard to assess, but appears to have been modest. It is clear that transplanting sicker patients leads to longer post-transplant hospitalization, increased complications and increased costs[8]. MELD scores greater than 30 are associated with increased post-transplant mortality (23% 1-year mortality, compared to ~13% for cirrhotic patients with MELD <30 or exceptional MELD scores). However, overall post-transplant 1-year mortality after implementation of MELD has not changed significantly (Figure 4). The contribution of 'sickest first' organ allocation to post-transplant mortality is obscured by a number of concurrent developments. Developments that favour better survival include continued technical improvements in transplantation and immunosuppression, transplantation of increasing numbers of patients under MELD exceptions unrelated to cirrhosis severity (e.g. HCC), better patient selection, and growing organ supply. Developments that adversely affect survival include increasing average recipient age at transplantation and increased use of extended criteria donor livers.

MELD – PROS AND CONS

Although MELD has always been described as a 'work in progress', it has not been modified since its adoption, and attempts to improve MELD must overcome considerable inertia. The relative weighting factors for INR, bilirubin, and creatinine have never been reassessed, despite the fact that the original coefficients were based on a relatively small, selected population and probably are not optimal. There is an unnecessary element of arithmetic complexity. Use of base 10 rather than natural logarithms and elimination of the constant component (both simple linear transformations with no effect on the model's predictive value) would make the index more intuitively accessible. It may be that logarithms can be eliminated altogether. We found that a logistic regression model employing simple arithmetic values of creatinine, INR and bilirubin, without logarithmic transformation, was as accurate as MELD for predicting short-term mortality (unpublished data).

The practice of using minimum MELD scores as threshold criteria for listing is not well justified by the data. Though a relationship of MELD to short-term mortality can be demonstrated at all scores above 14, the performance of MELD at the low end of the range (below 20) is poor. In patients with MELD scores ≤20, we found that only hyponatraemia and uncontrolled ascites were independent predictors of 6-month pre-transplant survival[9]. Incorporation of these factors into MELD might improve its prognostic accuracy. Studies from five continents have uniformly confirmed that low serum sodium is a predictor of short-term cirrhotic mortality independent of MELD[9-12]. Although there is reluctance to consider inclusion of 'subjective' measures of disease severity in the MELD model, we also found that inclusion of points for uncontrolled ascites improved the ability of MELD to predict 180-day survival for patients with MELD <21[9]. Hepatic encephalopathy likewise may have independent prognostic significance[13]. However, a consensus panel in 2006 discouraged the routine granting of MELD exceptions for hyponatraemia, ascites and encephalopathy[14].

While MELD is overall an objective measure of liver disease severity, each of the components of MELD can be altered by factors unrelated to cirrhotic prognosis[15]. Intrinsic renal disease, transient biliary ductal obstruction, and warfarin therapy each can increase MELD score to 20 or more in the absence of any chronic liver disease. Because it is logarithmic, MELD is particularly sensitive to changes at the low end of the scale, and fluctuations of 3–5 points can result when transient dehydration raises creatinine, or when fasting increases the bilirubin level (especially in patients with Gilbert's syndrome). Substantial variation in INR from laboratory to laboratory can occur because of differences in reagents used[16]. Physicians have learned to manipulate these factors to increase transplant priority for their patients. It is possible to circumvent some of these concerns. For example, a surrogate MELD score excluding the INR can give a reasonable approximation of true risk in patients treated with warfarin[17]. However, the organ allocation system remains blind to these nuances, and patients with artefactual elevations of MELD continue to receive enhanced priority for transplantation.

Finally, the current practice in 'sickest-first' organ allocation makes no allowance for the cumulative consequences of disability. The decision to define the 'sickest' patients solely in terms of short-term mortality risk was a reasonable response to the Final Rule, given the need for an objective endpoint around which to build a consensus. But many patients who are severely disabled by cirrhosis have stable MELD scores that are too low to permit transplantation. These patients now face an indefinite wait. Some are hospitalized repeatedly for complications such as encephalopathy, variceal bleeding or spontaneous bacterial peritonitis, and may die of these complications without ever achieving a transplantable MELD score. Many eventually will develop co-morbid conditions that preclude transplantation. Some who are unable to continue working will lose health insurance and may be dropped from the transplant list. Often they face personal bankruptcy. As MELD evolves, the inclusion of secondary 'quality of life' endpoints should be considered to address issues such as these.

CONCLUSIONS

The requirements of the Final Rule have been met, and MELD has eliminated much of the subjectivity from the process of organ allocation. Waiting time is no longer a factor. The transplant waiting list is no longer growing. Sicker patients are being transplanted sooner. Post-transplant mortality appears to be no worse, but pre-transplant mortality rate also has shown little improvement so far. MELD has proven to be a good but imperfect predictor of short-term survival in cirrhosis; it is subject to a number of extrahepatic influences, and it fails to fully capture the mortality risk associated with ascites and hyponatraemia.

References

1. Organ Procurement and Transplantation Network – HRSA. Final rule with comment period. Fed Regist. 1998;63:16296–338.
2. Malinchoc M, Kamath PS, Gordon FD, Peine CJ, Rank J, ter Borg PC. A model to predict poor survival in patients undergoing transjugular intrahepatic portosystemic shunts. Hepatology. 2000;31:864–71.
3. Kamath PS, Wiesner RH, Malinchoc M et al. A model to predict survival in patients with end-stage liver disease. Hepatology. 2001;33:464–70.
4. Wiesner RH. Evidence-based evolution of the MELD/PELD liver allocation policy. Liver Transplant. 2005;11:261–3.
5. Heuman DM, Mihas A. Utility of the MELD score for assessing 3-month survival in patients with liver cirrhosis: one more positive answer. Gastroenterology. 2003;125:992–3.
6. Pomfret EA, Fryer JP, Sima CS, Lake JR, Merion RM. Liver and intestine transplantation in the United States, 1996-2005. Am J Transplant. 2007;7:1376–89.
7. Brown RS Jr, Lake JR. The survival impact of liver transplantation in the MELD era, and the future for organ allocation and distribution. Am J Transplant. 2005;5:203–4.
8. Zapata R, Innocenti F, Sanhueza E et al. Predictive models in cirrhosis: correlation with the final results and costs of liver transplantation in Chile. Transplant Proc. 2004;36:1671–2.
9. Heuman DM, bou-Assi SG, Habib A et al. Persistent ascites and low serum sodium identify patients with cirrhosis and low MELD scores who are at high risk for early death. Hepatology. 2004;40:802–10.

10. Biggins SW, Rodriguez HJ, Bacchetti P, Bass NM, Roberts JP, Terrault NA. Serum sodium predicts mortality in patients listed for liver transplantation. Hepatology. 2005;41:32–9.
11. Ruf AE, Kremers WK, Chavez LL, Descalzi VI, Podesta LG, Villamil FG. Addition of serum sodium into the MELD score predicts waiting list mortality better than MELD alone. Liver Transplant. 2005;11:336–43.
12. Londono MC, Cardenas A, Guevara M et al. MELD score and serum sodium in the prediction of survival of patients with cirrhosis awaiting liver transplantation. Gut. 2007;56:1283–90.
13. Stewart CA, Malinchoc M, Kim WR, Kamath PS. Hepatic encephalopathy as a predictor of survival in patients with end-stage liver disease. Liver Transplant. 2007;13:1366–71.
14. Freeman RB, Gish RG, Harper A et al. Model for Endstage Liver Disease (MELD) exception guidelines: results and recommendations from the MELD exception study group and conference (MESSAGE) for the approval of patients who need liver transplantation with diseases not considered by the standard MELD formula, 12 edn. 2006:S128–36.
15. Biggins SW, Feng S. In a MELD-based economy, how can we fight off inflation? Liver Transplant. 2007;13:2–4.
16. Trotter JF, Brimhall B, Arjal R, Phillips C. Specific laboratory methodologies achieve higher model for endstage liver disease (MELD) scores for patients listed for liver transplantation. Liver Transplant. 2004;10:995–1000.
17. Heuman DM, Mihas AA, Habib A et al. MELD-XI: a rational approach to 'sickest first' liver transplantation in cirrhotic patients requiring anticoagulant therapy. Liver Transplant. 2007;13:30–7.

30
Emerging future therapies for portal hypertension

J. BOSCH and A. De GOTTARDI

KEY POINTS

1. Treatments for portal hypertension and selection of patients are still unsatisfactory.

2. We need better ways of assessing treatments and non-invasive methods to assess the response to therapy.

3. Advances in knowledge of pathophysiology translate into new targets for therapy that go beyond the classical paradigm based on the use of vasoactive agents.

TREATMENTS FOR PORTAL HYPERTENSION ARE STILL UNSATISFACTORY

Despite marked improvement in therapy during the past two decades, treatments for portal hypertension are still far from ideal. The following is a non-comprehensive list of the more important pending issues:

1. There is no proven therapy for preventing the formation of varices.

2. Medical treatments for the prophylaxis of first variceal bleeding are partly effective, but have many limitations and selection of patients and screening procedures are still under debate.

3. Very much the same applies with regard to the prevention of recurrent bleeding, where we still do not know if hepatic venous pressure gradient (HVPG) monitoring improves outcomes and if it is cost-effective, what to do with non-responders, and whether there is a role for transjugular intrahepatic portosystemic shunt (TIPS) outside rescue of medical failures.

4. Treatment of acute variceal bleeding is not adjusted for disease severity and other well-known risk factors.
5. Prevention of ascites, spontaneous bacterial peritonitis and hepatorenal syndrome is still being studied.
6. There is no medical treatment for hepatopulmonary syndrome and treatment for portopulmonary hypertension is only of limited efficacy.

NEW METHODS FOR ASSESSING NEW TREATMENTS

HVPG is a strong prognostic indicator in chronic liver disease and portal hypertension[1-7]. Moreover, changes in HVPG during therapy for portal hypertension closely correlate with clinical outcomes and survival. There is an increasing awareness that HVPG may be the best surrogate endpoint in the evaluation of new therapies for portal hypertension and its complications, as well as to assess progression of alcoholic, viral, metabolic, genetic (and perhaps cholestatic) cirrhosis[2]. The use of HVPG as a surrogate of clinical events in initial clinical trials will greatly facilitate research in treatments testing new paradigms. Procedures for HVPG measurement need to be standardized in internationally agreed guidelines to make its use reliable worldwide[2].

Methods for the non-invasive assessment of response to therapy

There is a need for new, reliable, objective and non-invasive methods for evaluating new treatments and to monitor the effects of therapy, especially in the context of pharmacological treatment. The current gold standard for assessing treatment response is the measurement of HVPG. Although this is a minimally invasive method (as endoscopic procedures require sedation) it would be desirable to have a less demanding substitute. However, available methods (Doppler ultrasound, Fibroscan, MRI, Varipress, etc.) are either unreliable or less accurate; some are equally invasive and none allows substituting the measurement of HVPG[2,8].

EMERGING THERAPIES

The old paradigm: use of vasoactive drugs

Up to now the medical treatment of portal hypertension has been based on the use of vasoactive drugs that decrease splanchnic blood flow and portal (and variceal) pressure[8] (Figure 1). These include terlipressin, somatostatin (and analogues) and non-selective beta-blockers, alone or in association with a low-dose vasodilator (to enhance the reduction in portal pressure and minimize systemic side-effects).

These treatments, however, have a number of limitations (see the list at the beginning of this chapter), the more important being that the maximal risk-reduction afforded is of about 50%. There is a subgroup of patients who benefit

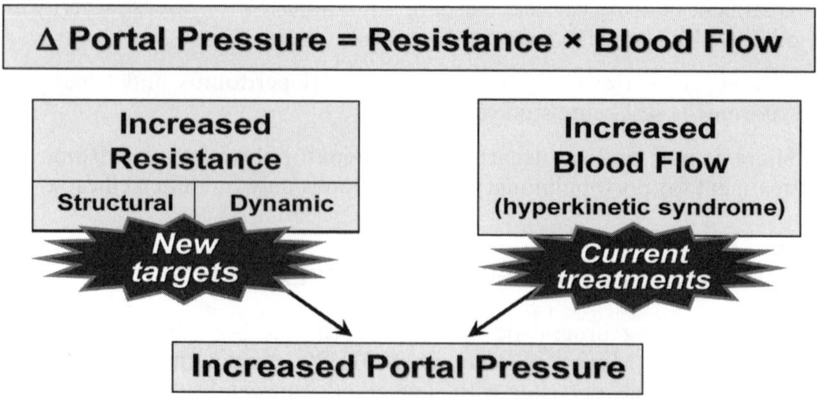

Figure 1 Current treatments for portal hypertension are based on the use of vasoactive agents that decrease portal pressure mainly by acting on the increased splanchnic blood flow and hyperkinetic circulation. Advances in knowledge of the basic mechanisms leading to portal hypertension have disclosed new targets for therapy, based on the correction of the structural and dynamic abnormalities that result in increased hepatic resistance

the most from these therapies. In the case of long-term therapy with non-selective β-blockers (associated or not to isosorbide mononitrate), measurement of the chronic HVPG response allows identifying these patients, as many studies and meta-analyses have demonstrated that the risk of bleeding is dramatically decreased when HVPG is decreased by ⩾20% from baseline or below 12 mmHg[1-7]. This 'responder' subgroup may have other beneficial effects, including prevention of spontaneous bacterial peritonitis[4,10], ascites[4] and portal hypertensive gastropathy[9], altogether resulting in improved survival.

New therapeutic developments based on the same paradigm use drugs or drug combinations with a more powerful portal pressure-decreasing effect. The two that have been shown to be more effective are carvedilol[11,12] (as single agent) and the combination of propranolol and prazosin[13]. Both have proved more powerful than propranolol/nadolol in randomized controlled trials testing its effects on portal pressure; however, both have significantly more frequent and severe side-effects than do non-selective β-blockers[12,13]. The more relevant are linked to development of systemic hypotension, which translates in worsening of renal function and of ascites. These limitations apply to all available vasodilators. Because of the adverse effects linked to systemic hypotension in patients with cirrhosis, it is widely accepted that these patients should not receive vasodilators as monotherapy[14], although these agents may be used associated with a vasoconstrictor or a non-selective β-blocker.

New paradigms in therapy

Emerging treatments for portal hypertension are testing new paradigms, for which objective evidence has been accumulating in recent years (Figures 1 and 2). These new targets for therapy include the following:

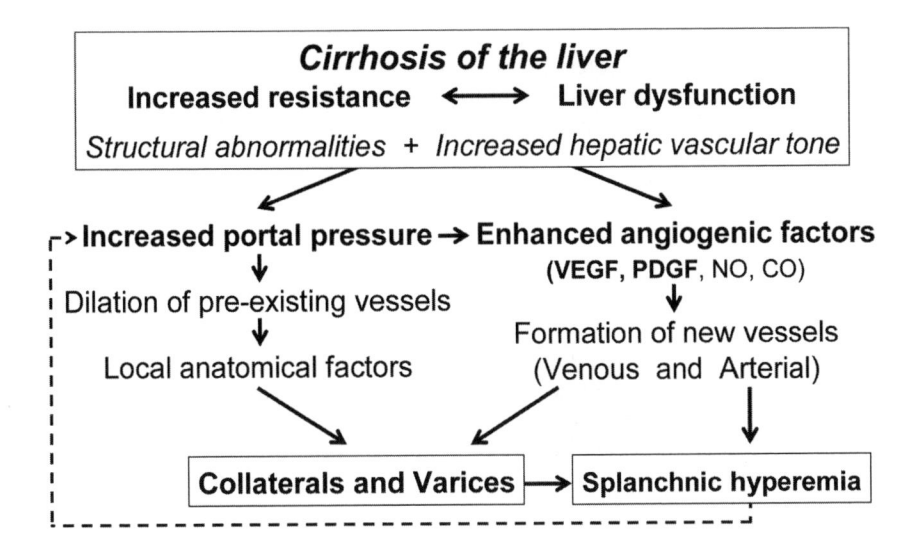

Figure 2 New concepts in the pathophysiology of portal hypertension are the basis for new therapeutic targets

Modification of the structural abnormalities increasing hepatic vascular resistance

This may be achieved using two different approaches. One is non-disease-specific, based on the use of drugs or cell therapy to prevent/reverse sinusoidal remodelling and fibrogenesis[15]. The second is based on specific treatments for the underlying liver disease (interferon and antivirals for chronic hepatitis C and B, iron depletion for haemochromatosis, copper chelation for Wilson's disease, and alcohol abstinence for alcoholism, etc.). For each of these treatments there is evidence showing reduction in portal pressure/HVPG with successful therapy[16,17].

Correction of the dynamic component of increased hepatic resistance

To date most efforts have been directed at improving intrahepatic NO availability. This has been attempted by means of either NOS[18], aAKT[19] or SOD gene-transfer[20]; by the development of liver-specific NO donors[21,22]; by post-translational up-regulation of eNOS using statins[23,24], and by increasing NO bioavailability by means of antioxidant[25] or tetrahydrobiopterin supplementation[26]. Another potential approach is the inhibition of COX-1/TXA2[27-29] or increasing H_2S[30].

Inhibition of VEGF- and PDGF-mediated angiogenesis

Recent studies have demonstrated that VEGF/PDGF/PlaGF-mediated angiogenesis plays a relevant role in sinusoidal remodelling and liver fibrogenesis, in the formation of portal-systemic collaterals and in the development of a hyperkinetic splanchnic circulation[31,32]. Since all these processes may contribute to portal hypertension and its complications, it has been proposed that anti-angiogenic therapies may represent a novel strategy for the treatment of portal hypertension[32]. These new paradigms are being tested in animal models.

Acknowledgements

The author is indebted to Ms Clara Esteva for expert secretarial support, and to the staff, nurses and fellows of the Hepatic Hemodynamic Laboratory for continuous help and stimulus.

This work was supported in part by grants from the Ministerio de Sanidad y Consumo and Instituto de Salud Carlos III (FIS 05/0519 and FIS 06/0623).

References

1. Merkel C, Bolognesi M, Bellon S et al. Prognostic usefulness of hepatic vein catheterization in patients with cirrhosis and esophageal varices. Gastroenterology. 1992;102:973–9.
2. Bosch J, García-Pagán JC, Berzigotti A, Abraldes JG. Measurement of portal pressure and its role in the management of chronic liver disease. Semin Liver Dis. 2006;26:348–62.
3. Feu F, García-Pagán JC, Bosch J et al. Relation between portal pressure response to pharmacotherapy and risk of recurrent variceal haemorrhage in patients with cirrhosis. Lancet. 1995;346:1056–9.
4. Abraldes JG, Tarantino I, Turnes J, García-Pagán JC, Rodes J, Bosch J. Hemodynamic response to pharmacological treatment of portal hypertension and long-term prognosis of cirrhosis. Hepatology. 2003;37:902–8.
5. D'Amico G, García-Pagán JC, Luca A, Bosch J. Hepatic vein pressure gradient reduction and prevention of variceal bleeding in cirrhosis: a systematic review. Gastroenterology. 2006;131:1611–24.
6. Groszmann RJ, Garcia-Tsao G, Bosch J et al. Beta-blockers to prevent gastroesophageal varices in patients with cirrhosis. N Engl J Med. 2005;353:2254–61.
7. Villanueva C, Lopez-Balaguer JM, Aracil C et al. Maintenance of hemodynamic response to treatment for portal hypertension and influence on complications of cirrhosis. J Hepatol. 2004;40:757–65.
8. Bosch J, Abraldes JG, Berzigotti A, García-Pagán JC. Portal hypertension and gastrointestinal bleeding. Semin Liver Dis. 2008;28:2–25.
9. Perez-Ayuso RM, Pique JM, Bosch J et al. Propranolol in prevention of recurrent bleeding from severe portal hypertensive gastropathy in cirrhosis. Lancet. 1991;337:1431–4.
10. Turnes J, García-Pagán JC, Abraldes JG, Hernandez-Guerra M, Dell'Era A, Bosch J. Pharmacological reduction of portal pressure and long-term risk of first variceal bleeding in patients with cirrhosis. Am J Gastroenterol. 2006;101:506–12.

11. Banares R, Moitinho E, Piqueras B et al. Carvedilol, a new nonselective beta-blocker with intrinsic anti-alpha1-adrenergic activity, has a greater portal hypotensive effect than propranolol in patients with cirrhosis [See comments]. Hepatology. 1999;30:79–83.
12. Banares R, Moitinho E, Matilla A et al. Randomized comparison of long-term carvedilol and propranolol administration in the treatment of portal hypertension in cirrhosis. Hepatology. 2002;36:1367–73.
13. Albillos A, García-Pagán JC, Iborra J et al. Propranolol plus prazosin compared with propranolol plus isosorbide-5- mononitrate in the treatment of portal hypertension. Gastroenterology. 1998;115:116–23.
14. Groszmann RJ. Beta-adrenergic blockers and nitrovasodilators for the treatment of portal hypertension: the good, the bad, the ugly. Gastroenterology. 1997;113:1794–7.
15. Friedman SL, Bansal MB. Reversal of hepatic fibrosis – fact or fantasy? Hepatology. 2006;43(Suppl. 1):S82–8.
16. Carrion JA, Navasa M, Garcia-Retortillo M et al. Efficacy of antiviral therapy on hepatitis c recurrence after liver transplantation: a randomized controlled study. Gastroenterology. 2007;132:1746–56.
17. Rincon D, Ripoll C, Iacono OL et al. Antiviral therapy decreases hepatic venous pressure gradient in patients with chronic hepatitis C and advanced fibrosis. Am J Gastroenterol. 2006;101:2269–74.
18. Yu Q, Shao R, Qian HS, George SE, Rockey DC. Gene transfer of the neuronal NO synthase isoform to cirrhotic rat liver ameliorates portal hypertension. J Clin Invest. 2000;105:741–8.
19. Morales-Ruiz M, Cejudo-Martin P, Fernandez-Varo G et al. Transduction of the liver with activated Akt normalizes portal pressure in cirrhotic rats. Gastroenterology. 2003;125:522–31.
20. Lavina B, Gracia-Sancho J, Rodriguez-Vilarrupla A et al. Extracellular superoxide dismutase gene transfer reduces portal pressure and improves intrahepatic endothelial dysfunction in cirrhotic rat livers by diminishing superoxide and incresing nitric oxide bioavailability. J Hepatol. 2007;46(Suppl. 1):51A.
21. Loureiro-Silva MR, Cadelina GW, Iwakiri Y, Groszmann RJ. A liver-specific nitric oxide donor improves the intra-hepatic vascular response to both portal blood flow increase and methoxamine in cirrhotic rats. J Hepatol. 2003;39:940–6.
22. Fiorucci S, Antonelli E, Brancaleone V et al. NCX-1000, a nitric oxide-releasing derivative of ursodeoxycholic acid, ameliorates portal hypertension and lowers norepinephrine-induced intrahepatic resistance in the isolated and perfused rat liver. J Hepatol. 2003;39:932–9.
23. Zafra C, Abraldes JG, Turnes J et al. Simvastatin enhances hepatic nitric oxide production and decreases the hepatic vascular tone in patients with cirrhosis. Gastroenterology. 2004;126:749–55.
24. Abraldes JG, Rodriguez-Vilarrupla A, Graupera M et al. Simvastatin treatment improves liver sinusoidal endothelial dysfunction in CCl_4 cirrhotic rats. J Hepatol. 2007;46:1040–6.
25. Hernandez-Guerra M, García-Pagán JC, Turnes J et al. Ascorbic acid improves the intrahepatic endothelial dysfunction of patients with cirrhosis and portal hypertension. Hepatology. 2006;43:485–91.
26. Matei V, Rodriguez-Vilarrupla A, Deulofeu R et al. The eNOS cofactor tetrahydrobiopterin improves endothelial dysfunction in livers of rats with CCl_4 cirrhosis. Hepatology. 2006;44:44–52.
27. Graupera M, March S, Engel P, Rodes J, Bosch J, García-Pagán JC. Sinusoidal endothelial COX-1-derived prostanoids modulate the hepatic vascular tone of cirrhotic rat livers. Am J Physiol Gastrointest Liver Physiol. 2005;288:G763–70.
28. Graupera M, García-Pagán JC, Pares M et al. Cyclooxygenase-1 inhibition corrects endothelial dysfunction in cirrhotic rat livers. J Hepatol. 2003;39:515–21.
29. Graupera M, García-Pagán JC, Abraldes JG et al. Cyclooxygenase-derived products modulate the increased intrahepatic resistance of cirrhotic rat livers. Hepatology. 2003;37:172–81.
30. Fiorucci S, Antonelli E, Mencarelli A et al. The third gas: H_2S regulates perfusion pressure in both the isolated and perfused normal rat liver and in cirrhosis. Hepatology. 2005;42:539–48.

31. Fernandez M, Mejias M, Angermayr B, García-Pagán JC, Rodes J, Bosch J. Inhibition of VEGF receptor-2 decreases the development of hyperdynamic splanchnic circulation and portal-systemic collateral vessels in portal hypertensive rats. J Hepatol. 2005;43:98–103.
32. Fernandez M, Mejias M, Garcia-Pras E, Mendez R, García-Pagán JC, Bosch J. Reversal of portal hypertension and hyperdynamic splanchnic circulation by combined vascular endothelial growth factor and platelet-derived growth factor blockade in rats. Hepatology. 2007;46:1208–17.

Index

A-II *see* angiotensin II
AASLD guidelines 217, 218, 220, 224–5
acetaminophen (AAP) 5, 6
acetylcholine 187, 188
acquired immunity mediation 132
activin A 55
activin receptor-like kinase (ALK) 46, 48, 49
acute variceal bleeding therapy 233–9
acute-phase signalling 38–9
adaptive immune system 19, 20, 22–6
adipokines 78–9, 135–6
adrenergic agonists 184–5
adrenergic blockers *see* β-adrenergic blockers
advanced fibrosis staging 164, 168–9
adverse effects
 diuretics 255
 non-selective β-adrenergic blockers 199, 200, 201
 repeat large volume paracentesis 252
 surgical treatments 243, 246
alarmins 8–9
albumin treatment 252–4, 257–8, 271–2, 284–7
alcohol-induced liver injury model 131, 132
alcohol-induced steatohepatitis (ASH) 77
ALK *see* activin receptor-like kinase
ALK1/Smad1 signalling pathway 49
ALK5/Smad3 signalling pathway 46, 49
allocation policy for liver transplantation 309–16
α-adrenergic agonists 184–5
alternative splicing of Krüppel-like factor-6 147, 148
ammonia role in hepatic encephalopathy 291–4
anandamide (arachidonyl ethanolamide) 186–7
anergy in T cells 22, 23
angiogenesis 112–27
 inhibition therapies 113–25, 322
 oxidative stress/haem oxygenase role 125–7
 PDGF mediation 113, 117, 120–5, 322
 platelet-derived growth factor 110
 VEGF mediation 113–27, 322
angiotensin II (A-II) 134–5, 186, 248–9
animal models
 angioinhibitor treatment 113–25
 antifibrotic therapies 177–8
 BXD recombinant inbred mice 70–3
 fibrogenesis 130–8
 fibrosis reversal 138–40
 liver injury methods 131–2
 non-alcoholic steatohepatitis 77, 79, 80
 profibrogenic susceptibility genes 70–3
anti-angiogenic therapies 113–25, 322
anti-apoptotic signalling pathway 34, 35, 36–8
anti-hepatitis C virus (anti-HCV) antibodies 24–5
anti-inflammatory cytokines 22
antibiotics 233–5, 271, 272–6
antibody-mediated liver damage 25
antifibrotic therapies 174–8
antigens in mucosal immune system 11–16
antimicrobial defence gene regulation 84, 86–8
antiviral pathways 20–6
apoptosis
 cytokine control 33, 34, 35–8
 fibrogenesis resolution 1, 3, 7, 9, 138–40
 fibrogenesis role 136–7
 mouse models 136–40
 oncotic necrosis distinction 7
 profibrotic signalling mechanisms 3–5, 7
apoptotic bodies 8
aquaretic agents (vaptans) 255–7, 258
arachidonyl ethanolamide (anandamide) 186–7
area under curve (AUC) 164–5
area under the receiving operating curve (AUROC) 157–8, 164–5
arterial effects *see* vasoactive drugs; vasoregulation
arterial oxygenation impairment 301–2
ascites 248–58
 albumin treatment 252–4, 257–8
 aquaretic vaptan treatment 255–7, 258
 development 248–52
 paracentesis/TIPS comparison 261–6
 refractory 251–8
 spontaneous bacterial peritonitis 267–76
 vasoconstrictor treatment 254–5, 258
ascitic cirrhosis 250–8

INDEX

ascitic fluid
  antimicrobial capacity 269
  bacterial count 270
  protein content 274–5
ASH *see* alcohol-induced steatohepatitis
astrocyte swelling 292, 293–4
AUC *see* area under curve
AUROC *see* area under the receiving operating curve
autoantibody formation 25
autoimmune hepatitis 13–14

B cell activation 24–5
bacteria, *see also* intestinal bacteria
bacterial infections
  acute variceal bleeding 234–5
  chronic immune responses 25
  hepatorenal syndrome 280, 281
  spontaneous bacterial peritonitis 267–76
balloon tamponade 238
band ligation *see* endoscopic band ligation
Bax translocation to mitochondria 3, 5
BB *see* β-adrenergic blockers
BDL *see* bile duct ligation
β-adrenergic agonists 185
β-adrenergic blockers (beta blockers; BB)
  adverse events 199, 200, 201
  $β_1$ versus $β_2$ blocking effects 198, 213
  other treatment comparison 244–5
  portopulmonary hypertension effects 198–202, 298
  predicting response 320
  selective versus non selective blockers 198, 213
  variceal bleeding prevention
    failure/non-response 222, 223, 224–6
    indications/guidelines 215–16, 217, 218, 219–20, 226–7
    pre-primary 198–202, 224–5
    primary 213–14
    secondary 224, 226, 243–5, 246
β-catenin-dependent Wnt signalling 95, 96, 98
Bid truncation apoptosis signalling 3, 5
bile acids 83–9
bile duct ligation (BDL) 88, 131, 132
biochemical marker tests 155–60, 164–5
biopsy *see* liver biopsy
bone morphogenetic proteins (BMP) 46, 55–8
bone-marrow-derived fibrocytes 130, 131
bosentan therapy 299–300
branched tube-like structure formation *in vitro* 95, 101, 102–3, 104
BXD recombinant inbred mice 70–3

calcium 249, 292
cannabinoids (endocannabinoids) 186–7
capsule endoscopy 207–8
carbon monoxide (CO) 189

carbon tetrachloride (CCl$_4$) challenge 71–3, 131, 132
carcinogenesis 144, 147–8
cardiac output insufficiency 280, 281
cardiopulmonary disease 301
carvedilol 214, 320
caspases 3–4, 5, 7, 34, 35–6
β-catenin-dependent Wnt signalling 95, 96, 98
CCl$_4$ *see* carbon tetrachloride
CCN2 *see* connective tissue growth factor
CD4$^+$ T cells 22–4, 133
CD8$^+$ T cells 22–4
CD31 overexpression 113, 115, 116
CD81 tetraspanin protein 21
CD133 expression 95–104
ceftriaxone 273, 274
cell death 3–9, 136–7
  see also apoptosis; oncotic necrosis
cell injury 7–9
cell morphology changes in apoptosis 4, 7
cell surface proteins 95–100
cell-mediated immunity to hepatitis C 22–4
cephalosporins 233–4, 235
cerebral oedema 292
chemotaxis of stellate cells 145
Child–Turcotte–Pugh (CTP) score 309, 310
children's organ allocation policy 310
cholangiocytes 130, 131
chronic intermittent hypoxia 79
chronic obstruction of the common bile duct 174
chronic viral hepatitis *see* hepatitis C virus
cirrhosis staging 164, 168–9
cirrhotic cardiomyopathy 251, 281
clinical evaluation
  disease progression 163–70
  hepatic venous pressure gradient 164, 204–5
  liver biopsy 155, 157–8, 163–4
  serum biomarker tests 155–60, 164–5
  test combinations 159, 165, 169, 170
  transient elastography 155, 159, 165–8, 169
clinical failure of variceal bleeding prevention 221, 224–5
clinical management of progressive liver fibrosis 153–80
clinical trials
  non-selective β-adrenergic blockers 199–200, 201
  variceal bleeding prevention therapies 214, 223, 224, 225, 227
  see also randomized controlled trials
clinically significant portal hypertension (CSPH) 204–5
CO *see* carbon monoxide
coeliac disease 12–13, 14
collagen 71, 72, 130
combined therapies
  ascites 252–3, 256–7, 258

326

INDEX

variceal bleeding prevention 223, 244–5
common bile duct chronic obstruction 174
complications of cirrhosis 231–304
  acute variceal bleeding 233–9
  ascites 248–66
  hepatic encephalopathy 291–5
  hepatopulmonary diseases 297–304
  hepatorenal syndrome 280–8
  hyperdynamic circulatory state 195
  spontaneous bacterial peritonitis 267–76
  see also gastro-oesophageal varices
conjugated bile acids 84
connective tissue growth factor (CTGF/CCN2) 50–1, 53, 54, 55
contractile cells 108, 109, 145, 183–90
conversion of treatment 223
cost effectiveness of treatment 215, 219
COX see cyclooxygenase
Crohn's disease 12, 13
cryoglobulinaemia (mixed) 25
CSE see cystathione-γ-lyase
CSPH see clinically significant portal hypertension
CT see cysteinyl leukotrienes
CTGF see connective tissue growth factor
CTL see cytolytic effector cells
CTP see Child–Turcotte–Pugh
cyclooxygenase (COX) 185, 190
cystathione-γ-lyase (CSE) 190
cysteinyl leukotrienes (CT) 185
cytochrome c 4, 5
cytokines
  acute phase disease/injury response 38–9
  apoptosis activation/control 34, 35–8
  differentiation of hepatic stellate cells 95, 101, 102–3, 104
  fibrogenesis role, mouse models 132–5
  hepatocellular signalling pathways 32–40
  inflammatory response in hepatic encephalopathy 292–3, 294
  receptors 32–5
  stellate cell activation 8–9, 45–6
cytolytic activity downregulation in chronic viral hepatitis 21–2
cytolytic effector cells (CTL) 21–2, 23

DC see dendritic cells
DC101 monoclonal antibody 114–15
death receptors 34, 37
death-inducing signalling complex (DISC) 3–4
dendritic cells (DC) 12, 21
diabetes 75, 77, 78, 80
dietary fat 79–80
differentiation potential of hepatic stellate cells 95–104
dimethylnitrosamine (DMN) 131, 132
DISC see death-inducing signalling complex
discordance in fibrosis biomarker tests 158, 159

distal splenorenal shunts 246
diuretics 251–4, 255–7, 258
DMN see dimethylnitrosamine
ductular reaction 104
dynamic modulation of intrahepatic vascular resistance 183–90
dyspnoea 297, 302

EBL see endoscopic band ligation
ECM see extracellular matrix
EDCF see endothelial-derived contracting factors
EGD see esophagogastroduodenoscopy
EIS see endoscopic injection sclerotherapy
elastography see transient elastography
ELF index 157, 159
embolization 303
emerging therapies 318–22
endogenous cannabinoids (endocannabinoids) 186–7
endoglin, BMP/TGF-β interactions 56
endoscopic band ligation (EBL) 214–15, 216, 237, 245, 246
endoscopic injection sclerotherapy (EIS) 237
endoscopic sclerotherapy 214, 244
endoscopic therapies 214–15, 223, 236–7, 244, 245–6
endoscopy, see also gastrointestinal endoscopy
endothelial dysfunction 183–4, 187, 188–90
endothelial liver sinusoidal cells 107–11
endothelial nitric oxide synthase (eNOS) 187–8
endothelial progenitor cells (EPC) 95, 98, 100, 101, 104
endothelial-derived contracting factors (EDCF) 187
endothelial-like cell formation in vitro 95, 101, 102–3, 104
endothelins (ET)
  ascites formation 251
  endothelin-1 (ET-1) 107, 109, 134
  fibrogenesis mouse models 134
  intrahepatic vascular resistance 186
  portal hypertension role 107, 109
endotoxins, intestinal permeability 77–8
eNOS see endothelial nitric oxide synthase
enteric bacteria see intestinal bacteria
enterohepatic lymphocyte migration 14–16
EPC see endothelial progenitor cells
epithelial cells 11–12
epithelial–mesenchymal transition 130, 131
ES see endoscopic sclerotherapy
escape mutations 23
esophagogastroduodenoscopy (EGD) 207–8
  see also gastrointestinal endoscopy
ET see endothelins
ethanol see alcohol-induced...; intragastric ethanol administration
experimental liver injury in animal models 131–2

INDEX

extracellular matrix (ECM) 46, 130, 138, 146
extrarenal arterial vasodilation 280, 281
extrinsic pathway of apoptotic cell death 3–4

Farnesoid X receptor (FXR) 84, 85–8
FAS receptors 3–4
FasL 34, 35–6
fats *see* alcohol-induced steatohepatitis; dietary fat; lipid...; non-alcoholic fatty liver disease; non-alcoholic steatohepatitis; steatosis
fatty acids 79–80
fibrogenesis
  genetic determinants 70–3
  HSC activation regulatory pathways 46–64
  initiation pathomechanisms 1–41
  mediators 43–91
  metabolic syndrome 75–81
  mouse models 130–40
    BXD recombinant inbred mice 70–3
    cellular/molecular processes 132–8
    insult methods 131–2
  non-alcoholic steatohepatitis 75–81
  profibrotic signalling mechanisms of cell death 3–9
FibroMeter 157, 158
Fibroscan 159, 165
fibrosis
  clinical management 153–80
  regression therapies 173–8
  reversal in mouse models 138–40
  serum biomarker tests 155–60
  stellate cell apoptosis 3, 7, 9
FibroSpect 157
FibroTest 157, 158, 159
Final Rule, USA organ allocation policy 309–10, 316
financial factors in organ allocation policy 313, 315
fluid retention *see* ascites
FXR *see* Farnesoid X receptor

GALT *see* gut-associated lymphoid tissue
gasotransmitters
  intrahepatic vascular resistance 190
  see also carbon monoxide; hydrogen sulphide; nitric oxide
gastro-oesophageal varices
  endoscopic prophylactic therapies 214–15
  endoscopic screening 214
  gastric 239
  identifying patients 205–6
  liver stiffness measurement 169
  natural history 195, 196, 197, 206–7
  pharmacological prophylaxis 213–14, 223
  portosystemic collateral vessels 112
  prevention/growth restriction 199–200, 201
  treatment combinations 223
  treatment options/guidelines 213–27

upper gastrointestinal endoscopy 205–8
  see also variceal bleeding
gastrointestinal..., *see also* intestinal bacteria; intestines
gastrointestinal bleeding 272–4
  see also variceal bleeding
gastrointestinal endoscopy
  portal hypertension 204–8
  screening for varices 214
  standard EGD versus capsule endoscopy 207–8
  variceal bleeding prevention therapies 214–15, 223, 236–7, 244, 245–6
gene transcription factors 146
gene transcription regulation 84, 88, 89
genetic factors 50–1, 53, 54, 55, 70–3
Gleevec 120, 121–5
glomerular filtration rate (GFR) 248, 251, 283, 284, 287
glue, variceal obturation 215, 239
glycaemic dysregulation effects 80
  see also diabetes
gold standards in clinical tests 157, 158, 159, 163–4, 170
graft-versus-host disease (GVHD) 15
Gram-negative bacteria 267–9, 271, 276
Gram-positive bacteria 271, 276
gut, *see also* gastrointestinal...; intestines
gut-associated lymphoid tissue (GALT) 12
gut-specific lymphocyte trafficking 12, 15–16
GVHD *see* graft-versus-host disease

H_2S *see* hydrogen sulphide
haem oxygenases (HO) 125–7, 189
haematopoietic system 100, 104
haemodynamics of hepatorenal syndrome 280, 281, 282
haemorrhage *see* variceal bleeding
HCC *see* hepatocellular carcinoma
HCV *see* hepatitis C virus
HE *see* hepatic encephalopathy
helicase receptors 20
HepaScore 157, 158
hepatic ammonia detoxification 291–2
hepatic encephalopathy (HE; portosystemic encephalopathy) 112, 246, 291–4
hepatic portal vein 107–11
hepatic stellate cells (HSC)
  activation/transdifferentiation 130, 131
  BMP signalling 55–8
  CTGF role 50–1, 53–5
  initiation 145
  PDGF isoform expression 58–61
  perpetuation 145–6
  regulatory pathways 45–64
  Smad signalling pathways 46, 48–9, 56, 58
  SRF interactions 61–4
  TGF-β role 46–50, 51, 53–8, 61–4
apoptosis to resolve fibrogenesis 3, 7, 9

INDEX

cell surface proteins 95–100
collagen deposition 130
contractility of active phenotype 108, 109, 183
cytolytic activity downregulation by hepatitis C virus 22
elimination therapies 138–40
embryonic origin 96, 104
endothelin-1 interactions 109
fibrogenesis mouse models 137–40
functions 45, 95, 96, 108
glycaemic dysregulation effects 80
in vitro differentiation 95, 101, 102–3, 104
inflammatory cell recruitment 130–1
inflammatory signalling 137–8
Krüppel-like factor-6 effects 147
nitric oxide interactions 108–9
non-alcoholic steatohepatitis 77
platelet-derived growth factor interactions 110
portal hypertension role 107–11
profibrotic signalling mechanisms 8–9
progenitor/stem cell nature 95–104
roles 45, 95, 96, 108
hepatic venous pressure gradient (HVPG)
  clinical evaluation 164, 204–5
  LSM comparison 168–9
  treatment assessment 198–200, 201–2, 234, 237, 319, 320
hepatitis B virus 147–8, 174–5
hepatitis C virus (HCV)
  chronic viral hepatitis 19–26, 168
  fibrogenesis risk, genetic factors 70
  hepatocellular carcinoma 147–8
  immune responses 19–26
  interferon therapy 174, 176
  interleukin-10 therapy 177
  serum biomarker evaluation 155–60, 165
  specific interventions 174–5
hepatocellular carcinoma (HCC) 144, 147–8
hepatocyte-like cell formation *in vitro* 95, 101, 102–3, 104
hepatocytes
  apoptotic cell death 3–4, 131, 136–7
  myofibroblast transformation 130, 131
hepatoprotective factors 38–9, 78–9
hepatopulmonary diseases 297–304
hepatopulmonary syndrome (HPS) 297, 301–4
hepatorenal reflex 250–1
hepatorenal syndrome (HRS) 280–8
histopathological analysis *see* liver biopsy
HO *see* haem oxygenase
HPS *see* hepatopulmonary syndrome
HRS *see* hepatorenal syndrome
HSC *see* hepatic stellate cells
HVPG *see* hepatic venous pressure gradient
hydrogen sulphide (H$_2$S) 190
hyperdynamic splanchnic circulatory state 112–25, 195
hyponatraemia 255–6, 258

I/R *see* ischaemia–reperfusion
IAP *see* inhibitors of apoptosis proteins
iatrogenic factors 270
IBD *see* inflammatory bowel disease
IFN *see* interferon
IκB kinase (IKK) complex 34, 36–8
IL *see* interleukins
iloprost 299
immune system
  gut mucosal 11–16, 84, 88
  hepatitis C response 19–26
in vitro cell differentiation 95, 101, 102–3, 104
individual patient data meta-analysis 265–6
infections
  gut mucosal T cells migrating to liver 15–16
  hepatic encephalopathy 291
  Th2 cytokine release mouse models 131–2
  see also bacterial infections; hepatitis C virus
inflammatory bowel disease (IBD) 11, 12, 13–15
inflammatory cell recruitment 130–1
inflammatory pathways
  cell death signalling 5, 7, 8–9, 34, 35–7
  fibrogenesis signalling cascade in mouse models 132–4
  hepatocellular cytokines/receptors 32–40
  IL-6 signalling 35, 38–9
  liver homeostasis/injury 32–40
  TNF-α/receptors 34, 35–7
inflammatory responses 21, 75–80, 292–3, 294
inhibitors of apoptosis proteins (IAP) 4
innate immune system 19, 20, 21–2, 84, 88
insulin resistance 80
interferons (IFN) 20, 133, 134, 174, 175–6
interleukins (IL) 25, 35, 38–9, 133–4, 176–7
intestinal bacteria
  non-alcoholic steatohepatitis 77, 78
  overgrowth 77, 78, 267, 268
  pathogen immune response 11, 15–16
  portal endotoxaemia 77, 78
  spontaneous bacterial peritonitis 267–9
  translocation 83–9, 267–9
intestines
  bile acid role 83–9
  decontamination 272–5
  diseases 12–14
  Farnesoid X receptor role 84, 85–9
  gut-associated lymphoid tissue 12
  gut-specific lymphocyte trafficking 12, 15–16
  immune system 11–16
  mucosal barrier 84, 88, 89
  portal endotoxaemia, non-alcoholic steatohepatitis 77–8
  spontaneous bacterial peritonitis 268
intragastric ethanol administration 131, 132

INDEX

intrahepatic cell populations in liver homeostasis 32, 33
intrahepatic vascular resistance 183–90
intrapulmonary vasodilation 301–2
intrinsic pathway of apoptotic cell death 5
invasive tests *see* hepatic venous pressure gradient; liver biopsy
ischaemia–reperfusion (I/R) liver injury 38
isosorbide mononitrate 214, 244–5

kidneys 248–9, 250–1, 280–8
Krüppel-like factors (KLF) 146–8
Kupffer cells 4, 8–9

large volume paracentesis 252, 261–6
latent transforming growth factor beta binding protein (LTBP) 49–50, 51, 52
LEC *see* liver sinusoidal endothelial cells
leptin 78–9, 135–6
ligation 236, 237
 see also endoscopic band ligation
lipids 75–6, 85
 see also non-alcoholic fatty liver disease; steatosis
lipopolysaccharide (LPS) 77, 291–2
liver biopsy
 avoidance by non invasive tests 159, 164, 165
 fibrosis biomarker test comparison 155, 157–80
 limitations 155, 158, 159, 163
 as reference standard 157, 158, 159, 163–4, 165
liver homeostasis 32–40
liver imaging 155
liver injury in experimental methods 131–2
liver regeneration 95, 104
liver sinusoidal endothelial cells (LEC) 107–11
liver stiffness measurement (LSM) 155, 159, 163, 165–9
liver transplantation (LT)
 allocation policy, USA 309–16
 ascitic cirrhosis 252
 hepatopulmonary syndrome 303
 hepatorenal syndrome 282
 paracentesis/TIPS comparison trials 264
 portopulmonary hypertension 300–1
 spontaneous bacterial peritonitis 272
loop of Henle 249
low protein ascites 274–5
LPS *see* lipopolysaccharide
LSM *see* liver stiffness measurement
LT *see* liver transplantation
LTBP *see* latent transforming growth factor beta binding protein
lungs *see* hepatopulmonary syndrome; portopulmonary hypertension
lymphatic circulation 267, 268
lymphocytes 12, 14–16

lymphoproliferative disorders 25

magnetic cell sorting 95, 96, 98, 99
major histocompatibility complex 20, 21
malignancy 25, 144, 147–8
matrix metalloprotease (MMP) 138–9
MCD *see* methionine choline-deficient
MDA-5 receptors 20
MELD *see* Model for Endstage Liver Disease
memory T cells 15–16
mesenteric lymph nodes (MLN) 12, 267, 268
meta-analysis of paracentesis/TIPS comparison trials 264–6
metabolic syndrome 75–81
metabolically induced liver injury in mouse models 77, 131
methionine choline-deficient (MCD) 77, 131, 132
MFB *see* myofibroblasts
microcirculatory effects 134–5
midodrine 254–5
mitochondria 3–7
mitogens 110
mixed cryoglobulinaemia 25
MLN *see* mesenteric lymph nodes
MMP *see* matrix metalloprotease
Model for Endstage Liver Disease (MELD) 265, 266, 309–16
molecular markers of stem cells 95–100
mortality
 organ allocation policy effects 311–13, 314
 paracentesis/TIPS comparison trials 261–6
mouse models 130–40, 177
mucosal immune system 11–16
myofibroblast-like cells formation *in vitro* 95, 101, 102–3, 104
myofibroblasts (MFB)
 cell transformation in other organs 130, 131
 contraction 108, 109, 183
 mouse models 137–40
 multicell transformations 130, 131
 transdifferentiation regulatory pathways 45–64
 see also hepatic stellate cells

N-methyl-D-aspartate (NMDA) receptors 292
nadolol combination therapy 320
NAFLD *see* non-alcoholic fatty liver disease
NASH *see* non-alcoholic steatohepatitis
natural killer (NK) cells 21–2, 138, 139–40
necrosis 3–9, 75–6, 80
neovascularization 117, 120
 see also angiogenesis
NF-κB
 evolution 33
 hepatocellular apoptosis inhibition 34, 35, 36–8

INDEX

inhibition in NASH antifibrotic
    therapy 177–8
ischaemia–reperfusion liver injury
    interactions 38
nicotinamide adenine dinucleotide phosphatase
    (NADPH) oxidases 126–7, 135
nitrate therapy 214, 244–5
nitric oxide (NO)
    ascites formation 251
    bioavailability 187–9, 321–2
    hepatopulmonary syndrome
        pathophysiology 302
    portal hypertension role 107, 108–9, 187–9
nitric oxide synthase (NOS) 134, 187–8
nitrosative stress 292–4
NK *see* natural killer
NMDA *see* N-methyl-D-aspartate
NO *see* nitric oxide
NOD *see* nucleotide-binding oligomerization
    domain
non-alcoholic fatty liver disease
    (NAFLD) 75–81
non-alcoholic steatohepatitis (NASH) 75–81,
    131, 177–8
non-Hodgkin's lymphoma 25
non-invasive clinical tests
    advanced fibrosis/cirrhosis staging 168–9
    combinations 159, 165, 169, 170
    invasive method integration 163–70
    oesophageal varices prediction 205–6
    serum biomarkers 155–60, 164–5
    transient elastography 155, 159, 165–8, 169
    treatment assessment 319
non-response, variceal bleeding
    prevention 221, 224
non-selective β-adrenergic blockers
    adverse events 199, 200, 201
    predicting response 320
    versus selective B1 blockers 198, 213
    see also β-adrenergic blockers
non-specific antifibrotic interventions 175–8
norepinephrine 184–5
norfloxacin 272–4, 276
NOS *see* nitric oxide synthase
nuclear factors *see* NF-κB
nuclear receptors 84, 85–9
nucleotide-binding oligomerization domain
    (NOD) molecules 12

O_2 therapy, hepatopulmonary syndrome 303
obesity 77–9
obstructive sleep apnoea 79
octreotide 236
oesophageal varices *see* gastro-oesophageal
    varices
oesophageal videocapsule endoscopy system
    (PillCam ESO) 207–8
OLT *see* orthotopic liver transplantation
oncotic necrosis 3, 5–7, 8–9
opsonic activity of ascitic fluid 269

organ allocation policy, USA 309–16
orthotopic liver transplantation (OLT) 300–1,
    303
oxidative stress
    fibrogenesis role 135
    hepatic encephalopathy 292–4
    intrahepatic vascular resistance 189
    mouse models 135
    oncotic necrosis 5, 7, 9
    VEGF induced angiogenesis role 125–7
oxygen therapy, hepatopulmonary
    syndrome 303

paediatric organ allocation policy, USA 310
PAH *see* pulmonary arterial hypertension
paracentesis 252, 261–6
pathogen-associated molecular pattern
    (PAMP) receptors 20
PBC *see* primary biliary cirrhosis
PBR *see* peripheral benzodiazepine receptor
PDGF *see* platelet-derived growth factor
pericyte contraction 183
peripheral benzodiazepine receptor
    (PBR) 292
perisinusoidal space of Disse 183
peritonitis *see* spontaneous bacterial peritonitis
peroxisome proliferators-activated receptor-α
    (PPARα) 177–8
peroxynitrite 5
Peyer's patches 12
PG *see* prostaglandin
pharmacological therapy
    acute variceal bleeding 233–5, 236, 237
    antibiotics 233–5, 271, 272–6
    ascites 251–8
    combined therapies 223
    hepatopulmonary syndrome 303
    portopulmonary hypertension 298–301
    variceal bleeding prevention 213–14, 243–
        5, 246
    see also β-adrenergic blockers; vasoactive
        drugs
PillCam ESO (oesophageal videocapsule
    endoscopy system) 207–8
plasma renin activity (PRA) 281, 284, 287
platelet-derived growth factor (PDGF)
    blockade 113, 120–5
    isoform expression 58–61, 63, 64
    neovascularization role 117, 120
    portal hypertension role 107, 110
pluripotency maintenance of hepatic stellate
    cells 98, 104
portal endotoxaemia 77, 78
portal fibroblasts 130, 131
portal hypertension
    angiogenesis role 112–27
    clinical assessment 204–5
    clinical management 181–230
    emerging therapies 318–22
    endothelin-1 role 107, 109

gastro-oesophageal varices 195, 196
gastrointestinal endoscopy 204–8
hepatic venous pressure gradient
  measurement 164
intrahepatic vascular resistance dynamic
  modulation 183–90
liver stiffness measurement 168–9
natural history 212–13
nitric oxide role 107, 108–9
non-parenchymal cells role 107–11
non-selective β-adrenergic blockers 198–202
oxidative stress/haem oxygenase
  effects 125–7
pathophysiology 195–6
platelet-derived growth factor role 107, 110
preprimary prophylaxis 195–202
prevention by VEGF blockade 113–17
reversal by VEGF/PDGF blockade 117, 120–5
therapy problems 318–19
variceal bleeding prevention 212–27
portal venous inflow reduction 198–202
portopulmonary hypertension
  (PPHTN) 297–301
portosystemic collateral vessels 112–27, 195
portosystemic encephalopathy (PSE; hepatic
  encephalopathy) 112, 246, 291–4
portosystemic shunts see transjugular
  intrahepatic portosystemic shunts
post-transplantation outcomes of organ
  allocation policy 314
posture, sodium retention 248–9
PPARα see peroxisome proliferators-activated
  receptor-α
PPHTN see portopulmonary hypertension

PRA see plasma renin activity
pre-ascitic cirrhosis 248–9
pre-primary prevention of varices 197–202, 219, 224–5
pre-primary prophylaxis in portal
  hypertension 195–202
pre-transplantation mortality 311–13
prevention stages of variceal bleeding,
  definitions 219
prevention of therapeutic failure 221–3
primary biliary cirrhosis (PBC) 13
primary prevention of variceal bleeding 197, 212–27
primary sclerosing cholangitis (PSC) 13–15
proapoptotic signalling cascades 34, 35–6
profibrogenic susceptibility genes 70–3
profile performance test of fibrosis biomarker
  assessments 158
progenitor cells 95–104
prognostic indicators of acute variceal
  bleeding 233
prognostic value of fibrosis biomarker
  tests 159

proinflammatory cytokines 8–9
proliferation
  B cells 25
  hepatic stellate cells 145
  Krüppel-like factor-6 effects 147
  see also hepatocellular carcinoma;
    lymphoproliferative disorders
prophylaxis
  antibiotics 233–5, 271, 272–6
  portal hypertension 196–202
propranolol 213–14, 215–16, 320
prostacyclin 298–9
prostaglandin (PG) 185
prostanoid 190
protection from liver damage 38–9
protein tyrosine nitration (PTN) 292–3
proximal renal tubule 248, 251
PSC see primary sclerosing cholangitis
PSE see portosystemic encephalopathy
PTN see protein tyrosine nitration
pulmonary arterial hypertension (PAH) 297–301
pulmonary vascular complications 297–304
  see also hepatopulmonary syndrome;
    portopulmonary hypertension

quality-of-life factors in organ allocation 315
quantitative trait locus (QTL) analysis 70, 71, 73
quinolone-resistant bacteria 276
quinolones 233–4, 235

R-Smads see receptor-regulated Smads
RAAS see renin-angiotensin-aldosterone
  system
Rael expression 139–40
randomized controlled trials (RCT)
  acute variceal bleeding therapies 236–7, 239
  non-selective β-adrenergic blockers 199–200, 201
  paracentesis/TIPS comparison 261–6
  prophylactic antibiotics 235
  variceal bleeding prevention therapies 214, 224, 225, 227
  variceal rebleeding prevention
    treatments 244–5
rapamycin 116–17, 118–19, 120–5
RCT see randomized controlled trials
reactive metabolites 5, 7
reactive nitrogen species (RNS) 292–4
reactive oxygen species (ROS) 5, 7, 130–1, 135, 292–4
receiver operating characteristics (ROC) 164–5
  see also area under the receiving operating
    curve
receptor-mediated (extrinsic) pathway of
  apoptotic cell death 3–4
receptor-regulated Smads (R-Smads) 46

INDEX

recombinant coagulation factor VIIa (rFVIIa) 237
recombinant inbred mice 70–3
refractory ascites 251–7, 261–6
refractory rebleeding treatments 246
regulatory T cell (Treg) induction 22, 23–4
remodelling portal hypertension 195–202
renal failure 280–8
renal sodium/water retention 248–9, 250–1
renin-angiotensin-aldosterone system (RAAS) 248–9
  see also angiotensin
repeat large volume paracentesis 252, 261–6
reticuloendothelial system (RES) 267–8, 269
rFVIIa see recombinant coagulation factor VIIa
RIG-1, hepatitis C virus response 20
RNA mutation in chronic hepatitis C infection 23
RNA virus responses of helicase sensors 20
RNS see reactive nitrogen species
ROC see receiver operating characteristics
ROS see reactive oxygen species

satavaptan 256–7
SBP see spontaneous bacterial peritonitis
schistosomiasis infection 132
sclerotherapy 236–7
  see also endoscopic injection sclerotherapy
'scope' assessments see gastrointestinal endoscopy
secondary necrosis 5
secondary prophylaxis
  gastro-oesophageal varices 196, 197
  spontaneous bacterial peritonitis 275
  variceal rebleeding 213, 219, 224, 225–6, 243–6
selective β_1-adrenergic blockers 198, 213
self-expandable metallic stents 238
sepsis 112, 291
serum biomarker tests 155–60, 164–5
serum response factor (SRF) 61–4
shunts see distal splenorenal shunts; transjugular intrahepatic portosystemic shunts
sickest-first policy in organ allocation 314, 315
side effects see adverse effects
sildenafil 300
sinusoidal portal pressure 250–1
Smad signalling pathways 46, 48–9, 56, 58, 133
small oesophageal varices progressing to large 207
smooth muscle cell (SMC) marker genes 61–3
sodium retention 248–9, 251
somatostatin 236
splanchnic arteriolar resistance 198
splanchnic arteriolar vasodilation 195, 280, 281, 283

splanchnic hyperaemia see hyperdynamic splanchnic circulatory state
splenorenal shunts 246
spontaneous bacterial peritonitis (SBP) 267–76, 280, 281, 283
SRF see serum response factor
stages of fibrosis 158, 163, 164, 165, 168–9
steatosis 75–6, 79
  see also non-alcoholic fatty liver disease
stellate cells see hepatic stellate cells
stem cell marker expression 95–100
stents (self-expandable metallic) 238
stress responses see nitrosative stress; oxidative stress
structural abnormality modification 321
surgical treatments
  adverse effects 243, 246
  see also splenorenal shunts; transjugular intrahepatic portosystemic shunts
survival
  organ allocation policy effects 311–13, 314
  paracentesis/TIPS comparison trials 261–6
sympathetic nervous system 250–1
systemic circulation
  enteric bacterial translocation 267
  hepatorenal syndrome 280, 281, 282
  receiving hepatic portal blood 112

T cells 15–16, 22–4
TAA see thiocetamide
terlipressin 254, 284, 285–7
tertiary prevention of variceal bleeding 220, 225–6
tetraspanin protein CD81 21
TGF-β see transforming growth factor beta
Th1/2 cells 133–4
Th2 cytokine release 132
therapeutic endoscopy 214–15, 223, 236–7, 244, 245–6
therapeutic failures in variceal bleeding prevention 217, 221–7
thiocetamide (TAA) 131
thromboxane (TX) 185
TIPS see transjugular intrahepatic portosystemic shunts
tissue degeneration inhibition 138
tissue inhibitor of matrix metalloprotease-1/2 (TIMP-1/2) 138–9
TLR see toll-like receptors
TNF see tumour necrosis factor
TNF-α see tumour necrosis factor alpha
toll-like receptors (TLR) 9, 20
toxic liver injury animal models 131
transcription factors 146
transcription regulation 84, 88, 89
transforming growth factor beta (TGF-β)
  antifibrotic intervention target 175–6
  bioavailability regulation 49–50
  complex role in fibrogenesis 64
  CTGF interaction 51, 53, 54, 55

333

INDEX

fibrogenesis role 133
hepatic stellate cell activation/
    transdifferentiation 46–50, 51, 53–8, 61–4
matrix metalloprotease inhibition 138
mouse models 133, 138, 140
natural killer cell suppression 140
SRF interactions 61–4
transient elastography 155, 159, 165–8, 169
transjugular intrahepatic portosystemic shunts (TIPS)
  adverse effects 243, 246
  ascites reduction 251, 252
  hepatorenal syndrome 282, 287–8
  paracentesis comparison 261–6
  portopulmonary hypertension effects 298
  uncontrolled variceal bleeding 238
  variceal bleeding prevention 215, 220, 226, 245–6
transplants *see* liver transplantation
Treg *see* regulatory T cell
treprostinil 299
Tsukamoto–French model of alcohol-induced liver injury in mice 131
tumour necrosis factor alpha (TNF-α) 34, 35–8, 251, 293
tumour necrosis factors (TNF) 34, 36, 37, 77
TX *see* thromboxane

UDCA *see* ursodeoxycholic acid
ulcerative colitis 13
unconjugated bile acids 84–5
uncontrolled variceal bleeding 238
ursodeoxycholic acid (UDCA) 174
USA, liver transplantation allocation policy 309–16

validation of fibrosis biomarker tests 155–8
vaptans (aquaretic agents) 255–7, 258
variceal bleeding 196, 204, 205, 207
  acute therapy 233–9

natural history 196, 197
prevention treatments 212–27
rebleeding prevention 213, 219, 224, 225–6, 243–6
spontaneous bacterial peritonitis 272–4
therapy problems 318–19
uncontrolled 238
see also gastro-oesophageal varices
variceal obturation with glue 215
vascular endothelial growth factor (VEGF) 113–27
vascular remodelling *see* angiogenesis
vascular smooth muscle cells 183
vasoactive drugs
  acute variceal bleeding 236
  ascites therapy 254–5, 258
  hepatorenal syndrome 284–7
  portal hypertension therapy problems 319–20
  portopulmonary hypertension therapy 298–301
vasopressin receptor agonists 255–7, 258
vasoregulation
  ascites formation 251
  ascitic cirrhosis 250
  endothelial dysfunction 183–4, 187–90
  fibrosis regulation in mouse models 134–5
  hepatopulmonary syndrome pathophysiology 301–2
  hepatorenal syndrome 280, 281
  intrahepatic vascular resistance moderation 183–90
  normal liver vs. portal hypertension 109
  splanchnic/peripheral 195
VEGF *see* vascular endothelial growth factor
viruses *see* hepatitis B virus; hepatitis C virus

water retention, ascites formation 250–1
whole genome QTL scans 71, 73

zinc finger transcription factors 146

334

Falk Symposium Series

100. Blum HE, Bode Ch, Bode JCh, Sartor RB, eds. *Gut and the Liver.* Falk Symposium 100. 1998   ISBN 0-7923-8736-8
101. Rachmilewitz D, ed. *V International Symposium on Inflammatory Bowel Diseases.* Falk Symposium 101. 1998   ISBN 0-7923-8743-0
102. Manns MP, Boyer JL, Jansen PLM, Reichen J, eds. *Cholestatic Liver Diseases.* Falk Symposium 102. 1998   ISBN 0-7923-8746-5
102B. Manns MP, Chapman RW, Stiehl A, Wiesner R, eds. *Primary Sclerosing Cholangitis.* International Falk Workshop. 1998.   ISBN 0-7923-8745-7
103. Häussinger D, Jungermann K, eds. *Liver and Nervous System.* Falk Symposium 102. 1998   ISBN 0-7924-8742-2
103B. Häussinger D, Heinrich PC, eds. *Signalling in the Liver.* International Falk Workshop. 1998   ISBN 0-7923-8744-9
103C. Fleig W, ed. *Normal and Malignant Liver Cell Growth.* International Falk Workshop. 1998   ISBN 0-7923-8748-1
104. Stallmach A, Zeitz M, Strober W, MacDonald TT, Lochs H, eds. *Induction and Modulation of Gastrointestinal Inflammation.* Falk Symposium 104. 1998
     ISBN 0-7923-8747-3
105. Emmrich J, Liebe S, Stange EF, eds. *Innovative Concepts in Inflammatory Bowel Diseases.* Falk Symposium 105. 1999   ISBN 0-7923-8749-X
106. Rutgeerts P, Colombel J-F, Hanauer SB, Schölmerich J, Tytgat GNJ, van Gossum A, eds. *Advances in Inflammatory Bowel Diseases.* Falk Symposium 106. 1999
     ISBN 0-7923-8750-3
107. Špičák J, Boyer J, Gilat T, Kotrlik K, Mareček Z, Paumgartner G, eds. *Diseases of the Liver and the Bile Ducts – New Aspects and Clinical Implications.* Falk Symposium 107. 1999   ISBN 0-7923-8751-1
108. Paumgartner G, Stiehl A, Gerok W, Keppler D, Leuschner U, eds. *Bile Acids and Cholestasis.* Falk Symposium 108. 1999   ISBN 0-7923-8752-X
109. Schmiegel W, Schölmerich J, eds. *Colorectal Cancer – Molecular Mechanisms, Premalignant State and its Prevention.* Falk Symposium 109. 1999
     ISBN 0-7923-8753-8
110. Domschke W, Stoll R, Brasitus TA, Kagnoff MF, eds. *Intestinal Mucosa and its Diseases – Pathophysiology and Clinics.* Falk Symposium 110. 1999
     ISBN 0-7923-8754-6
110B. Northfield TC, Ahmed HA, Jazwari RP, Zentler-Munro PL, eds. *Bile Acids in Hepatobiliary Disease.* Falk Workshop. 2000   ISBN 0-7923-8755-4
111. Rogler G, Kullmann F, Rutgeerts P, Sartor RB, Schölmerich J, eds. *IBD at the End of its First Century.* Falk Symposium 111. 2000   ISBN 0-7923-8756-2
112. Krammer HJ, Singer MV, eds. *Neurogastroenterology: From the Basics to the Clinics.* Falk Symposium 112. 2000   ISBN 0-7923-8757-0
113. Andus T, Rogler G, Schlottmann K, Frick E, Adler G, Schmiegel W, Zeitz M, Schölmerich J, eds. *Cytokines and Cell Homeostasis in the Gastrointestinal Tract.* Falk Symposium 113. 2000   ISBN 0-7923-8758-9
114. Manns MP, Paumgartner G, Leuschner U, eds. *Immunology and Liver.* Falk Symposium 114. 2000   ISBN 0-7923-8759-7
115. Boyer JL, Blum HE, Maier K-P, Sauerbruch T, Stalder GA, eds. *Liver Cirrhosis and its Development.* Falk Symposium 115. 2000   ISBN 0-7923-8760-0
116. Riemann JF, Neuhaus H, eds. *Interventional Endoscopy in Hepatology.* Falk Symposium 116. 2000   ISBN 0-7923-8761-9

Falk Symposium Series

116A. Dienes HP, Schirmacher P, Brechot C, Okuda K, eds. *Chronic Hepatitis: New Concepts of Pathogenesis, Diagnosis and Treatment*. Falk Workshop. 2000
ISBN 0-7923-8763-5
117. Gerbes AL, Beuers U, Jüngst D, Pape GR, Sackmann M, Sauerbruch T, eds. *Hepatology 2000 – Symposium in Honour of Gustav Paumgartner*. Falk Symposium 117. 2000 ISBN 0-7923-8765-1
117A. Acalovschi M, Paumgartner G, eds. *Hepatobiliary Diseases: Cholestasis and Gallstones*. Falk Workshop. 2000 ISBN 0-7923-8770-8
118. Frühmorgen P, Bruch H-P, eds. *Non-Neoplastic Diseases of the Anorectum*. Falk Symposium 118. 2001 ISBN 0-7923-8766-X
119. Fellermann K, Jewell DP, Sandborn WJ, Schölmerich J, Stange EF, eds. *Immunosuppression in Inflammatory Bowel Diseases – Standards, New Developments, Future Trends*. Falk Symposium 119. 2001 ISBN 0-7923-8767-8
120. van Berge Henegouwen GP, Keppler D, Leuschner U, Paumgartner G, Stiehl A, eds. *Biology of Bile Acids in Health and Disease*. Falk Symposium 120. 2001
ISBN 0-7923-8768-6
121. Leuschner U, James OFW, Dancygier H, eds. *Steatohepatitis (NASH and ASH)*. Falk Symposium 121. 2001 ISBN 0-7923-8769-4
121A. Matern S, Boyer JL, Keppler D, Meier-Abt PJ, eds. *Hepatobiliary Transport: From Bench to Bedside*. Falk Workshop. 2001 ISBN 0-7923-8771-6
122. Campieri M, Fiocchi C, Hanauer SB, Jewell DP, Rachmilewitz R, Schölmerich J, eds. *Inflammatory Bowel Disease – A Clinical Case Approach to Pathophysiology, Diagnosis, and Treatment*. Falk Symposium 122. 2002 ISBN 0-7923-8772-4
123. Rachmilewitz D, Modigliani R, Podolsky DK, Sachar DB, Tozun N, eds. *VI International Symposium on Inflammatory Bowel Diseases*. Falk Symposium 123. 2002 ISBN 0-7923-8773-2
124. Hagenmüller F, Manns MP, Musmann H-G, Riemann JF, eds. *Medical Imaging in Gastroenterology and Hepatology*. Falk Symposium 124. 2002 ISBN 0-7923-8774-0
125. Gressner AM, Heinrich PC, Matern S, eds. *Cytokines in Liver Injury and Repair*. Falk Symposium 125. 2002 ISBN 0-7923-8775-9
126. Gupta S, Jansen PLM, Klempnauer J, Manns MP, eds. *Hepatocyte Transplantation*. Falk Symposium 126. 2002 ISBN 0-7923-8776-7
127. Hadziselimovic F, ed. *Autoimmune Diseases in Paediatric Gastroenterology*. Falk Symposium 127. 2002 ISBN 0-7923-8778-3
127A. Berr F, Bruix J, Hauss J, Wands J, Wittekind Ch, eds. *Malignant Liver Tumours: Basic Concepts and Clinical Management*. Falk Workshop. 2002
ISBN 0-7923-8779-1
128. Scheppach W, Scheurlen M, eds. *Exogenous Factors in Colonic Carcinogenesis*. Falk Symposium 128. 2002 ISBN 0-7923-8780-5
129. Paumgartner G, Keppler D, Leuschner U, Stiehl A, eds. *Bile Acids: From Genomics to Disease and Therapy*. Falk Symposium 129. 2002 ISBN 0-7923-8781-3
129A. Leuschner U, Berg PA, Holtmeier J, eds. *Bile Acids and Pregnancy*. Falk Workshop. 2002 ISBN 0-7923-8782-1
130. Holtmann G, Talley NJ, eds. *Gastrointestinal Inflammation and Disturbed Gut Function: The Challenge of New Concepts*. Falk Symposium 130. 2003
ISBN 0-7923-8783-X
131. Herfarth H, Feagan BJ, Folsch UR, Schölmerich J, Vatn MH, Zeitz M, eds. *Targets of Treatment in Chronic Inflammatory Bowel Diseases*. Falk Symposium 131. 2003
ISBN 0-7923-8784-8

Falk Symposium Series

132. Galle PR, Gerken G, Schmidt WE, Wiedenmann B, eds. *Disease Progression and Carcinogenesis in the Gastrointestinal Tract.* Falk Symposium 132. 2003
ISBN 0-7923-8785-6
132A. Staritz M, Adler G, Knuth A, Schmiegel W, Schmoll H-J, eds. *Side-effects of Chemotherapy on the Gastrointestinal Tract.* Falk Workshop. 2003
ISBN 0-7923-8791-0
132B. Reutter W, Schuppan D, Tauber R, Zeitz M, eds. *Cell Adhesion Molecules in Health and Disease.* Falk Workshop. 2003   ISBN 0-7923-8786-4
133. Duchmann R, Blumberg R, Neurath M, Schölmerich J, Strober W, Zeitz M. *Mechanisms of Intestinal Inflammation: Implications for Therapeutic Intervention in IBD.* Falk Symposium 133. 2004   ISBN 0-7923-8787-2
134. Dignass A, Lochs H, Stange E. *Trends and Controversies in IBD – Evidence-Based Approach or Individual Management?* Falk Symposium 134. 2004
ISBN 0-7923-8788-0
134A. Dignass A, Gross HJ, Buhr V, James OFW. *Topical Steroids in Gastroenterology and Hepatology.* Falk Workshop. 2004   ISBN 0-7923-8789-9
135. Lukáš M, Manns MP, Špičák J, Stange EF, eds. *Immunological Diseases of Liver and Gut.* Falk Symposium 135. 2004   ISBN 0-7923-8792-9
136. Leuschner U, Broomé U, Stiehl A, eds. *Cholestatic Liver Diseases: Therapeutic Options and Perspectives.* Falk Symposium 136. 2004   ISBN 0-7923-8793-7
137. Blum HE, Maier KP, Rodés J, Sauerbruch T, eds. *Liver Diseases: Advances in Treatment and Prevention.* Falk Symposium 137. 2004   ISBN 0-7923-8794-5
138. Blum HE, Manns MP, eds. *State of the Art of Hepatology: Molecular and Cell Biology.* Falk Symposium 138. 2004   ISBN 0-7923-8795-3
138A. Hayashi N, Manns MP, eds. *Prevention of Progression in Chronic Liver Disease: An Update on SNMC (Stronger Neo-Minophagen C).* Falk Workshop. 2004
ISBN 0-7923-8796-1
139. Adler G, Blum HE, Fuchs M, Stange EF, eds. *Gallstones: Pathogenesis and Treatment.* Falk Symposium 139. 2004   ISBN 0-7923-8798-8
140. Colombel J-F, Gasché C, Schölmerich J, Vucelic C, eds. *Inflammatory Bowel Disease: Translation from Basic Research to Clinical Practice.* Falk Symposium 140. 2005.   ISBN 1-4020-2847-4
141. Paumgartner G, Keppler D, Leuschner U, Stiehl A, eds. *Bile Acid Biology and its Therapeutic Implications.* Falk Symposium 141. 2005   ISBN 1-4020-2893-8
142. Dienes H-P, Leuschner U, Lohse AW, Manns MP, eds. *Autoimmune Liver Disease.* Falk Symposium 142. 2005   ISBN 1-4020-2894-6
143. Ammann RW, Büchler MW, Adler G, DiMagno EP, Sarner M, eds. *Pancreatitis: Advances in Pathobiology, Diagnosis and Treatment.* Falk Symposium 143. 2005
ISBN 1-4020-2895-4
144. Adler G, Blum AL, Blum HE, Leuschner U, Manns MP, Mössner J, Sartor RB, Schölmerich J, eds. *Gastroenterology Yesterday – Today – Tomorrow: A Review and Preview.* Falk Symposium 144. 2005   ISBN 1-4020-2896-2
145. Henne-Bruns D, Buttenschön K, Fuchs M, Lohse AW, eds. *Artificial Liver Support.* Falk Symposium 145. 2005   ISBN 1-4020-3239-0
146. Blumberg RS, Gangl A, Manns MP, Tilg H, Zeitz M, eds. *Gut–Liver Interactions: Basic and Clinical Concepts.* Falk Symposium 146. 2005   ISBN 1-4020-4143-8
147. Jewell DP, Colombel JF, Peña AS, Tromm A, Warren BS, eds. *Colitis: Diagnosis and Therapeutic Strategies.* Falk Symposium 147. 2006   ISBN 1-4020-4315-5

Falk Symposium Series

148. Kruis W, Forbes A, Jauch K-W, Kreis ME, Wexner SD, eds. *Diverticular Disease: Emerging Evidence in a Common Condition.* Falk Symposium 148. 2006
    ISBN 1-4020- 4317-1
149. van Cutsem E, Rustgi AK, Schmiegel W, Zeitz M, eds. *Highlights in Gastrointestinal Oncology.* Falk Symposium 149. 2006.   ISBN 1-4020-5108-5
150. Galle PR, Gerken G, Schmidt WE, Wiedenmann B, eds. *Disease Progression and Disease Prevention in Hepatology and Gastroenterology.* Falk Symposium 150. 2006
    ISBN 1-4020-5109-3
151. Fraser A, Gibson PR, Hibi T, Qian J-M, Schölmerich, eds. *Emerging Issues in Inflammatory Bowel Disease.* Falk Symposium 151. 2006
    ISBN-13 978-1-4020-5701-4
152. Not published.
153. Dignass A, Rachmilewitz D, Stange E-F, Weinstock JV, eds. *Immunoregulation in Inflammatory Bowel Diseases – Current Understanding and Innovation.* Falk Symposium 153. 2007   ISBN-13 978-1-4020-5888-2
154. Adler G, Fiocchi C, Lazebnik LB, Vorobiev GI, eds. *Inflammatory Bowel Disease – Diagnostic and Therapeutic Strategies.* Falk Symposium 154. 2007
    ISBN-13 978-1-4020-6115-8
155. Keppler D, Beuers U, Leuschner U, Stiehl A, Trauner M, Paumgartner G, eds. *Bile Acids: Biological Actions and Clinical Relevance.* Falk Symposium 155. 2007
    ISBN 978-1-4020-6251-3
156. Blum HE, Cox DW, Häussinger D, Jansen PLM, Kullak-Ublick GA, eds. *Genetics in Liver Diseases.* Falk Symposium 156. 2007   ISBN 978-14020-6393-0
157. Diehl AM, Hayashi N, Manns MP, Sauerbruch T, eds. *Chronic Hepatitis: Metabolic, Cholestatic, Viral and Autoimmune.* Falk Symposium 157. 2007
    ISBN 978-1-4020-6522-4
158. Gasche G, Herrerías Gutiérrez JM, Gassull M, Monterio E, eds. *Intestinal Inflammation and Colorectal Cancer.* Falk Symposium 158. 2007
    ISBN 978-1-4020-6825-6
159. Tözün N, Mantzaris G, Dağlı Ü, Schölmerich J, eds. *IBD 2007 – Achievements in Research and Clinical Practice.* Falk Symposium 159. 2008
    ISBN 978-1-4020-6986-4
160. Ferkolj I, Gangl A, Galle PR, Vucelic B, eds. *Pathogenesis and Clinical Practice in Gastroenterology.* Falk Symposium 160. 2008
161. Carey MC, Gabryelewicz A, Díte P, Keim V, Mössner J, eds. *Future Perspectives in Gastroenterology.* Falk Symposium 161. 2008
162. Bosch J, Lammert F, Burroughs AK, Lebrec D, Sauerbruch T, eds. *Liver Cirrhosis: From Pathophysiology to Disease Management.* Falk Symposium 162. 2008
    ISBN 978-1-4020-8655-7